Mastocytosis

Editor

MARIANA C. CASTELLS

IMMUNOLOGY AND ALLERGY CLINICS OF NORTH AMERICA

www.immunology.theclinics.com

Consulting Editor
STEPHEN A. TILLES

August 2018 • Volume 38 • Number 3

ELSEVIER

1600 John F. Kennedy Boulevard • Suite 1800 • Philadelphia, Pennsylvania, 19103-2899

http://www.theclinics.com

IMMUNOLOGY AND ALLERGY CLINICS OF NORTH AMERICA Volume 38, Number 3

August 2018 ISSN 0889-8561, ISBN-13: 978-0-323-61392-7

Editor: Jessica McCool

Developmental Editor: Kristen Helm

Immunology and Allergy Clinics of North America (ISSN 0889–8561) is published quarterly by Elsevier Inc., 360 Park Avenue South, New York, NY 10010-1710. Months of issue are February, May, August, and November. Periodicals postage paid at New York, NY and additional mailing offices. Subscription prices are $333.00 per year for US individuals, $565.00 per year for US institutions, $100.00 per year for US students and residents, $411.00 per year for Canadian individuals, $220.00 per year for Canadian students, $717.00 per year for Canadian institutions, $445.00 per year for international individuals, $717.00 per year for international institutions, $220.00 per year for international students. To receive student/resident rate, orders must be accompanied by name of affiliated institution, date of term, and the *signature* of program/residency coordinator on institution letterhead. Orders will be billed at individual rate until proof of status is received. Foreign air speed delivery is included in all *Clinics* subscription prices. All prices are subject to change without notice. **POSTMASTER**: Send address changes to *Immunology and Allergy Clinics of North America,* Elsevier Health Sciences Division, Subscription Customer Service, 3251 Riverport Lane, Maryland Heights, MO 63043. **Customer Service: 1-800-654-2452 (U.S. and Canada); 314-447-8871 (outside U.S. and Canada). Fax: 314-447-8029. E-mail: journalscustomerservice-usa@elsevier.com (for print support); journalsonlinesupport-usa@elsevier.com (for online support).**

Reprints. For copies of 100 or more, of articles in this publication, please contact the Commercial Reprints Department, Elsevier Inc., 360 Park Avenue South, New York, New York 10010-1710. Tel. 212-633-3874, Fax: 212-633-3820, E-mail: reprints@elsevier.com.

Immunology and Allergy Clinics of North America is covered in MEDLINE/PubMed (Index Medicus), Current Contents/Life Sciences, Science Citation Index, ISI/BIOMED, Chemical Abstracts, and EMBASE/Excerpta Medica.

Contributors

CONSULTING EDITOR

STEPHEN A. TILLES, MD
Executive Director, ASTHMA Inc. Clinical Research Center, Partner, Northwest Asthma and Allergy Center, Clinical Professor of Medicine, University of Washington, Seattle, Washington, USA

EDITOR

MARIANA C. CASTELLS, MD, PhD
Director, Drug Hypersensitivity and Desensitization Center, Professor, Department of Medicine, Division of Rheumatology, Immunology, and Allergy, Director, Mastoctytosis Center, Brigham and Women's Hospital, Professor in Medicine, Harvard Medical School, Boston, Massachusetts, USA

AUTHORS

LONE AGERTOFT, MD, PhD
Mastocytosis Centre Odense University Hospital (MastOUH), Hans Christian Andersen Children's Hospital, Odense University Hospital, Odense, Denmark

CEM AKIN, MD, PhD
Division of Allergy and Clinical Immunology, Professor, Department of Internal Medicine, University of Michigan, Ann Arbor, Michigan, USA

IVÁN ALVAREZ-TWOSE, MD, PhD
Instituto de Estudios de Mastocitosis de Castilla La Mancha, Hospital Virgen del Valle, Toledo, Spain; Spanish Network on Mastocytosis (REMA)

MICHEL AROCK, PharmD, PhD
Cellular and Molecular Oncology, LBPA CNRS UMR8113, Ecole Normale Supérieure de Paris Saclay, Cachan, France; Laboratory of Hematology, Pitié-Salpêtrière Hospital, Paris, France

MARCELO VIVOLO AUN, MD, PhD
Associate Researcher, Clinical Immunology and Allergy Division, University of São Paulo, Assistant Professor, Faculdade Israelita de Ciências da Saúde Albert Einstein, São Paulo, São Paulo, Brazil

JOSÉ MANUEL AZAÑA, MD, PhD
Department of Dermatology, Complejo Hospitalario Universitario de Albacete, Hospital General Universitario de Albacete, Albacete, Spain

SIHAM BIBI, PhD
Cellular and Molecular Oncology, LBPA CNRS UMR8113, Ecole Normale Supérieure de Paris Saclay, Cachan, France

CARSTEN BINDSLEV-JENSEN, MD, PhD, DMSc
Mastocytosis Centre Odense University Hospital (MastOUH), Department of Dermatology
and Allergy Centre, Odense Research Centre for Anaphylaxis (ORCA), Odense University
Hospital, Odense, Denmark

PATRIZIA BONADONNA, MD
Allergy Unit, Multidisciplinary Outpatients Clinic for Mastocytosis (GISM), Azienda
Ospedaliera Universitaria Integrata di Verona, Verona, Italy

RAFAEL BONAMICHI-SANTOS, MD
PhD Candidate, Clinical Immunology and Allergy Division, University of São Paulo,
São Paulo, São Paulo, Brazil

MASSIMILIANO BONIFACIO, MD
Hematology Unit, University of Verona, Verona, Italy

SIGURD BROESBY-OLSEN, MD
Mastocytosis Centre Odense University Hospital (MastOUH), Department of Dermatology
and Allergy Centre, Odense Research Centre for Anaphylaxis (ORCA), Odense University
Hospital, Odense, Denmark

JOSEPH H. BUTTERFIELD, MD, FACP, FAAAAI
Consultant, Division of Allergic Diseases, Mayo Clinic, Rochester, Minnesota, USA

MELODY CARTER, MD
Laboratory of Allergic Diseases, National Institute of Allergy and Infectious Diseases,
National Institutes of Health, Bethesda, Maryland, USA

MARIANA C. CASTELLS, MD, PhD
Director, Drug Hypersensitivity and Desensitization Center, Professor, Department of
Medicine, Division of Rheumatology, Immunology, and Allergy, Director, Mastoctytosis
Center, Brigham and Women's Hospital, Professor in Medicine, Harvard Medical School,
Boston, Massachusetts, USA

TRACY I. GEORGE, MD
Professor, Department of Pathology, University of Utah, Salt Lake City, Utah, USA

PEDRO GIAVINA-BIANCHI, MD, PhD
Associate Professor, Clinical Immunology and Allergy Division, University of São Paulo,
São Paulo, São Paulo, Brazil

MATTHEW J. HAMILTON, MD
Assistant Professor, Division of Gastroenterology, Hepatology, and Endoscopy, Harvard
Medical School, Brigham and Women's Hospital, Boston, Massachusetts, USA

ANA FILIPA HENRIQUES, BSc, PhD
Instituto de Estudios de Mastocitosis de Castilla La Mancha, Hospital Virgen del Valle,
Toledo, Spain; Spanish Network on Mastocytosis (REMA)

FRED H. HSIEH, MD
Staff Physician, Allergy and Immunology, Respiratory Institute, Cleveland Clinic,
Cleveland, Ohio, USA

SUSAN V. JENNINGS, PhD
Chair, Research Committee, The Mastocytosis Society, Inc, Sterling, Massachusetts,
USA

LORENZO FALCHI, MD
Division of Hematology/Oncology, Columbia University Irving Medical Center, New York, New York, USA

HENRIK FOMSGAARD KJAER, MD, PhD
Mastocytosis Centre Odense University Hospital (MastOUH), Department of Dermatology and Allergy Centre, Odense Research Centre for Anaphylaxis (ORCA), Odense University Hospital, Odense, Denmark

THOMAS KIELSGAARD KRISTENSEN, PhD
Mastocytosis Centre Odense University Hospital (MastOUH), Department of Pathology, Odense University Hospital, Odense, Denmark

PHILINA LEE, PhD
Blueprint Medicines, Cambridge, Massachusetts, USA

JONATHAN J. LYONS, MD
Assistant Clinical Investigator, Laboratory of Allergic Diseases, National Institute of Allergy and Infectious Diseases, National Institutes of Health, Bethesda, Maryland, USA

MICHAEL BOE MØLLER, MD, DMSc
Mastocytosis Centre Odense University Hospital (MastOUH), Department of Pathology, Odense University Hospital, Odense, Denmark

ALMUDENA MATITO, MD, PhD
Instituto de Estudios de Mastocitosis de Castilla La Mancha, Hospital Virgen del Valle, Toledo, Spain; Spanish Network on Mastocytosis (REMA)

CHARLOTTE GOTTHARD MORTZ, MD, PhD
Mastocytosis Centre Odense University Hospital (MastOUH), Department of Dermatology and Allergy Centre, Odense Research Centre for Anaphylaxis (ORCA), Odense University Hospital, Odense, Denmark

GIOVANNI ORSOLINI, MD
Rheumatology Unit, University of Verona, Verona, Italy

THANAI PONGDEE, MD, FAAAAI
Consultant, Division of Allergic Diseases, Mayo Clinic, Rochester, Minnesota, USA

ANUPAMA RAVI, MD, FAAAAI
Senior Associate Consultant, Division of Pediatric Allergy and Immunology, Mayo Clinic, Rochester, Minnesota, USA

MAURIZIO ROSSINI, MD, PhD
Professor, Rheumatology Unit, University of Verona, Verona, Italy

LAURA SÁNCHEZ-MUÑOZ, MD, PhD
Instituto de Estudios de Mastocitosis de Castilla La Mancha, Hospital Virgen del Valle, Toledo, Spain; Spanish Network on Mastocytosis (REMA)

LUIGI SCAFFIDI, MD
Multidisciplinary Outpatients Clinic for Mastocytosis (GISM), Department of Medicine, Section of Hematology, Azienda Ospedaliera Universitaria Integrata di Verona, Verona, Italy

CHARLES F. SCHULER IV, MD
Division of Allergy and Clinical Immunology, Fellow, Department of Internal Medicine, University of Michigan, Ann Arbor, Michigan, USA

HONGLIANG SHI, MS
Blueprint Medicines, Cambridge, Massachusetts, USA

VALERIE M. SLEE, RN, BSN
Chair, Board of Directors, The Mastocytosis Society, Inc, Sterling, Massachusetts, USA

ANTONIO TORRELO, MD, PhD
Department of Dermatology, Hospital Infantil Universitario del Niño Jesús, Madrid, Spain

SRDAN VERSTOVSEK, MD, PhD
Professor, Department of Leukemia, The University of Texas MD Anderson Cancer Center, Houston, Texas, USA

OMBRETTA VIAPIANA, MD, PhD
Rheumatology Unit, University of Verona, Verona, Italy

SOFIJA VOLERTAS, MD
Division of Allergy and Clinical Immunology, Fellow, Department of Internal Medicine, University of Michigan, Ann Arbor, Michigan, USA

KELLY YOSHIMI-KANAMORI, MD
PhD Candidate, Clinical Immunology and Allergy Division, University of São Paulo, São Paulo, São Paulo, Brazil

RACHEL M. ZACK, ScD, SM
Member, Research Committee, The Mastocytosis Society, Inc, Sterling, Massachusetts, USA

ROBERTA ZANOTTI, MD
Hematology Unit, University of Verona, Verona, Italy

Contents

Mastocytosis is a heterogeneous group of neoplasms that involve the clonal expansion of mast cells into one or more organ systems, which typically involves the skin and hematopoietic systems. Systemic mastocytosis consists of a multifocal infiltration of mast cells into various noncutaneous tissue sites, especially the bone marrow. Diagnosis requires tissue confirmation, and algorithms have been developed to assist clinicians in this process. The current classification system focuses on delineating prognostic categories. Therapeutic approaches include symptomatic management, prevention of complications, and, in advanced disease, cytoreductive therapy.

The skin is one of the most frequent tissues affected in patients with mastocytosis, but cutaneous lesions are highly heterogeneous in shape, size, color, number, localization, and distribution. The World Health Organization recognizes 3 subtypes of cutaneous mastocytosis (CM): maculopapular CM (MPCM), diffuse CM, and mastocytoma of skin. An international task force of experts in mastocytosis has recently proposed subdividing MPCM into monomorphic and polymorphic, which could predict the duration of the disease in children. More research is warranted to develop an improved classification of CM that ideally should incorporate robust factors with prognostic impact on disease behavior.

Mast cell activation disorders is a term proposed to cover diseases and conditions related to the activation of mast cells and effects of mast cell mediators. In its broadest sense, the term encompasses a wide range of diseases from allergic asthma to rhinoconjunctivitis, urticaria, food allergy, anaphylaxis, mastocytosis, and other conditions in which MC activation contributes to the pathogenesis. This article focuses on clinical presentations,

challenges, and controversies in pediatric mastocytosis and gives an overview of current knowledge and areas in need of further research.

Mast cell disorders comprise a heterogeneous group of rare diseases, the
diagnosis of which still remains a challenge. Bone marrow analysis
constitutes the most appropriate site for screening systemic involvement
in mastocytosis. Morphologic, immunohistochemical, flow cytometric immunophenotyping, and molecular studies should be routinely performed
for diagnostic/prognostic purposes in experienced reference centers during the diagnostic workup in suspected systemic mastocytosis. The
authors review the most relevant characteristics of bone marrow expression of mast cell disorders as well as the different methodological approaches to be applied to perform an objective and reproducible
diagnosis and classification of mastocytosis and other mast cell disorders.

Mast cells leave evidence, a "fingerprint," of their participation in acute and
chronic clinical events. That fingerprint is an elevation, either chronic or
acute, in levels of their secreted mediators or their metabolites. Of these,
only serum tryptase is currently one of the diagnostic criteria for systemic
mastocytosis or mast cell activation. Combinations of easily obtained and
quantified urinary mast cell mediator metabolite levels correlate well with
bone marrow findings of systemic mastocytosis. By inhibiting synthesis
of or blockading receptors to the elevated mast cell mediator, relief of clinical symptoms can often be achieved.

Mastocytosis is a World Health Organization–defined clonal mast cell disorder characterized by significant clinicopathologic heterogeneity. Despite
this diversity, a mutation of the *KIT* gene, most commonly D816V, is found
in almost all cases and believed to be a driver lesion. Peripheral blood
allele-specific oligonucleotide polymerase chain reaction can reliably
detect *KIT* D816V and is used for the initial screening of adults with suspected systemic mastocytosis. The discovery of *KIT* mutations as central
to the pathobiology of mastocytosis has prompted development of KIT-
targeted agents, including imatinib and midostaurin (approved medications for patients with advanced systemic mastocytosis), and drugs in
development, such as KIT D816V-specific inhibitor avapritinib.

Gastrointestinal (GI) symptoms are commonly reported in patients with
mast cell disease. GI involvement in systemic mastocytosis is heterogeneous, and symptoms may be caused by infiltration of abnormal mast cells

in the GI tract and/or by the downstream effect of mast cell mediators on GI tissues. GI symptoms that described the monoclonal mast cell activation syndrome are best characterized in the context of acute anaphylaxis. The presence of GI symptoms and a subjective response of symptoms to anti–mast cell mediator therapy are considered qualifying criteria in the diagnosis of the idiopathic mast cell activation syndrome. Antimediator therapy may help alleviate GI symptoms in mast cell disease.

Systemic mastocytosis can give very different bone pictures: from osteosclerosis to osteoporosis. Osteoporosis is one of the most frequent manifestations particularly in adults and the most clinically relevant. It is often complicated by a high recurrence of mainly vertebral fragility fractures. The main factor of bone loss is the osteoclast with a relative or absolute predominance of bone resorption. The RANK-RANKL pathway seems of key importance, but histamine and other cytokines also play a significant role in the process. The predominance of resorption made bisphosphonates, as antiresorptive drugs, the most rational treatment of bone involvement in systemic mastocytosis.

Up to 7% of adult patients with Hymenoptera venom allergy may suffer from a clonal mast cell disease. Patients with clonal mast cell disease and Hymenoptera venom anaphylaxis are commonly males, without skin lesions, and anaphylaxis is characterized by hypotension and syncope in the absence of urticaria and angioedema. A normal value of tryptase does not exclude a mastocytosis. The diagnosis of a mast cell disease leads to several therapeutic consequences concerning the treatment of Hymenoptera venom allergy; as matter of fact, these patients have to undergo long-term venom immunotherapy to prevent further, potentially fatal severe reactions.

Patients who present with typical features of mast cell activation with laboratory confirmation and without evidence of a clonal mast cell disorder or other medical condition should be initiated on medical treatment to block mast cells and their mediators. If a major response is achieved, a diagnosis of nonclonal mast cell activation syndrome (NC-MCAS) is likely and treatment should be optimized, including management of any associated conditions. In this article, the latest evidence with regard to the diagnosis and treatment of NC-MCAS is presented.

Hereditary alpha tryptasemia is an autosomal dominant genetic trait caused by increased germline copies of *TPSAB1* encoding alpha-tryptase.

Individuals with this trait have elevated basal serum tryptase and may present with associated multisystem complaints. Both basal serum tryptase levels and severity of clinical symptoms display a gene-dose relationship with *TPSAB1*, whereby higher tryptase levels and greater symptom severity are correlated with increasing numbers of alpha-encoding *TPSAB1*. As the functional effects of increased basal serum tryptase and/or altered tryptase gene expression are elucidated, greater insights will be gained into the symptoms associated with hereditary alpha tryptasemia and their potential therapy.

Mast cell activation disorders (MCADs) consist of episodic systemic symptoms due to mast cell mediator release. Diagnosis is based on clinical presentation and determination of high levels of tryptase or histamine. Ehlers-Danlos syndrome (EDS) and postural tachycardia syndrome (POTS) frequently coexist. It has been described that individuals with these syndromes can even present symptoms compatible to MCADs, which could represent a new specific phenotype. Preliminary genetic data suggest a role for tryptase in the pathogenesis of MCADs, EDS, and POTS association. Studies with larger samples evaluating clinics, genetics, and histopathology are required to define the real correlation between these 3 clinical entities.

Understanding experiences, perceptions, and perspectives of patients with a mast cell disorder (MCD), including cutaneous mastocytosis, systemic mastocytosis, mast cell activation syndromes, and hereditary α-tryptasemia, is an important aspect of successful care, treatment, and informed development of novel therapies. This article reviews existing studies and presents new data on MCD patient perceptions regarding medical care, symptoms, allergies/sensitivities, triggers, future health/disease progression, treatment, impact on daily living, quality of life, support needs, and concerns regarding possible familial disease. Discussion includes aspects affecting the MCD community that require further consideration and development.

Mastocytosis is a group of rare disorders characterized by abnormal accumulation of mast cells in one or several organs. Mastocytosis can be seen at any age; but, in adults, the disease is usually systemic and chronic. Patients with indolent systemic mastocytosis (SM) are usually treated symptomatically, but cytoreductive treatments are needed in more advanced SM. In most patients with SM, an activating *KIT* D816V mutation is found. Thus, patients with advanced SM benefit from treatment with KIT-targeting tyrosine kinase inhibitors. However, none of these drugs are curative; new targeted drugs or combinations are still needed to improve patients' outcome.

IMMUNOLOGY AND ALLERGY CLINICS OF NORTH AMERICA

THE CLINICS ARE AVAILABLE ONLINE!
Access your subscription at:
www.theclinics.com

Foreword

The Many Faces of Mast Cell Disorders

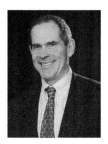

Stephen A. Tilles, MD
Consulting Editor

Mast cells were discovered more than 100 years ago, and the interaction between allergens, IgE, and mast cells in type I hypersensitivity immune responses has been a core part of the medical school curriculum for decades. Yet the absence of mature mast cells in circulating blood has prevented researchers from easily accessing mast cells for study, and to this day we are still not certain the full extent of mast cell heterogeneity. Fortunately, our understanding of mast cell function has improved significantly in recent years, including the critical roles mast cells play in both adaptive and innate immune responses. This has led to advances in our understanding of mast cell disorders.

This issue of *Immunology and Allergy Clinics of North America* comprehensively highlights up-to-date concepts involving the pathophysiology, diagnosis, and management of clonal and nonclonal mast cell disorders. With an international team of authors representing a wide range of perspectives, I am certain this *Immunology and Allergy Clinics of North America* issue will be an invaluable resource for practicing allergists and clinical immunologists.

Stephen A. Tilles, MD
ASTHMA Inc. Clinical Research Center
Northwest Asthma and Allergy Center
University of Washington
9725 3rd Avenue Northeast, Suite 500
Seattle, WA 98115, USA

E-mail address:
stilles@nwasthma.com

Immunol Allergy Clin N Am 38 (2018) xiii
https://doi.org/10.1016/j.iac.2018.05.002
0889-8561/18/© 2018 Published by Elsevier Inc.

immunology.theclinics.com

Preface

Mastocytosis: Moving the Field to Precision and Personalized Medicine

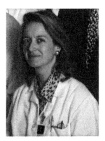

Mariana C. Castells, MD, PhD
Editor

This issue is dedicated to the new, recent, and groundbreaking advances in the field of Mastocytosis, a rare but important overlooked field, with the contributing authors scattered around the world and being the experts driving the field.

Mastocytosis encompasses a spectrum of rare disorders associated with the clonal expansion of mast cells in the skin and/or other tissues, most commonly the bone marrow, gastrointestinal tract, lymph nodes, liver, and spleen. Clonal mast cells typically carry somatic activating mutations in KIT proto-oncogene, which drives expansion and activation, with the Aspartate 816 Valine mutation being the most common. The new classification of maculopapular monomorphic versus polymorphic cutaneous mastocytosis has helped better define children and adult disease presentations, providing diagnostic and prognostic guidelines. Cutaneous mastocytosis has been generally considered a benign condition due to the favorable outcomes in a majority of children, but recent data indicate that skin mast cell can carry KIT-activating and nonactivating mutations, and the presence of these mutations may determine the progression to adult disease. Patients with low mast cell burden or absence of tryptase alpha genes can present normal tryptase with bone marrow mast cell aggregates, CD25 expression, and KIT D816V mutation, qualifying for WHO criteria for systemic mastocytosis. It is now possible to query KIT mutations in peripheral leukocytes with great sensitivity and specificity, helping improve the evaluation of mastocytosis in patients with episodes of hypotension and/or anaphylaxis. In the last 10 years, an increasing population of patients presenting with symptoms of mast cell activation with negative BMB for mast cell aggregates and elevated mast cell mediators has been diagnosed with nonclonal/idiopathic mast cell activation syndrome (**MCAS); treatment with mast cell controller medications has improved the outcomes, but the

Immunol Allergy Clin N Am 38 (2018) xv–xvii
https://doi.org/10.1016/j.iac.2018.05.001
0889-8561/18/© 2018 Published by Elsevier Inc.

immunology.theclinics.com

molecular causes and mechanisms of mast cell activation are lagging. More recently, the breakthrough description of familial tryptasemia in families with several members presenting with elevated tryptases and atypical symptoms of mast cell activation is the first advance in further understanding the causes of MCAS. In 2016, the description of the mast cell transcriptome with unique surface membrane and granular components, apart from basophils, eosinophils, dendritic, B cells, T cells, and other cells, indicates an unappreciated complexity for mast cell heterogeneity, which could also contribute to explain MCAS. New tyrosine kinase inhibitors such as midostaurin have been shown recently to extend the lives of patients with severe mastocytosis and should be explored for milder forms of mastocytosis for patients for whom their quality of life is not satisfactory with antihistamines, leukotriene blockers, or mast cell stabilizers. Anaphylaxis is a common presentation of clonal and nonclonal mast cell activation disorders, and omalizumab, a monoclonal antibody against IgE, is a promising approach that may contribute to mast cell stabilization. Of paramount importance is to listen to the other side: what are the patients feeling, how are their lives, how do they cope with mastocytosis?

Sofija Volertas, Charles F. Schuler IV, and Cem Akin introduce the classification of mast cell activation disorders: primary (due to intrinsic mast cells proliferation or clonal expansion and typically associated with KIT mutations), secondary or associated with allergic conditions and other inflammatory and autoimmune disorders, and idiopathic when no evidence for clonal expansion or proliferation is found but symptoms are compatible with mast cell activation. Whether patients present with skin-limited expansion of mast cells or have systemic involvement is of critical importance for their treatment and prognosis. Almudena Matito, José Manuel Azaña, Antonio Torrelo, and Iván Alvarez-Twose describe the new classification of cutaneous mastocytosis in adults and children and provide much needed prognostic factors. Children are particularly vulnerable to delayed or misdiagnosis; Sigurd Broesby-Olsen, Melody Carter, Henrik Fomsgaard Kjaer, Charlotte Gotthard Mortz, Michael Boe Møller, Thomas Kielsgaard Kristensen, Carsten Bindslev-Jensen, and Lone Agertoft describe the symptoms, presentation, associated morbidities, and natural history of pediatric mast cell disorders. Mast cell tissue aggregates are the hallmark of mastocytosis, and other features of mast cell activation are frequently overlooked; Laura Sanchez-Muñoz, Ana Filipa Henriques, Iván Alvarez-Twose, and Almudena Matito present the wide heterogeneity of bone marrow expression of mastocytosis. Mast cell mediators are present in blood and urine of patients with mast cell activation and provide important clinical clues for targeted therapies, as described by Joseph H. Butterfield, Anupama Ravi, and Thanai Pongdee. Whether proliferation of mast cells is generally driven by KIT mutations is explored by Lorenzo Falchi and Srdan Verstovsek, who describe new clinically relevant and pathogenic mutations. The consequences of mast cell activation and proliferation result in gastrointestinal symptoms, described by Fred H. Hsieh, and in bone disorders, described by Giovanni Orsolini, Ombretta Viapiana, Maurizio Rossini, Massimiliano Bonifacio, and Roberta Zanotti. Recent evidence indicates that more than 20% of patients with life-threatening hymenoptera anaphylaxis may carry a mast cell disorder, as described by Patrizia Bonadonna and Luigi Scaffidi. Idiopathic nonclonal mast cell activation MCAS affecting mostly women, but also seen in men and children, has surfaced as the new disease of the century; Matthew J. Hamilton provides a glimpse of its presentation, manifestations, and response to targeted therapies. The recent discovery of familial tryptasemia due to multiple copies of alpha tryptase genes without mast cell aggregates in tissues and atypical symptoms of mast cell activation is presented by Jonathan J. Lyons. The intriguing associations of familial tryptasemia and MCAS with postural tachycardia syndrome and Ehlers-Danlos syndrome are described by Rafael Bonamichi-Santos, Kelly Yoshimi-Kanamor, Pedro Giavina-Bianchi, and Marcelo Vivolo Aun. Importantly, patients' perceptions of their diseases and well-being are described by Susan V. Jennings, Valerie Slee, Rachel M. Zack, Srdan Verstovsek, Tracy I. George, Hongliang Shi, and Philina Lee. Current and future treatments for mastocytosis heavily rely on modifying KIT signaling, which is described by Siham Bibi and Michel Arock.

Giant advances have occurred in the last 5 years, and future research is needed in defining better biomarkers, newer mast cell stabilization strategies, and targeted/personalized treatment options, as in precision medicine. Most importantly, our efforts are geared to an early diagnosis, improving the quality of life of patients with cutaneous and systemic mastocytosis and MACSs, and finding a cure.

Mariana C. Castells, MD, PhD
Drug Hypersensitivity and
Desensitization Center
Mastoctytosis Center
Brigham and Women's Hospital
Harvard Medical School
60 Fenwood Road, Room 5002
Boston, MA 02115, USA

850 Boylston Street
Brookline, MA 02445, USA

E-mail addresses:
mcastells@partners.org; mcastells@bwh.harvard.edu

New Insights into Clonal Mast Cell Disorders Including Mastocytosis

Sofija Volertas, MD[1], Charles F. Schuler IV, MD[1],
Cem Akin, MD, PhD*

KEYWORDS

- Mastocytosis • Mast cell • Clonal mast cell disorders
- Monoclonal mast cell activation syndrome • Mast cell leukemia • Mast cell sarcoma
- Tryptase

KEY POINTS

- Mastocytosis is a heterogeneous grouping of neoplasms with clonal expansion of mast cells in one or more organ systems, typically including the skin and hematopoietic system.
- Systemic mastocytosis consists of a multifocal infiltration of mast cells into various organs, including the bone marrow.
- The diagnosis of mastocytosis requires tissue confirmation. Diagnostic algorithms have been established to guide the approach to patients with suspected mastocytosis.
- The mainstays of therapy for mastocytosis are symptomatic management, prevention of complications, and cytoreductive therapies for advanced disease.

Mast cells are an integral cell in the immune system, and disorders of regulation of mast cell production and activation have various presentations. Mastocytosis is a heterogeneous grouping of neoplasms with clonal expansion of mast cells in one or more organ systems, typically including the skin and hematopoietic system.[1–3] Mast cells are not found in the blood under normal circumstances but rather are present in most tissues. Abnormal mast cell expansion in clonal mast cell disorders tends to be focused in the skin, bone marrow, spleen, lymph nodes, and gastrointestinal tract, causing symptoms related to mast cell degranulation and less frequently symptoms of

Disclosure Statement: Dr C. Akin has consultancy agreements with Novartis, Blueprint Medicines, and Deciphera. Dr S. Volertas and Dr C.F. Schuler have no conflicts to report.
Division of Allergy and Clinical Immunology, Department of Internal Medicine, University of Michigan, 24 Frank Lloyd Wright Drive, PO Box 442, Suite H-2100, Ann Arbor, MI 48106-0442, USA
[1] Co–first authors.
* Corresponding author.
E-mail addresses: cemakin@med.umich.edu; cemakin@umich.edu

Immunol Allergy Clin N Am 38 (2018) 341–350
https://doi.org/10.1016/j.iac.2018.04.014
0889-8561/18/© 2018 Elsevier Inc. All rights reserved.

immunology.theclinics.com

organ dysfunction. Mast cell activation can cause various symptoms in all organ systems, such as cardiovascular (hypotension, syncope, light-headedness, tachycardia), cutaneous (flushing, pruritus, urticaria, angioedema), digestive (abdominal cramps, diarrhea, esophageal reflux, nausea and vomiting), musculoskeletal (aches, bone pain, osteopenia and osteoporosis), neurologic (anxiety, depression, decreased concentration and memory, insomnia and migraines), respiratory (nasal congestion, nasal pruritus, shortness of breath, throat swelling, and wheezing), and systemic (fatigue, general malaise and weight loss).[4] Notably, there is an increased risk of anaphylaxis in patients with mastocytosis; this risk is higher in males, in the absence of mastocytosis in the skin, presence of atopy, immunoglobulin E (IgE) levels of 15 kU/L or greater, and baseline tryptase levels less than 40 ng/mL.[5]

Significant advancements over the past decade in understanding the cause, prognosis, diagnosis, and potential targets for treatment changed the understanding of mast cell disease and, thus, can guide physicians in appropriate care of patients with clonal mast cell disorders.

HISTORICAL PERSPECTIVE

The first urticaria pigmentosa (UP) lesion was described by Nettleship and Tay[6] in 1869, and mast cells were discovered by Paul Ehrlich in 1879.[1] A short 8 years later, it was noted that mast cells were present in these UP lesions by Paul Unna[7] in 1887. However, systemic disease was not described for another 60 years until Ellis[8] in 1949. There were further categories described; the modern criteria for diagnosis were established in the 2000s, with the World Health Organization's (WHO) first classification in 2001.[9] In 2016, the WHO adopted changes to these categories of mastocytosis and have brought us to our current state of understanding.

CLASSIFICATION OF CLONAL MAST CELL DISORDERS AND WORLD HEALTH ORGANIZATION'S RECENT UPDATES

The WHO's previous classification of mast cell disorders from 2001 focused on dividing mast cell disorders into cutaneous mastocytosis (CM), systemic mastocytosis (SM), and solid mast cell tumors.[9] This framework has remained the same, with changes within the individual categories to reflect increasing knowledge of prognosis (**Box 1**). Notably, extracutaneous mastocytomas as a category were removed, as this is so rare and very few cases have been described in the past 20 years.[10]

Localized Mast Cell Tumors

Mast cell sarcomas (MCS) are extremely rare and remain as a separate category. There have been various reports of localized MCS that were present intracranially,[11] in the lung,[10] in the larynx,[12] and in the colon.[13] However, the data are too scarce to make any clear prognostic statement. Usually, MCS transform into a form of SM called mast cell leukemia (MCL).

Cutaneous Mastocytosis

Mast cell expansion within the skin has varying degrees of cutaneous involvement. CM can develop as a localized mastocytoma of the skin, maculopapular CM, also known as UP, or the most involved form of diffuse CM. Major and minor criteria to diagnose CM have been proposed. The major criterion is presence of typical skin lesions of mastocytosis associated with the Darier sign.[14] Minor criteria include increased numbers of mast cells in the biopsy of lesional skin and an activating KIT mutation in the lesional skin tissue.[14]

Box 1
World Health Organization's updated classification of mastocytosis in 2016

CM
- Maculopapular CM = UP
- Diffuse CM
- Mastocytoma of skin

SM
- Indolent SM
- Smoldering SM
- SM with associated hematologic neoplasm[a]
- Aggressive SM
- Mast cell leukemia

Mast cell sarcoma

[a] The previous term *SM with clonal hematologic non–mast cell–lineage disease* and the new term *SM with associated hematologic neoplasm* can be used synonymously.
Adapted from Valent P, Akin C, Hartmann K, et al. Advances in the classification and treatment of mastocytosis: current status and outlook toward the future. Cancer Res 2017;77(6):1263; with permission.

Systemic Mastocytosis

SM consists of a multifocal infiltration of mast cells into various organs, including the bone marrow.[15] Diagnosis of SM is reviewed in **Table 1**, with the requirement of 1 major criterion and 1 minor criterion OR 3 minor criteria.[3,9] The major criterion for diagnosis is a multifocal accumulation of clustered mast cells ($\geq$15 per cluster) in the bone marrow or other extracutaneous organ. Minor criteria are as follows:

- Abnormal mast cell morphology (such as spindle-shaped cells)
- CD2 and/or CD25 expression on mast cells in extracutaneous organs
- Activating KIT mutation in codon 816 (typically D816 V) in extracutaneous mast cells
- Serum tryptase greater than 20 ng/mL in a basal state[3,9]

Monoclonal Mast Cell Activation Syndrome

Some patients with limited clonal mast cell expansion may come to clinical attention because of symptoms of mast cell activation and anaphylaxis. These patients do not have skin lesions and typically have tryptase levels less than 20 ng/mL. They are

---

Table 1
Diagnosis of systemic mastocytosis

SM: Diagnosis Met with 1 Major + 1 Minor or 3 Minor Criteria	
Major criterion	Multifocal accumulation of clustered mast cells ($\geq$15 per cluster) in the bone marrow or other extracutaneous organ
Minor criteria	Abnormal mast cell morphology (such as spindle-shaped cells) CD2 and/or CD25 expression in mast cells in extracutaneous organs Activating KIT mutation in codon 816 (typically D816 V) in extracutaneous mast cells Serum tryptase >20 ng/mL in basal state

Adapted from Valent P, Horny HP, Escribano L, et al. Diagnostic criteria and classification of mastocytosis: a consensus proposal. Leuk Res 2001;25(7):611; with permission.

determined to have monoclonal mast cell activation syndrome (MMAS) if the pathologic evaluation meets 1 or 2 minor clonality criteria (aberrant CD25 expression on mast cells and/or codon 816 KIT mutation in lesional tissue or peripheral blood) without fulfilling the full criteria for SM.[16,17] MMAS is not an official category of the WHO's current classification but is mentioned in the text of the document.[18]

Well-Differentiated Systemic Mastocytosis

Well-differentiated systemic mastocytosis (WDSM) is a histopathologic variant of SM with compact mast cell infiltrates in bone marrow but with a round morphology and absence of aberrant CD25 or CD2 expression.[19,20] Most of these patients also typically lack the D816 V KIT mutation and may be candidates for imatinib therapy (see therapy section later). Patients with WDSM may present as any category of SM.

SUBTYPES OF SYSTEMIC MASTOCYTOSIS

The WHO's updates in 2016 apply to the categories of mastocytosis and are based on a newer understanding of the prognosis and natural course of the various presentations (**Table 2**). Adverse prognostic factors for survival of patients with SM overall include advanced age, weight loss, anemia, thrombocytopenia, hypoalbuminemia, and excess bone marrow blasts.[16]

After diagnosis of SM by major and/or minor criteria, SM is then subdivided into 5 types:

1. Indolent SM (ISM)
2. Smoldering SM (SSM)
3. SM with associated hematologic neoplasm (SM-AHN)
4. Aggressive SM (ASM)
5. MCL

Table 2
Subtypes of systemic mastocytosis and criteria for diagnosis

Indolent SM	Criteria for SM No C Findings	Provisional Subtype Bone Marrow Mastocytosis
Smoldering SM	Criteria for SM 2 or more B findings and no C findings	
SM with associated hematologic neoplasm	Criteria for SM MDS, MPN, AML, lymphoma, or other hematologic neoplasm	
ASM	Criteria SM 1 or more C findings	*Subtypes of ASM* Untransformed ASM ASM-t: mast cells in bone marrow $\geq$5% but <20%
MCL	Mast cells in bone marrow $\geq$20% Chronic MCL: no C findings Acute MCL: 1 or more C findings	*Subtypes of MCL* Classic MCL: $\geq$10% mast cells in peripheral blood Aleukemia MCL: <10% mast cells in peripheral blood

Abbreviations: ASM, aggressive SM; ASM-t, aggressive SM in transformation; AML, acute myelogenous leukemia; MDS, myelodysplastic syndromes; MPD, myeloproliferative disorders.

Data from Horny HP, Akin C, Arber D, et al. Mastocytosis. In: WHO classification of tumors of haematopoietic and lymphoid tissues. Revised 4th edition. Lyon (France): IARC Press; 2017.

SSM was added as a separate category, whereas previously it was considered a subtype of ISM. This change occurred because the prognosis of SSM is more favorable than ASM and MCL but distinctly less favorable than ISM.[17] The subcategory of SM-AHN was simplified from the terminology of associated clonal hematologic non–mast cell lineage disease (AHNMD) to SM-AHN.[3] Additionally, a provisional subtype of ISM was added as bone marrow mastocytosis, which is characterized by a low burden of mast cells, absence of cutaneous disease, and a good prognosis.[9]

Indolent Systemic Mastocytosis

ISM is a limited clonal expansion of mast cells. These patients tend to have normal or near-normal survival but may have mast cell mediator–related symptoms.[16] The disease progression rate is also very low at 1.7% in 5 years.[21] However, some do progress to a more aggressive form of the disease. The most powerful independent factors for predicting transformation are the presence of KIT mutation in all hematopoietic lineages and an increased serum beta2-microglobulin.[21]

Smoldering Systemic Mastocytosis

SSM presents with a KIT-associated neoplastic process expanding into other myeloid lineages. There is a high burden of mast cells in non–bone marrow organs as well. To diagnose SSM, there must be 2 or more B findings and no C findings (**Table 3**). There is a lower survival rate in SSM that may be age independent.[17] Additionally, each B finding (organomegaly, tryptase >200 ng/mL, and clonal involvement of non–mast cell lineages) as well a KIT D816 V mutation burden independently suggest a poorer prognosis.[21–26]

Systemic Mastocytosis with Associated Hematologic Neoplasm

SM-AHN is the presence of a different, non–mast cell neoplasm in the setting of SM. It is clinically more useful to consider each group of specific hematologic neoplasms as individual entities, as they have different prognoses. For example, SM-MPN seems to

Table 3	
B and C findings in systemic mastocytosis	
B findings	1. Bone marrow biopsy showing >30% infiltration by mast cells (focal, dense aggregates) and/or serum total tryptase level >200 ng/mL
	2. Signs of dysplasia or myelo-proliferation in non-mast cell lineages (insufficient criteria for definitive diagnosis of hematopoietic neoplasm)
	3. Hepatomegaly without impairment of function, and/or palpable spleno-megaly without hypersplenism, and/or lymphadenopathy
C findings	1. Bone marrow dysfunction: one or more cytopenias (ANC <1.0 × 10⁹/L, hemoglobin <10 g/dL, or platelets <100 × 10⁹/L), and no obvious non–mast cell hematopoietic malignancy
	2. Palpable hepatomegaly WITH impairment of liver function, ascites, and/or portal hypertension
	3. Skeletal involvement with large osteolytic lesions and/or pathologic fractures
	4. Palpable splenomegaly with hypersplenism
	5. Malabsorption with weight loss caused by gastrointestinal mast cell infiltrates

Data from Horny HP, Akin C, Arber D, et al. Mastocytosis. In: WHO classification of tumors of haematopoietic and lymphoid tissues. Revised 4th edition. Lyon (France): IARC Press; 2017.

have a better life expectancy than the others, and SM-MDS has a higher rate of leukemic transformation.[27]

Aggressive Systemic Mastocytosis

ASM is defined by meeting the criteria for SM as well as 1 C finding indicating organ damage (see **Table 3**). ASM is newly divided by the WHO's updates into an untransformed variant and "in transformation to MCL" (ASM in transformation [ASM-t]). The percentage of mast cells in the bone marrow smear is of prognostic significance; thus, if the percentage of mast cells in bone marrow smears 5% or greater but less than 20%, it is considered ASM-t.[28,29] When the percentage of mast cells in the bone marrow reaches 20%, the diagnosis changes from ASM-t to MCL.[29]

Mast Cell Leukemia

MCL is diagnosed in patients with bone marrow smears that contain 20% or greater mast cells.[29] Previously, MCL was further divided into a classic variant with at least 10% of circulating white blood cells as mast cells and an aleukemic MCL variant with less than 10% mast cells circulating.[9] This division still applies; however, the WHO's updated guidelines also categorize MCL into a chronic and an acute (more aggressive) form. Chronic MCL has no obvious organ damage with no C findings present, and acute MCL has organ damage (C findings).[3]

DIAGNOSING MASTOCYTOSIS

Mastocytosis diagnosis requires tissue confirmation. In some patients, there are typical skin lesions which can aid in the diagnosis of mastocytosis. In other patients, these lesions are not present, and thus take further investigation for diagnosis. Diagnostic algorithms have been established to delineate an approach to patients with suspected mastocytosis.[30] These algorithms are divided by the presence or absence of mastocytosis in the skin, and use tryptase levels and a Spanish Mastocytosis Network (REMA) score to further stratify patients. A REMA score is used to assess the risk of mast cell clonality or SM in patients presenting with mast cell activation symptoms. It consists of positive or negative points for male (+1), female (−1), serum baseline tryptase less than 15 mcg/L(−1) or greater than 25 mcg/L (+2), presence (−2) or absence (+1) of pruritus, hives or angioedema and presence (+3) of presyncope or syncope.[31] A score greater than 2 would indicate a higher risk with a sensitivity and specificity at 84% and 74% for mast cell clonality and 86% and 73% for SM.[31]

In adult patients with typical lesions of mastocytosis in the skin, complete staging, including bone marrow investigation, is recommended. Based on the presence or absence of criteria of SM as outlined previously, patients will be categorized as SM or CM. In children with mastocytosis in the skin, no bone marrow investigation is required unless clinical and/or laboratory data suggest the development of a hematopoietic neoplasm (such as organomegaly). Serum tryptase and complete blood counts should be monitored at least yearly for the potential progression of disease.[30]

In adults with suspected mastocytosis without typical skin lesions, serum tryptase should be measured. It is very rare to have children with mastocytosis without skin lesions; thus, there is no algorithm for this scenario. The algorithm for adults without typical skin lesions uses the patients' tryptase level and a REMA score to further decide on bone marrow investigation or follow-up. If the tryptase level is 25 to 30 ng/mL or greater, then one should proceed directly to bone marrow studies and staging of mastocytosis. If the tryptase is less than 15 ng/mL, a decision for continued follow-up or using REMA scoring should be made by the physician. In patients with serum tryptase of 15 to 25 ng/mL, a REMA score should be used. If the REMA score is 2 or greater, and typical symptoms of SM are present or KIT D816 V is detectable in peripheral blood cells, then bone marrow biopsy should be performed. If the REMA score is not 2 or greater, there are no typical clinical signs, and no KIT D816 V mutation in peripheral blood cells, then continued follow-up is recommended with tryptase and assessment of symptoms yearly.[30]

THERAPIES

Once the diagnosis and staging of mastocytosis is established, the mainstay of treatment is either symptomatic management or cytoreductive therapies based on the subtype of SM. Currently the treatment of ISM, SSM, or mast cell activation syndrome (MCAS) is symptomatic management with antihistamines (both H1 and H2 receptor blockade), antileukotriene drugs, and mast cell stabilizers, such as cromolyn. Self-injectable epinephrine is usually prescribed because of the increased risk of anaphylaxis. For patients with SM-AHN, ASM, and MCL, cytoreductive therapy can be considered to reduce the mast cell burden.

Currently, there is no standard therapy for cytoreduction for patients with SM-AHN, ASM or MCL. These patients have been typically treated with cladribine or interferon-alpha until the recent approval of midostaurin (see later discussion).[32,33] Chemotherapy agents, such as cladribine, do induce a meaningful response in 50% of patients with SM-AHN, ASM, or MCL; but patients often develop resistance.[34] Stem cell transplants have also been used, but most reports have been in the setting of SM-AHN.[35] Hematopoietic stem cell transplants seem to be more favorable in patients with ASM and SM-AHN rather than MCL, and myeloablative conditioning is more effective with better outcomes compared with reduced intensity.[35]

Future directions for research are focusing on targets specific to mast cell proliferation, such as KIT and mutations of KIT, KIT-downstream molecules, KIT-independent oncogenic drivers of mast cells, epigenetic targets, immunogenic cell-surface targets on mast cells, and leukemic stem cells. The most studied of these targets are KIT tyrosine kinase inhibitors.

KIT Tyrosine Kinase Inhibitors

Midostaurin (PKC412) seems to be one of the most promising new treatments available for advanced SM, such as ASM, SM-AHN, and MCL. It blocks wild-type KIT as well as D816 V mutant KIT kinase activity. In this way, it opposes KIT-dependent growth of mast cells and inhibits IgE-dependent mediator secretion from mast cells.[36] It has shown an overall response rate of 60%, improved overall and relapse-free survival, and improved quality of life in a recent open-label phase II trial.[36,37] Interestingly, those patients on midostaurin who have a reduction in alkaline phosphatase by 50% have an independently increased survival.[38] As D816 V is a codriver of cell proliferation and survival of mast cells, and oncogenic KIT mutations are detected in greater than 80% of patients with SM, and in greater than 90% of all cases of indolent SM, there is significant promise for this drug.[39] It is currently recommended as a the first-line treatment approach for patients in need of cytoreductive therapy. The use of the drug in ISM, SSM, or MCAS has not been studied in detail.

The KIT D816V mutation confers resistance to multiple KIT-targeting drugs, such as imatinib and masitinib.[40] However, imatinib can target non–D816 V-mutant patients, which are usually present in well-differentiated SM. In one case report, a patient with a transmembrane c-KIT mutation received therapy with imatinib, which decreased mast cell burden and symptoms.[19] However, this is not broadly applicable to most patients who do not have this same transmembrane c-KIT mutation. There are other mutant forms of KIT, such as K509I or F522 C, which can be sensitive to imatinib as well.[41,42] There is also a small subset of patients with SM that express a wild-type KIT that may respond to imatinib.[41] Masitinib can be used to inhibit wild-type KIT and LIN kinases. It does not affect D816 V; but it has been shown to decrease the total symptom burden despite no cytoreductive effects.[40] This drug is currently in a phase III randomized placebo controlled trial in severely symptomatic patients with ISM.

SUMMARY

Clonal mast cell diseases, including mastocytosis, have been divided into prognostically relevant subtypes; exciting new treatments are in development that directly target the mechanisms of disease. Tyrosine kinase inhibitors are currently a major area of investigation; relevance to the most common mutation, KIT D816 V, seems to be most important in this pathway. There are future potential targets at earlier stages of exploration that might likely change the field further.

REFERENCES

1. Valent P, Akin C, Hartmann K, et al. Advances in the classification and treatment of mastocytosis: current status and outlook toward the future. Cancer Res 2017; 77:1261–70.
2. Valent P, Akin C, Metcalfe DD. Mastocytosis: 2016 updated WHO classification and novel emerging treatment concepts. Blood 2017;129:1420–7.
3. Arber DA, Orazi A, Hasserjian R, et al. The 2016 revision to the World Health Organization classification of myeloid neoplasms and acute leukemia. Blood 2016;127:2391–405.
4. Theoharides TC, Valent P, Akin C. Mast cells, mastocytosis, and related disorders. N Engl J Med 2015;373:163–72.
5. Gulen T, Ljung C, Nilsson G, et al. Risk factor analysis of anaphylactic reactions in patients with systemic mastocytosis. J Allergy Clin Immunol Pract 2017;5: 1248–55.
6. Nettleship E, Tay W. Rare forms of urticaria. Br Med J 1869;2:323–30.
7. Unna PG. Bëitrage zur anatomie und pathogenese der urticaria simplex und pigmentosa Mschr. Prakt. Dermatol. Suppl. Dermatol. Stud., 3 1887. p. 9.
8. Ellis JM. Urticaria pigmentosa; a report of a case with autopsy. Arch Pathol (Chic) 1949;48:426–35.
9. Valent P, Horny HP, Escribano L, et al. Diagnostic criteria and classification of mastocytosis: a consensus proposal. Leuk Res 2001;25:603–25.
10. Ayadi L, Abid N, Makni S, et al. An unusual tumour of the lung. Pathologica 2015; 107:14–8.
11. Guenther PP, Huebner A, Sobottka SB, et al. Temporary response of localized intracranial mast cell sarcoma to combination chemotherapy. J Pediatr Hematol Oncol 2001;23:134–8.
12. Horny HP, Parwaresch MR, Kaiserling E, et al. Mast cell sarcoma of the larynx. J Clin Pathol 1986;39:596–602.
13. Schwaab J, Horny HP, Jonescheit J, et al. Mast cell sarcoma mimicking metastatic colon carcinoma. Ann Hematol 2014;93:1067–9.
14. Hartmann K, Escribano L, Grattan C, et al. Cutaneous manifestations in patients with mastocytosis: consensus report of the European Competence Network on Mastocytosis; the American Academy of Allergy, Asthma & Immunology; and

the European Academy of Allergology and Clinical Immunology. J Allergy Clin Immunol 2016;137:35–45.

15. Valent P, Akin C, Sperr WR, et al. Diagnosis and treatment of systemic mastocytosis: state of the art. Br J Haematol 2003;122:695–717.

16. Lim KH, Tefferi A, Lasho TL, et al. Systemic mastocytosis in 342 consecutive adults: survival studies and prognostic factors. Blood 2009;113:5727–36.

17. Pardanani A, Lim KH, Lasho TL, et al. WHO subvariants of indolent mastocytosis: clinical details and prognostic evaluation in 159 consecutive adults. Blood 2010; 115:150–1.

18. Horny HP, Akin C, Arber D, et al. Mastocytosis. In: Swerdlow SH, Campo E, Harris NL, editors. WHO classification of tumors of haematopoietic and lymphoid tissues. Revised 4th edition. Lyon (France): IARC Press; 2017. p. 61–9.

19. Akin C, Fumo G, Yavuz AS, et al. A novel form of mastocytosis associated with a transmembrane c-kit mutation and response to imatinib. Blood 2004;103:3222–5.

20. Alvarez-Twose I, Jara-Acevedo M, Morgado JM, et al. Clinical, immunophenotypic, and molecular characteristics of well-differentiated systemic mastocytosis. J Allergy Clin Immunol 2016;137:168–78.e1.

21. Escribano L, Alvarez-Twose I, Sanchez-Munoz L, et al. Prognosis in adult indolent systemic mastocytosis: a long-term study of the Spanish Network on Mastocytosis in a series of 145 patients. J Allergy Clin Immunol 2009;124:514–21.

22. Matito A, Morgado JM, Alvarez-Twose I, et al. Serum tryptase monitoring in indolent systemic mastocytosis: association with disease features and patient outcome. PLoS One 2013;8:e76116.

23. Erben P, Schwaab J, Metzgeroth G, et al. The KIT D816V expressed allele burden for diagnosis and disease monitoring of systemic mastocytosis. Ann Hematol 2014;93:81–8.

24. Hoermann G, Gleixner KV, Dinu GE, et al. The KIT D816V allele burden predicts survival in patients with mastocytosis and correlates with the WHO type of the disease. Allergy 2014;69:810–3.

25. Jawhar M, Schwaab J, Hausmann D, et al. Splenomegaly, elevated alkaline phosphatase and mutations in the SRSF2/ASXL1/RUNX1 gene panel are strong adverse prognostic markers in patients with systemic mastocytosis. Leukemia 2016;30:2342–50.

26. Garcia-Montero AC, Jara-Acevedo M, Alvarez-Twose I, et al. KIT D816V-mutated bone marrow mesenchymal stem cells in indolent systemic mastocytosis are associated with disease progression. Blood 2016;127:761–8.

27. Pardanani A, Lim KH, Lasho TL, et al. Prognostically relevant breakdown of 123 patients with systemic mastocytosis associated with other myeloid malignancies. Blood 2009;114:3769–72.

28. Sperr WR, Escribano L, Jordan JH, et al. Morphologic properties of neoplastic mast cells: delineation of stages of maturation and implication for cytological grading of mastocytosis. Leuk Res 2001;25:529–36.

29. Valent P, Sotlar K, Sperr WR, et al. Refined diagnostic criteria and classification of mast cell leukemia (MCL) and myelomastocytic leukemia (MML): a consensus proposal. Ann Oncol 2014;25:1691–700.

30. Valent P, Escribano L, Broesby-Olsen S, et al. Proposed diagnostic algorithm for patients with suspected mastocytosis: a proposal of the European Competence Network on Mastocytosis. Allergy 2014;69:1267–74.

31. Alvarez-Twose I, Gonzalez-de-Olano D, Sanchez-Munoz L, et al. Validation of the REMA score for predicting mast cell clonality and systemic mastocytosis in

patients with systemic mast cell activation symptoms. Int Arch Allergy Immunol 2012;157:275–80.

32. Casassus P, Caillat-Vigneron N, Martin A, et al. Treatment of adult systemic mastocytosis with interferon-alpha: results of a multicentre phase II trial on 20 patients. Br J Haematol 2002;119:1090–7.

33. Lim KH, Pardanani A, Butterfield JH, et al. Cytoreductive therapy in 108 adults with systemic mastocytosis: outcome analysis and response prediction during treatment with interferon-alpha, hydroxyurea, imatinib mesylate or 2-chlorodeoxyadenosine. Am J Hematol 2009;84:790–4.

34. Barete S, Lortholary O, Damaj G, et al. Long-term efficacy and safety of cladribine (2-CdA) in adult patients with mastocytosis. Blood 2015;126:1009–16 [quiz: 1050].

35. Ustun C, Gotlib J, Popat U, et al. Consensus opinion on allogeneic hematopoietic cell transplantation in advanced systemic mastocytosis. Biol Blood Marrow Transplant 2016;22:1348–56.

36. Valent P, Akin C, Hartmann K, et al. Midostaurin: a magic bullet that blocks mast cell expansion and activation. Ann Oncol 2017;28:2367–76.

37. Gotlib J, Kluin-Nelemans HC, George TI, et al. Efficacy and safety of midostaurin in advanced systemic mastocytosis. N Engl J Med 2016;374:2530–41.

38. Jawhar M, Schwaab J, Naumann N, et al. Response and progression on midostaurin in advanced systemic mastocytosis: KIT D816V and other molecular markers. Blood 2017;130:137–45.

39. Arock M, Sotlar K, Akin C, et al. KIT mutation analysis in mast cell neoplasms: recommendations of the European Competence Network on Mastocytosis. Leukemia 2015;29:1223–32.

40. Lortholary O, Chandesris MO, Bulai Livideanu C, et al. Masitinib for treatment of severely symptomatic indolent systemic mastocytosis: a randomised, placebo-controlled, phase 3 study. Lancet 2017;389:612–20.

41. Alvarez-Twose I, Gonzalez P, Morgado JM, et al. Complete response after imatinib mesylate therapy in a patient with well-differentiated systemic mastocytosis. J Clin Oncol 2012;30:e126–9.

42. de Melo Campos P, Machado-Neto JA, Scopim-Ribeiro R, et al. Familial systemic mastocytosis with germline KIT K509I mutation is sensitive to treatment with imatinib, dasatinib and PKC412. Leuk Res 2014;38:1245–51.

Cutaneous Mastocytosis in Adults and Children

New Classification and Prognostic Factors

Almudena Matito, MD, PhD[a], José Manuel Azaña, MD, PhD[b],
Antonio Torrelo, MD, PhD[c], Iván Alvarez-Twose, MD, PhD[a],*

KEYWORDS

- Mastocytosis • Mast cell • Cutaneous mastocytosis • Urticaria pigmentosa
- Classification • Prognosis • WHO

KEY POINTS

- Cutaneous mastocytosis is a highly heterogeneous subtype of mastocytosis. Heterogeneity mainly depends on the age at disease onset and the clinical form of presentation.
- The classification of cutaneous mastocytosis has recently been redefined by the World Health Organization and an international consensus task force.
- A subset of children with mastocytosis shows persistence of the disease into adulthood, usually as the classic indolent systemic mastocytosis or as well-differentiated systemic mastocytosis.

INTRODUCTION

Mastocytosis is a heterogeneous disease characterized by the clonal expansion and accumulation of mast cells (MCs) in different organs and tissues.[1–3] The clonal nature of the disease can be established by the demonstration of activating mutations of the c-kit gene in most patients, provided that highly sensitive diagnostic methods are used.[4–7] This proto-oncogene encodes for a receptor in the membrane of MCs called *KIT*, a tyrosine-kinase protein that regulates growth and differentiation of MCs. In mastocytosis, *KIT* mutations induce a ligand-independent hyperactivation state of the receptor that leads to an increased survival of MCs, resulting in their accumulation in tissues.

Depending on the sites of organ involvement, 2 main forms of mastocytosis are recognized: (1) cutaneous mastocytosis (CM), when the skin is the only tissue affected, and (2) systemic mastocytosis (SM), characterized by MC infiltrates in

Disclosure Statement: The authors declare that they have no conflict of interest.
[a] Instituto de Estudios de Mastocitosis de Castilla La Mancha (CLMast), Hospital Virgen del Valle, Ctra. Cobisa s/n, Toledo 45071, Spain; [b] Department of Dermatology, Complejo Hospitalario Universitario de Albacete, Hospital General Universitario de Albacete, C/Hermanos Falcó no 37, Albacete 02006, Spain; [c] Department of Dermatology, Hospital Infantil Universitario del Niño Jesús, Av/Menéndez Pelayo, no 65, Madrid 28009, Spain
* Corresponding author.
E-mail address: ivana@sescam.jccm.es

Immunol Allergy Clin N Am 38 (2018) 351–363
https://doi.org/10.1016/j.iac.2018.04.001
0889-8561/18/© 2018 Elsevier Inc. All rights reserved.

immunology.theclinics.com

extracutaneous organs, mostly the bone marrow (BM), with or without concomitant skin involvement.[1,8–10] The heterogeneity of mastocytosis is evidenced by the fact that the disease can develop both in children, supposedly as CM that tends to spontaneously regress by adolescence, and in adults, in whom mastocytosis is often systemic and shows a chronic course. More rarely, mastocytosis can exhibit an aggressive behavior with high cell proliferation rates and shortened survival.

In this article, we focus on the dermatologic aspects of mastocytosis, including a brief review through the different terminologies, concepts, and classification approaches that have been used along the history, with special emphasis on the most modern vision of the disease.

HISTORIC OVERVIEW

In 1869, Nettleship and Tay[11] described the case of a 2-year-old girl who presented with what looked like a rare form of chronic urticaria leaving brownish stains, which is widely thought to be the first case of mastocytosis reported in the literature, 10 years before the discovery of MCs by Paul Ehrlich.[12] The term *urticaria pigmentosa* (UP) was coined in 1878 by Sangster[13] to refer to a skin eruption found in a child that was described as "an anomalous mottled rash accompanied by pruritus, factitious urticaria and pigmentation." Nine years later, Unna[14] documented the presence of MCs in skin lesions of UP, but it was not until 1936 when the term mastocytosis was first used.[15]

Early attempts for classification of CM date from the first quarter of the twentieth century. At that time, 3 main forms of UP were already distinguished:

1. Macular
2. Nodular (xanthelasmoid form)
3. Mixed type (maculonodular)[16,17]

Later, more uncommon forms of UP with peculiar characteristics, such as bullous UP,[18,19] diffuse erythrodermic mastocytosis,[20,21] and *telangiectasia macularis eruptiva perstans* (TMEP)[22] were described, becoming rapidly recognized as novel cutaneous variants of UP.

By the mid-twentieth century, the systemic nature of mastocytosis was first established on the basis of histopathological findings in an autopsy carried out in a fatal case of UP that showed MC infiltrates not only in the skin but also in internal organs.[23] Within the following years, the concept of mastocytosis as a systemic disease in nature was rapidly spread out in parallel to increasing numbers of reports showing extracutaneous involvement,[24–29] but also cases purely restricted to the skin were described,[24,25] a dual vision of the disease that still remains today.

In the 1960s, Caplan[26,27] proposed to classify UP cases into 3 categories according to the number of skin lesions and the age at disease onset:

1. Solitary lesion (group I)
2. Multiple lesions appearing in infancy and early childhood (group II)
3. Multiple lesions appearing in late childhood, adolescence, and adulthood (group III)

Noteworthy, this classification provided pioneer information in terms of prognosis of the different categories of the disease. Thus, whereas solitary lesions tended to involute completely with time, some cases in group II and most cases in group III seemed to persist indefinitely; moreover, a correlation was found between late onset of skin lesions (group III) and the existence of a systemic MC disease.

The first comprehensive classification of mastocytosis in which both CM and SM were incorporated together was developed by Lennert and Parwaresch in 1979.[28]

The investigators divided MC neoplasms into 2 main categories: (1) benign MC neo-plasms, which included mastocytoma, CM (diffuse or localized variants), and SM with skin involvement, and (2) malignant (systemic) MC neoplasms, which included malignant mastocytosis (also called MC reticulosis), MC sarcoma, and MC leukemia. Here, the investigators emphasized the poor prognosis in terms of survival of patients with malignant MC tumors.

In early 1990s, a consensus classification of mastocytosis was agreed on at an interdisciplinary meeting.[29] The new classification was adapted from previous classi-fication schemes developed at the Mayo Clinic[30] and at the National Institutes of Health,[31] and recognized 4 categories of the disease:

1. Category I (indolent mastocytosis)
2. Category II (mastocytosis associated with a hematologic disorder)
3. Category III (aggressive mastocytosis)
4. Category IV (mastocytic leukemia)

In this revised classification, cutaneous lesions of mastocytosis, including UP, mas-tocytoma, diffuse and erythrodermic mastocytosis, and TMEP, were grouped under the general term of "cutaneous disease" and included within the category of indolent mastocytosis together with other manifestations, such as syncope, ulcer disease, malabsorption, BM MC aggregates, skeletal involvement, hepatosplenomegaly, and lymphadenopathy.[29]

Over the following decade, major advances were made in the understanding of MC physiopathology that contributed to provide more specific diagnostic criteria for SM. Such criteria were used as a basis for a new consensus classification of mastocytosis formulated in the year 2000,[32] which was adopted by the World Health Organization (WHO) in 2001.[33] In this classification, CM was considered as a separate entity defined by the presence of skin lesions (with histologic demonstration of MC infiltrates in the dermis) in the absence of diagnostic criteria for SM, and included 3 main variants:

1. UP
2. Diffuse CM (DCM)
3. Mastocytoma of skin

Within the UP variant, for which the investigators proposed also the term "maculo-papular CM (MPCM)," several subvariants were recognized, including a plaque form, a nodular form, and a telangiectatic subvariant (also referred to as TMEP). However, other investigators were aligned with the idea of considering the subvariants of UP as separate entities of CM on the basis of their different macroscopic appearance and prognosis; accordingly, a modified classification of CM including 5 variants also was proposed:

1. MPCM
2. Plaque-type CM
3. Nodular CM/mastocytoma (solitary or multiple)
4. DCM
5. Telangiectatic CM[34]

The 2001 WHO classification of mastocytosis remained substantially unchanged in terms of CM variants in the updated versions of the WHO classification in 2008[1] and 2016.[8,9] However, an international task force involving experts from Europe (EU) and the United States has recently recommended that MPCM/UP should be subdivided into 2 variants: (1) monomorphic variant, characterized by small maculopapular le-sions that typically arise in the adulthood, and (2) polymorphic variant, which shows large and heterogeneous lesions that can be macular, plaque-type, or nodular and is almost exclusively seen in children.[10] The rationale for this proposal is a potential prognostic impact in terms of duration of the disease in children, because polymorphic lesions tend to spontaneously regress by adolescence, whereas in children with the monomorphic variant of MPCM, mastocytosis frequently persists into adulthood usually as a systemic disease. Other recommendations supported by the EU/US consensus group are to consider a maximum of 3 cutaneous lesions under the term mastocytoma, which should be no longer referred to as solitary mastocytoma, and to remove TMEP from the classification of CM.[10]

THE SKIN IN MASTOCYTOSIS

The skin is the most frequently affected tissue in patients with mastocytosis. Overall, virtually all children and more than 80% of adult patients with mastocytosis show cutaneous lesions, but their macroscopic and microscopic characteristics as well as their localization and distribution strongly differ from one patient to another.

Subtypes of Mastocytosis in the Skin/Cutaneous Mastocytosis

The WHO currently recognizes 3 main subforms of CM, which include MPCM/UP, DCM, and mastocytoma of skin.[8,9]

In the MPCM subform, skin lesions are typically brownish to reddish oval or round macules and papules, but in some cases large plaques or nodules can coexist or even predominate. According to the EU/US consensus group, MPCM can be divided into 2 variants[10]:

1. Monomorphic MPCM, characterized by homogeneous, small skin lesions that are highly variable in number and usually show a central body distribution with centrifugal spread (**Fig. 1**A).
2. Polymorphic MPCM, in which the skin lesions are heterogeneous and show different shapes and sizes, but are generally larger than those from the monomorphic variant (**Fig. 1**B).

Overall, the monomorphic MPCM variant is more commonly seen in adult-onset mastocytosis, in which the skin involvement usually coexists with SM. By contrast,

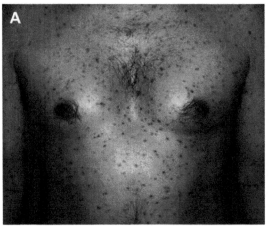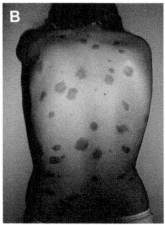

Fig. 1. MPCM. (*A*) MPCM monomorphic variant (EU/US consensus classification). (*B*) MPCM polymorphic variant (EU/US consensus classification).

polymorphic MPCM typically occurs in children in whom the disease is generally restricted to the skin and tends to show spontaneous regression by puberty in most cases.

DCM is defined by a generalized thickening of almost the entire skin in the absence of individual hyperpigmented cutaneous lesions.[10] Although as per definition the term DCM implies an extensive cutaneous involvement, it should be emphasized that not all patients showing extensive cutaneous disease correspond to DCM.[35] The typical macroscopic appearance of the skin in DCM has been traditionally referred to as "peau d'orange," "crocodile-like pachydermia," or "elephant skin" (**Fig. 2**A). Overall, this subform of CM is rare and generally develops at birth or shortly after.[10] Children with DCM usually show recurrent episodes of generalized blistering (**Fig. 2**B) often associated with systemic symptoms, such as flushing, gastrointestinal symptoms, and, in most severe cases, hypotension requiring epinephrine or other life-threatening complications.[36–38] Elevated serum tryptase (sT) levels (frequently higher than 100 μg/L) are typically detected at early stages of the disease, as a reflection of both the high MC burden in the skin and an increased MC-mediator releasability, but generally decline over time in parallel with gradual improvement of MC-mediator release symptoms.[10,37,39] Because of the high density of skin MCs that characterize DCM, it is not recommended to perform the Darier sign in these cases, to avoid a potentially massive MC desgranulation that could result in severe symptoms. Despite the extent of cutaneous involvement and the severity of clinical symptoms at onset, DCM usually resolves by adolescence, frequently leaving a *cutis laxa*–like residual appearance of the skin, although in some patients the disease persists into adulthood. In many of these later cases, the BM is infiltrated by round, fully granulated MCs in the absence of aberrant expression of CD25 and CD2 and frequently lacking *KIT* mutations or carrying germline mutations located at exons 8 or 9 of *KIT* (eg, del D419, K509I); altogether, these findings are consistent with the diagnosis of well-differentiated SM.[40–43]

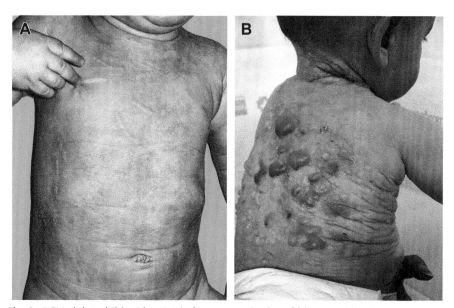

Fig. 2. DCM. (*A*) A child with DCM in between episodes of blistering showing "peau d'orange" skin and dermographism. (*B*) A child with DCM suffering an episode of extensive blistering.

Cutaneous mastocytoma usually consists of a solitary brown to yellowish nodular lesion that frequently involves the trunk or extremities, although any part of the body can be affected (**Fig. 3**). In the last consensus report by the EU/US task force, it was agreed to consider under the term mastocytoma all those cases showing a maximum of 3 cutaneous lesions, whereas patients with 4 or more lesions would be categorized as MPCM.[10] In most cases, cutaneous mastocytoma is often already present at birth or develops within the first months of life, and is extremely rare in adults. The histologic picture of mastocytoma is often undistinguishable from that found in DCM, with a massive MC infiltration occupying the whole dermis[44]; therefore, the Darier sign should not be elicited in such cases either. An important feature of mastocytoma is the dynamic pattern of the skin lesion/s, which initially may increase in size (but not in number) to further develop into other types of lesion (eg, nodule into papule) and finally regressing after variable periods of time.[45,46] In clinical daily practice, mastocytoma is often diagnosed exclusively on the basis of its characteristic clinical features, skin biopsy being not necessary in most cases.

It should be noted that some patients with mastocytosis show skin lesions that do not perfectly fit with any of the currently accepted subforms and variants. More rarely, patients can present with skin lesions confined to a segment or area of the body[47,48]; these cases might represent a mosaic manifestation of the disease (ie, type 1 mosaicism) in which the mutational event, albeit unconfirmed, would be limited to the part of the body affected.[49]

Diagnosis of Cutaneous Mastocytosis

At present, CM is defined by the presence of skin lesions resulting from the accumulation of MCs within the dermis in the absence of criteria for SM.[1,2,8–10] This means that BM examination would become necessary for the distinction between CM and SM, both entities being mutually exclusive, although many patients with SM can present with cutaneous involvement. For this reason, the concept of "mastocytosis in the skin" (MIS) has emerged in recent years as a provisional diagnosis for patients with mastocytosis skin lesions in the absence of a BM study that, when done, will provide the definitive diagnosis (eg, CM or SM).[2] As a general rule, the prediagnostic checkpoint MIS should be established in all adult patients and in children with persistently increased sT levels, until the BM study is performed. By contrast, it is generally accepted that in children with sT <20 µg/L, the diagnosis of CM can be assumed without BM examination.[2]

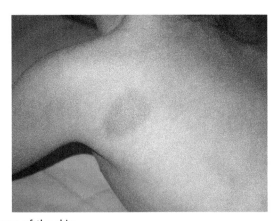

Fig. 3. Mastocytoma of the skin.

According to the recommendations of the EU/US consensus group, the diagnosis of MIS would require the presence of typical skin lesions (major criterion) together with at least 1 of the following minor criteria:

1. Increased MC numbers in a biopsy from lesional skin
2. Activating *KIT* mutations in lesional skin tissue[10]

Neoplastic infiltrates of dermal MCs can be identified by immunohistochemistry using specific stains (eg, tryptase or c-kit −CD117−) as spindle-shaped or spherical/cuboidal cells that may show different histologic patterns:

1. Perivascular
2. Interstitial
3. Nodular
4. Diffuse (sheetlike)[44]

In addition, recent studies have suggested that the aberrant expression of CD25 on skin MCs in patients with MIS might indicate a higher risk of having a systemic MC disease.[50–52]

Similar to BM MCs in patients with SM, the clonal neoplastic nature of MCs in MIS/CM can be established in most cases by the demonstration of activating *KIT* mutations in skin biopsies, with remarkable differences between adults and children. Thus, the *KIT* D816V mutation can be detected in virtually all adult patients using a sensitive polymerase chain reaction technique,[53] but only in 27% to 36% of children[54,55]; by contrast, other mutant variants involving codon 816 of *KIT* or mutations in regions of the *KIT* receptor other than codon 816 are detected in up to 50% of patients with childhood-onset mastocytosis.[55] Altogether, these findings support the notion that pediatric MIS is a clonal disease associated with *KIT* mutations that are often different from the classic D816V *KIT* mutation. Despite this, the identification of *KIT* mutations in children with MIS does not necessarily result into an increased risk for persistence of the disease into adulthood, as demonstrated by a previous study showing spontaneous regression of skin lesions in several children who carried the D816V *KIT* mutation.[54]

PROGNOSTIC FACTORS IN CUTANEOUS MASTOCYTOSIS

The clinical significance of the presence of MIS differs according to the age of the patients at disease onset. In most children, MIS emerges during the first 2 years of life, frequently within the first 6 months, and some patients show skin lesions already at birth.[10,37,56] In adults with MIS, although the peak of disease onset occurs at ages between 20 and 50 years,[10,57] cases evolving from pediatric-onset MIS also can be occasionally observed.[40,41,43,58–61] According to the current 2016 WHO classification of mastocytosis,[8,9] the most frequent subtype of MIS found in children is MPCM (~40%–75%), followed by cutaneous mastocytoma (~20%–50%), and DCM (~3%–8%),[10,37,44,62,63] whereas in adults, the vast majority of patients (eg, >95%) who present with skin involvement show the MPCM subform, mastocytoma and DCM being extremely rare in adulthood.[10] Interestingly, skin biopsies from patients with the polymorphic variant of pediatric MPCM often show findings highly suggestive of the so-called well-differentiated CM. These histologic findings consist of a variable degree of abnormally increased numbers of dermal MCs with a predominantly round or polygonal shape and fully granulated cytoplasm, frequently coexisting with dermal binucleated or polynucleated promastocytes, which tend to be disposed forming strands or rows between collagen bundles.[40] This same histologic picture of mature-appearing MCs infiltrating the skin also can be seen in mastocytoma and in some cases of DCM, where MC numbers are particularly increased and usually show a sheetlike pattern involving the whole dermis and eventually extending deep into the subcutaneous cellular tissue. In contrast to polymorphic MPCM lesions, MCs in skin lesions of patients with the monomorphic MPCM variant tend to be spindle shaped and their numbers appear to be lower.[10]

Itch and redness of skin lesions are common local MC-mediator symptoms in both adults and children with MIS. By contrast, blistering is restricted to pediatric patients, and it is particularly frequent in children with early disease onset (eg, <2 years) who present with extensive cutaneous involvement (eg, DCM)[36,37,56,64]; moreover, extensive blistering disease is an indicator of massive MC activation and has been regarded as a predictor of severe complications in children with mastocytosis.[35] Blisters also can be frequently observed in children with large skin lesions (eg, nodular lesions), especially when affecting the scalp or body sites exposed to repeated friction or pressure.[37] Flushing is another symptom that often occurs in patients with MIS. Although it has been classically considered as a cutaneous manifestation in patients with mastocytosis, flushing actually results from increased blood flow through the skin caused by vasoactive substances released from MCs (eg, histamine), and it can precede the development of hypotensive collapse; for this reason, the presence of flushing in a patient with mastocytosis should alert about the potential development of serious, life-threatening complications.[35] Patients with MIS also can suffer from a wide range of other (systemic) symptoms, including abdominal cramping, diarrhea, bone pain, dyspnea, headache, and anaphylaxis, among others.[37,56,63] Although systemic symptoms are more frequently observed in adults as a consequence of the presumably systemic nature of the disease,[65] systemic symptoms also can occur in pediatric mastocytosis, in which the disease is mostly restricted to the skin; in these latter cases, systemic symptoms result from the effect of a wide variety of mediators massively produced by huge numbers of cutaneous MCs that are released into the bloodstream; accordingly, systemic symptoms in pediatric mastocytosis are particularly common in patients with DCM and in those with very extensive MPCM.[37,38,65–67] The most common triggers of symptoms in patients with MIS are skin rubbing and exposition to extreme temperatures (eg, heat and/or hot water, more rarely cold).[37] Other frequent elicitors are stress, some drugs, insect venoms, and premenstrual stages in adults, and fever, irritability, teething, and vaccines among children, especially those with extended cutaneous involvement.[37,66,68]

Some features have been identified as potential predictors for the severity of MC-mediator release symptoms in patients with MIS. Total sT levels have been shown to correlate quite well with the burden of neoplastic MCs in patients with mastocytosis,[69,70] and also with the extent of skin involvement and the risk for severe MC activation events, including anaphylaxis in pediatric mastocytosis.[37,66,71] In contrast to children, the extent of cutaneous involvement in adult patients with MIS seems to correlate with the presence of pruritus and flushing,[36] but not with the risk for anaphylaxis.[66] The extent and the activity of mastocytosis cutaneous lesions together with the assessment of subjective symptoms have been incorporated into a scoring model called the SCORMA Index, which has shown to be useful as a tool for evaluating the severity of the disease in both adults and children with MIS.[71–73]

The current consensus classification, which divides MPCM into monomorphic and polymorphic variants, has been suggested to show prognostic impact, because most (but not all) children with the polymorphic MPCM variant usually display normal sT levels and show spontaneous regression by puberty, whereas those with the monomorphic MPCM variant more frequently have increased sT levels and higher probability of persistence of the disease in adulthood.[10,74] Other factors that have been strongly associated with disease resolution in pediatric-onset mastocytosis include a lower age at onset (eg, <2 years),[75,76] a lower extent of skin affected,[76] and a normal BM examination.[75]

By contrast, the potential persistence of childhood-onset MIS beyond adolescence is closely related to the presence of concomitant (underlying) systemic involvement[75,77] that can be demonstrated on the basis of BM findings. However, it should be noted that the probability of SM in children with MIS is low, particularly if sT levels are lower than 20 µg/L. However, a recent study including 105 patients with childhood-onset mastocytosis has shown that 19 of 53 patients who were selected for BM examination had SM, the presence of organomegalies being the best predictor of SM in this pediatric population, especially when increased sT levels were also detected.[39]

THE NEED FOR FURTHER CLASSIFICATION OF MASTOCYTOSIS

The current classification and categories of CM are not fully satisfactory. Some old-fashioned terms are now outdated, but others, such as "urticaria pigmentosa" are still used and need to be reevaluated. Other terms, such as "maculo-papular" or "nodular" are being inaccurately used according to their definition in dermatologic terminology. In children, the precise incidence of systemic involvement has not been established and, thus, a classification based on the number of lesions is not useful in terms of disease severity or prognosis. Regarding solitary lesions, also named mastocytomas, their clinical appearance is heterogeneous and it remains not clear if patients with 2 or 3 lesions should be included in this category.

Despite the great relevance of the 2016 WHO classification of mastocytosis and the recent consensus classification of CM by the EU/US task force in showing the heterogeneity of skin lesions in mastocytosis, a more accurate classification of the different patterns of cutaneous involvement in mastocytosis, probably incorporating histopathological and genetic profiles of the disease that could have prognostic impact, is warranted in the near future.

REFERENCES

1. Horny HP, Metcalfe DD, Bennet JM, et al. Mastocytosis. In: Swerdlow SH, Campo E, Harris NL, et al, editors. WHO classification of tumours of haematopoietic and lymphoid tissues. Lyon (France): IARC; 2008. p. 54–63.
2. Valent P, Akin C, Escribano L, et al. Standards and standardization in mastocytosis: consensus statements on diagnostics, treatment recommendations and response criteria. Eur J Clin Invest 2007;37(6):435–53.
3. Theoharides TC, Valent P, Akin C. Mast cells, mastocytosis, and related disorders. N Engl J Med 2015;373(19):1885–6.
4. Garcia-Montero AC, Jara-Acevedo M, Teodosio C, et al. KIT mutation in mast cells and other bone marrow haematopoietic cell lineages in systemic mast cell disorders. A prospective study of the Spanish Network on Mastocytosis (REMA) in a series of 113 patients. Blood 2006;108(7):2366–72.
5. Kristensen T, Vestergaard H, Moller MB. Improved detection of the KIT D816V mutation in patients with systemic mastocytosis using a quantitative and highly sensitive real-time qPCR assay. J Mol Diagn 2011;13(2):180–8.
6. Jara-Acevedo M, Teodosio C, Sanchez-Muñoz L, et al. Detection of the KIT D816V mutation in peripheral blood of systemic mastocytosis: diagnostic implications. Mod Pathol 2015;28(8):1138–49.
7. Arock M, Sotlar K, Akin C, et al. KIT mutation analysis in mast cell neoplasms: recommendations of the European competence network on mastocytosis. Leukemia 2015;29(6):1223–32.

8. Arber DA, Orazi A, Hasserjian R, et al. The 2016 revision to the World Health Organization classification of myeloid neoplasms and acute leukemia. Blood 2016; 127(20):2391–405.

9. Valent P, Akin C, Hartmann K, et al. Advances in the classification and treatment of mastocytosis: current status and outlook toward the future. Cancer Res 2017; 77(6):1261–70.

10. Hartmann K, Escribano L, Grattan C, et al. Cutaneous manifestations in patients with mastocytosis: consensus report of the European Competence Network on Mastocytosis; the American Academy of Allergy, Asthma & Immunology; and the European Academy of Allergology and Clinical Immunology. J Allergy Clin Immunol 2016;137(1):35–45.

11. Nettleship E, Tay W. Rare forms of urticaria. Br Med J 1869;2:323–30.

12. Ehrlich P. Beiträge zur Theorie und Praxis der histologischen Färbung. Leipzig University; 1878.

13. Sangster A. An anomalous mottled rash, accompanied by pruritus, factitious urticaria and pigmentation, "urticaria pigmentosa"? Trans Med Soc Lond 1878;11: 161–3.

14. Unna P. Beitrage zur anatomic und pathogenese der urticaria simplex und pigmentosa. Mscch Prakt Dermatol Suppl Dermatol Stud 1887;3:9.

15. Sézary A, Levy-Coblentz G, Chauvillon P. Dermographisme et mastocytose. Bull Soc Fr Dermatol Syphiligr 1936;43:359–61.

16. Little EG. Contribution on the study of urticaria pigmentosa. Br J Dermatol Syph 1905;17:355–73, 393–411, 427–47.

17. Finnerud CW. Urticaria pigmentosa (nodular type) with a summary of the literature: report of a case. Arch Dermatol Syphilol 1923;8(3):344–58.

18. Stuhmer A. Urticaria pigmentosa pemphigoides mit wechselnder Lokalisation. Dermatol Wochenschr 1939;109:939.

19. Robbins JG. Bullous urticaria pigmentosa: report of an unusual case. AMA Arch Derm Syphilol 1954;70(2):232–5.

20. Hissard R, Moncourier L, Jacquet J. Etude d'un cas de mastocytose. Bull Mem Soc Med Hop Paris 1951;52(6):583–607.

21. Degos R, Lortat-Jacob E, Mallarme J, et al. Mast cell reticulosis. Bull Soc Fr Dermatol Syphiligr 1951;58(4):435–40.

22. Weber FP. Telangiectasia macularis eruptiva perstans—probably a telangiectatic variety of urticaria pigmentosa in an adult. Proc R Soc Med 1930;24(2):96–7.

23. Ellis JM. Urticaria pigmentosa: a report of a case with autopsy. Arch Pathol 1949; 48(5):426–35.

24. Davis RJ, Waisman M. Urticaria pigmentosa: report of a case with autopsy examination. AMA Arch Derm 1959;79(6):649–50.

25. Yasuda T, Kukita A. A fatal case of purely cutaneous form of diffuse mastocytosis. Proc XIIth Int Cong Derm 1963;11:1558.

26. Caplan RM. The natural course of urticaria pigmentosa. Analysis and follow-up of 112 cases. Arch Dermatol 1963;87:146–57.

27. Caplan RM. Urticaria pigmentosa and systemic mastocytosis. JAMA 1965; 194(10):1077–80.

28. Lennert K, Parwaresch MR. Mast cells and mast cell neoplasia: a review. Histopathology 1979;3(5):349–65.

29. Metcalfe DD. Classification and diagnosis of mastocytosis: current status. J Invest Dermatol 1991;96(3):2S–4S.

30. Travis WD, Li CY, Bergstralh EJ, et al. Systemic mast cell disease. Analysis of 58 cases and literature review. Medicine (Baltimore) 1988;67(6):345–68.

31. Tauber AI, Wintroub BU, Simon AS, editors. Biochemistry of the acute allergic reactions: Fifth International Symposium: proceedings of the biochemistry of the acute allergic reactions–fifth international symposium, held in Boston, Massachusetts, June 20–21, 1988. New York: A.R. Liss; 1989. p. 350.
32. Valent P, Horny HP, Escribano L, et al. Diagnostic criteria and classification of mastocytosis: a consensus proposal. Leuk Res 2001;25(7):603–25.
33. Valent P, Horny HP, Li CY, et al. Mastocytosis. In: Jaffe ES, Harris NL, Stein H, et al, editors. World Health Organization (WHO) classification of tumours pathology and genetics tumours of haematopoietic and lymphoid tissues. Lyon (France): IARC Press; 2001. p. 291–302.
34. Hartmann K, Henz BM. Classification of cutaneous mastocytosis: a modified consensus proposal. Leuk Res 2002;26(5):483–4.
35. Brockow K, Ring J, Alvarez-Twose I, et al. Extensive blistering is a predictor for severe complications in children with mastocytosis. Allergy 2012;67(10):1323–4.
36. Brockow K, Akin C, Huber M, et al. Assessment of the extent of cutaneous involvement in children and adults with mastocytosis: relationship to symptomatology, tryptase levels, and bone marrow pathology. J Am Acad Dermatol 2003;48(4):508–16.
37. Alvarez-Twose I, Vañó-Galván S, Sánchez-Muñoz L, et al. Increased serum baseline tryptase levels and extensive skin involvement are predictors for the severity of mast cell activation episodes in children with mastocytosis. Allergy 2012;67(6): 813–21.
38. Lange M, Niedoszytko M, Nedoszytko B, et al. Diffuse cutaneous mastocytosis: analysis of 10 cases and a brief review of the literature. J Eur Acad Dermatol Venereol 2012;26(12):1565–71.
39. Carter MC, Clayton ST, Komarow HD, et al. Assessment of clinical findings, tryptase levels, and bone marrow histopathology in the management of pediatric mastocytosis. J Allergy Clin Immunol 2015;136(6):1673–9.
40. Alvarez-Twose I, Jara-Acevedo M, Morgado JM, et al. Clinical, immunophenotypic, and molecular characteristics of well-differentiated systemic mastocytosis. J Allergy Clin Immunol 2016;137(1):168–78.
41. Hartmann K, Wardelmann E, Ma Y, et al. Novel germline mutation of KIT associated with familial gastrointestinal stromal tumors and mastocytosis. Gastroenterology 2005;129(3):1042–6.
42. de Melo Campos P, Machado-Neto JA, Scopim-Ribeiro R, et al. Familial systemic mastocytosis with germline KIT K509I mutation is sensitive to treatment with imatinib, dasatinib and PKC412. Leuk Res 2014;38(10):1245–51.
43. Chan EC, Bai Y, Kirshenbaum AS, et al. Mastocytosis associated with a rare germline KIT K509I mutation displays a well-differentiated mast cell phenotype. J Allergy Clin Immunol 2014;134(1):178–87.
44. Wolff K, Komar M, Petzelbauer P. Clinical and histopathological aspects of cutaneous mastocytosis. Leuk Res 2001;25(7):519–28.
45. Azaña JM, Velasco E, Torrelo A, et al. Mastocitomas: revisión de 33 casos infantiles. Actas Dermosifiliogr 1993;84:559–62.
46. Webber NK, Ponnampalam J, Grattan CEH. How reliable is blood tryptase as a marker of systemic disease in an infant with cutaneous mastocytomas? Clin Exp Dermatol 2008;33(2):198–9.
47. Merika EE, Bunker CB, Francis N, et al. A segmental rash in a young male: a quiz. Naevoid urticaria pigmentosa. Acta Derm Venereol 2014;94(2):253–4.
48. Gonzalez-Castro U, Luelmo-Aguilar J, Castells-Rodellas A. Unilateral facial telangiectasia macularis eruptiva perstans. Int J Dermatol 1993;32(2):123–4.

49. Happle R. Mosaic manifestation of autosomal dominant skin disorders. In: Happle R, editor. Mosaicism in human skin. Heidelberg (Germany): Springer; 2014. p. 122–59.

50. Hollmann TJ, Brenn T, Hornick JL. CD25 expression on cutaneous mast cells from adult patients presenting with urticaria pigmentosa is predictive of systemic mastocytosis. Am J Surg Pathol 2008;32(1):139–45.

51. Morgado J, Sanchez-Muñoz L, Matito A, et al. Patterns of expression of CD25 and CD30 on skin mast cells in pediatric mastocytosis. J Contemp Immunol 2014;1(2):46–56.

52. Lange M, Żawrocki A, Nedoszytko B, et al. Does the aberrant expression of CD2 and CD25 by skin mast cells truly correlate with systemic involvement in patients presenting with mastocytosis in the skin? Int Arch Allergy Immunol 2014;165(2):104–10.

53. Kristensen T, Broesby-Olsen S, Vestergaard H, et al. KIT D816V mutation-positive cell fractions in lesional skin biopsies from adults with systemic mastocytosis. Dermatology 2013;226(3):233–7.

54. Sotlar K, Escribano L, Landt O, et al. One-step detection of c-kit point mutations using peptide nucleic acid-mediated polymerase chain reaction clamping and hybridization probes. Am J Pathol 2003;162(3):737–46.

55. Bodemer C, Hermine O, Palmérini F, et al. Pediatric mastocytosis is a clonal disease associated with D816V and other activating c-KIT mutations. J Invest Dermatol 2010;130(3):804–15.

56. Ben-Amitai D, Metzker A, Cohen HA. Pediatric cutaneous mastocytosis: a review of 180 patients. Isr Med Assoc J 2005;7(5):320–2.

57. Brockow K. Epidemiology, prognosis, and risk factors in mastocytosis. Immunol Allergy Clin North Am 2014;34(2):283–95.

58. Tang X, Boxer M, Drummond A, et al. A germline mutation in KIT in familial diffuse cutaneous mastocytosis. J Med Genet 2004;41(6):e88.

59. Zhang LY, Smith ML, Schultheis B, et al. A novel K509I mutation of KIT identified in familial mastocytosis—in vitro and in vivo responsiveness to imatinib therapy. Leuk Res 2006;30(4):373–8.

60. Wasag B, Niedoszytko M, Piskorz A, et al. Novel, activating KIT-N822I mutation in familial cutaneous mastocytosis. Exp Hematol 2011;39(8):859–65.

61. Huang L, Wang SA, Konoplev S, et al. Well-differentiated systemic mastocytosis showed excellent clinical response to imatinib in the absence of known molecular genetic abnormalities: a case report. Medicine (Baltimore) 2016;95(41):e4934.

62. Hannaford R, Rogers M. Presentation of cutaneous mastocytosis in 173 children. Australas J Dermatol 2001;42(1):15–21.

63. Méni C, Bruneau J, Georgin-Lavialle S, et al. Paediatric mastocytosis: a systematic review of 1747 cases. Br J Dermatol 2015;172(3):642–51.

64. Azaña JM, Torrelo A, Mediero IG, et al. Urticaria pigmentosa: a review of 67 pediatric cases. Pediatr Dermatol 1994;11(2):102–6.

65. Berezowska S, Flaig MJ, Ruëff F, et al. Adult-onset mastocytosis in the skin is highly suggestive of systemic mastocytosis. Mod Pathol 2014;27(1):19–29.

66. Brockow K, Jofer C, Behrendt H, et al. Anaphylaxis in patients with mastocytosis: a study on history, clinical features and risk factors in 120 patients. Allergy 2008; 63(2):226–32.

67. Barnes M, Van L, DeLong L, et al. Severity of cutaneous findings predict the presence of systemic symptoms in pediatric maculopapular cutaneous mastocytosis. Pediatr Dermatol 2014;31(3):271–5.

68. Torrelo A, Alvarez-Twose I, Escribano L. Childhood mastocytosis. Curr Opin Pediatr 2012;24(4):480–6.
69. Schwartz LB, Sakai K, Bradford TR, et al. The alpha form of human tryptase is the predominant type present in blood at baseline in normal subjects and is elevated in those with systemic mastocytosis. J Clin Invest 1995;96(6):2702–10.
70. Sperr WR, Jordan J-H, Fiegl M, et al. Serum tryptase levels in patients with mastocytosis: correlation with mast cell burden and implication for defining the category of disease. Int Arch Allergy Immunol 2002;128(2):136–41.
71. Lange M, Niedoszytko M, Renke J, et al. Clinical aspects of paediatric mastocytosis: a review of 101 cases. J Eur Acad Dermatol Venereol 2013;27(1):97–102.
72. Heide R, van Doorn K, Mulder PG, et al. Serum tryptase and SCORMA (SCORing MAstocytosis) Index as disease severity parameters in childhood and adult cutaneous mastocytosis. Clin Exp Dermatol 2009;34(4):462–8.
73. Schena D, Galvan A, Tessari G, et al. Clinical features and course of cutaneous mastocytosis in 133 children. Br J Dermatol 2016;174(2):411–3.
74. Wiechers T, Rabenhorst A, Schick T, et al. Large maculopapular cutaneous lesions are associated with favorable outcome in childhood-onset mastocytosis. J Allergy Clin Immunol 2015;136(6):1581–90.
75. Uzzaman A, Maric I, Noel P, et al. Pediatric-onset mastocytosis: a long term clinical follow-up and correlation with bone marrow histopathology. Pediatr Blood Cancer 2009;53(4):629–34.
76. Heinze A, Kuemmet TJ, Chiu YE, et al. Longitudinal study of pediatric urticaria pigmentosa. Pediatr Dermatol 2017;34(2):144–9.
77. Lanternier F, Cohen-Akenine A, Palmerini F, et al. Phenotypic and genotypic characteristics of mastocytosis according to the age of onset. PLoS One 2008;3(4): e1906.

Pediatric Expression of Mast Cell Activation Disorders

Sigurd Broesby-Olsen, MD[a,b,*], Melody Carter, MD[c],
Henrik Fomsgaard Kjaer, MD, PhD[a,b], Charlotte Gotthard Mortz, MD, PhD[a,b],
Michael Boe Møller, MD, DMSc[a,d], Thomas Kielsgaard Kristensen, PhD[a,d],
Carsten Bindslev-Jensen, MD, PhD, DMSc[a,b], Lone Agertoft, MD, PhD[a,e]

KEYWORDS

- Mastocytosis • Mast cell activation • Mast cell activation disorders • *KIT* mutations
- Urticaria pigmentosa • Tryptase • Anaphylaxis

KEY POINTS

- Symptoms in pediatric mastocytosis are often limited to the skin, and presence of skin lesions (urticaria pigmentosa) is the key feature for diagnosis.
- In most affected children, a somatic mutation in the *KIT* gene can be found; however, the *KIT* D816V mutation is only detected in one-third of pediatric patients.
- Extracutaneous symptoms, including anaphylaxis, are rare as opposed to in adult disease and mainly reported in children with very extensive skin involvement, bullous lesions, and high mast cell burden.
- Frequent triggers for exacerbations include friction, heat, fever, and insect stings; however, counseling in regard to avoidance of other potential mast cell activation triggers should be individualized after careful evaluation.
- In approximately 70% to 80% of children, the disease resolves by adulthood and risk for persistent disease may be related to the presence of small, monomorphic skin lesions; disease onset after 3 years of age; detection the *KIT* D816V mutation; high mast cell burden; and systemic disease. Further research is, however, needed including long-term follow-up studies.

Conflicts of Interest: Authors declare no relevant conflicts of interest in relation to this article.
Funding: M. Carter is supported by the Division of Intramural Research, National Institute of Allergy and Infectious Diseases, National Institutes of Health.
[a] Mastocytosis Centre Odense University Hospital (MastOUH), Søndre Boulevard 29, 5000 Odense C, Denmark; [b] Department of Dermatology and Allergy Centre, Odense Research Centre for Anaphylaxis (ORCA), Odense University Hospital, Søndre Boulevard 29, 5000 Odense C, Denmark; [c] Laboratory of Allergic Diseases, National Institute of Allergy and Infectious Diseases, National Institutes of Health, Bethesda, MD 20892, USA; [d] Department of Pathology, Odense University Hospital, J.B. Winsløws Vej 15, 5000 Odense C, Denmark; [e] Hans Christian Andersen Children's Hospital, Odense University Hospital, Kløvervænget 23C, 5000 Odense C, Denmark
* Corresponding author. Department of Dermatology and Allergy Centre, Odense Research Centre for Anaphylaxis (ORCA), Odense University Hospital, Søndre Boulevard 29, 5000 Odense C, Denmark.
E-mail address: sigurd.broesby-olsen@rsyd.dk

INTRODUCTION

Mast cell activation disorders (*MCADs*) is a term proposed to cover diseases and conditions related to activation of mast cells (MCs) and effects of released MC mediators. In its broadest sense, the term, therefore, encompasses a wide range of diseases from allergic asthma to rhinoconjunctivitis, urticaria, food allergy, and anaphylaxis, among many other conditions where MC activation (MCA) may contribute to the pathogenesis.[1]

This article focuses on mastocytosis and gives an overview of its presentations, challenges, and controversies from a pediatric perspective. Mastocytosis is an unusual, heterogeneous group of diseases characterized by the proliferation and accumulation of MCs in body tissues.[2,3] Clinical manifestations depend on the localization of MC infiltration and effects of mediators released from activated MCs, that is, MCA.

The World Health Organization (WHO) classifies mastocytosis into 7 subcategories, including cutaneous mastocytosis (CM)—where MC accumulation is limited to the skin—and systemic mastocytosis (SM)—where internal organs are involved.[3-5] Although most adults (>95%) with mastocytosis are diagnosed with SM when fully investigated, with diverse clinical manifestations ranging from mild to very severe or potentially life-threatening, the disease manifestations in pediatric mastocytosis are typically limited to the skin, that is, CM, and symptoms are often mild (**Table 1**), although gastrointestinal (GI) symptoms are encountered.[6]

Several areas of pediatric mastocytosis are in need of research, including the elucidation of mechanisms involved in the peculiar spontaneous disease resolution observed in approximately 70% to 80% of affected children during adolescence as opposed to adult-onset mastocytosis, which is a chronic disease.[7,8]

EPIDEMIOLOGY

Epidemiologic aspects of pediatric mastocytosis have not been studied in detail. In a population-based study, the prevalence of adult mastocytosis was found to be 10 in 100.000 with a slight female predominance.[9] The incidence and prevalence of pediatric mastocytosis are estimated to be overall similar to or higher than adult mastocytosis.[10] In the adult population, the disease is likely highly underdiagnosed due to a lack

Table 1
Comparison of adult mastocytosis and pediatric mastocytosis

	Pediatric Mastocytosis	Adult Mastocytosis
Most frequent disease category	CM	SM
KIT D816V mutation	20%–30%. Other *KIT* mutations (exons 8, 9, 11) frequent.[14]	>90%–95%
Skin lesions	Always present	May be absent
Typical tryptase level (ng/mL)	<11.4 (normal)	>20, but may be normal
Typical course of the disease	Resolution in 70%–80% before adulthood	Chronic
Symptoms	Often limited to the skin and controllable by anti-MC mediator therapy	Very heterogeneous, may be severe and difficult to control
Extracutaneous manifestations	Rare, but GI symptoms may be encountered	Frequent, including osteoporosis
Risk for anaphylaxis	Low (1%–9%)	High (35%–50%)
Advanced/aggressive disease	Exceedingly rare	5%–10% of patients

of awareness and the very heterogeneous clinical presentations. Although symptoms in pediatric mastocytosis are more homogeneous and often limited to skin and GI tract, the pediatric population is also facing a lack of awareness and experience with the disease among medical care providers and likely a similar under-recognition.

A majority of children (60%–90%) present with mastocytosis skin lesions within the first 2 years of life[11] and in approximately 10% to 20% the skin lesions are already present at birth.[12] When presenting later than the age of 15 years, the disease is likely to represent early-onset adult SM. In pediatric mastocytosis, a slight male predominance has been reported by some groups,[8,11] whereas others have not found any clear gender discrepancies in pediatric mastocytosis.[12]

Although adult disease is almost always equal to SM, invasive tests (ie, bone marrow examinations) to rule out systemic involvement are not routinely performed in pediatric mastocytosis and, thus, the exact frequency of SM in affected children is largely unknown.[3] Among those children who are diagnosed with systemic disease, virtually all have indolent SM (ISM) and advanced disease categories are exceedingly rare in the pediatric population.[11,13]

In general, mastocytosis is a sporadic-appearing disease; however, familial cases of mastocytosis are well documented, most often related to germline KIT mutations,[14] although cases of familial mastocytosis related to somatic KIT D816V mutations have been reported.[15,16]

PATHOGENESIS

In contrast to earlier assumptions, it has been shown that in a majority (approximately 80%) of children with mastocytosis, a somatic gain-of-function point mutation in the KIT gene can be found, at least in lesional skin MCs,[14] leading to a stem cell factor–independent constitutive activation and autophosphorylation of KIT with subsequent clonal accumulation of MCs through up-regulated recruitment from progenitor cells and defective apoptosis.

By far, the most frequent KIT mutation in adult-onset disease (ie, SM) involves codon 816, resulting in the replacement of an aspartic acid by a valine residue (D816V) in exon 17 involved in the kinase activity of KIT. The KIT D816V mutation can be detected in more than 90% of adult mastocytosis patients, not only in MCs in lesional skin and bone marrow but also in peripheral blood.[17–20] In pediatric mastocytosis, the KIT D816V mutation is only detected in approximately 25% to 35% of affected children,[8] and KIT mutations in exons 8, 9, and 11 are much more prevalent in the pediatric population compared with adult SM (**Fig. 1**).[8,14,21]

Thus, overall there is increasing evidence that pediatric mastocytosis is a clonal disease in line with adult-onset mastocytosis; however, the mechanisms involved in the apparent spontaneous resolution observed in approximately 70% to 80% of children before adulthood have not yet been elucidated.

The symptoms in mastocytosis are caused by the localization of MCs and effects of mediators released from activated MCs. MCs may excrete numerous preformed as well as de novo synthesized mediators, including histamine, tryptase, platelet-activating factor, leukotrienes, prostaglandins, and cytokines, with a wide range of potential effects and related symptoms.[22] Although the classic allergic IgE-mediated MC degranulation is a well described cellular reaction, MCA may also occur by non–IgE-mediated mechanisms and be induced by several different immunologic as well as nonimmunologic triggering factors. In childhood disease, MC accumulation and symptoms are often limited to the skin. The mechanisms involved in the hyperpigmentation of skin lesions in mastocytosis are not known in detail but involve the interaction

Pediatric mastocytosis   ## Adult mastocytosis

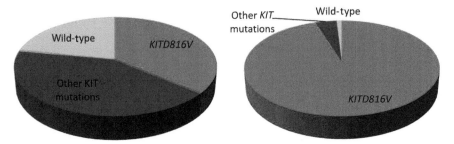

Fig. 1. Mutational profiles in pediatric mastocytosis (*left*) and adult mastocytosis (*right*). (*Data from* Bibi S, Langenfeld F, Jeanningros S, et al. Molecular defects in mastocytosis: *KIT* and beyond *KIT*. Immunol Allergy Clin North Am 2014;34(2):239–62.)

between clonal MCs in the skin and adjacent melanocytes, resulting in increased melanogenesis and melanin deposition in epidermis.[23] In adult SM, cytoreductive therapies have been shown to be able to reduce or clear skin lesions but so far no mediator-targeted therapy has been able to do so, although, for example, histamine has been shown to stimulate melanocytes.[24] Further studies are needed to clarify how the MC accumulation results in pigmented spots and furthermore why the clinical appearance of these skin lesions in pediatric mastocytosis is often more polymorphic compared with adult disease.

CLINICAL FEATURES
Skin Manifestations

The classic presentation of mastocytosis in children is the gradual onset of skin lesions within the first 2 years of life.[8,12] These demarcated, reddish-brown, maculopapular skin lesions have traditionally been named urticaria pigmentosa (UP); however, in recent literature the term, *maculopapular CM*, is applied.[4] Symptoms from the skin include pruritus, flushing, and whealing, which may be triggered by physical stimuli, such as heat, cold, sunlight, and friction as well as infections/fever. The number of skin lesions may vary from few to widespread skin involvement. Some children exhibit classic, small (up to 5 mm in diameter) monomorphic UP skin lesions as in adults (**Fig. 2**), whereas others have larger, polymorphic lesions (**Fig. 3**).[25,26] These skin lesions typically exhibit a wheal-and-flare reaction on friction—called the Darier sign. In clinical practice, a useful approach to elicit this sign is to apply 5 strokes with a wooden tongue spatula with a moderate pressure over the skin lesions—and wait 3 minutes to 5 minutes (up to 15 minutes) to evaluate response. False-negative results may be encountered due to intake of H_1-receptor blockers and individual thresholds. Dermographism (stripes of whealing in the normal skin on scratching) may be seen in mastocytosis but are also seen in inducible urticaria and should not be confused with the Darier sign.

A common type of CM almost exclusively seen in the pediatric population is mastocytoma of the skin, presenting as a solitary, itchy, and swollen or sometimes bullous pigmented lesion, with a diameter of typically 1 cm to 2 cm. In the vast majority of children with a mastocytoma, symptoms are limited to the affected skin area; however, generalized flushing and hypotensive episodes may rarely occur in relation to physical provocation of the mastocytoma.[12]

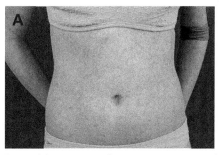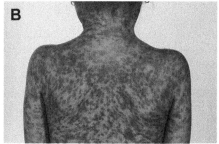

Fig. 2. (*A*) Monomorphic UP in cutaneous disease (CM). (*B*) Monomorphic UP in systemic disease (ISM).

Another special pediatric subtype is diffuse CM (DCM), in which the entire skin integument is infiltrated by MCs. Thus, children with DCM do not present with individual skin lesions but instead exhibit generalized erythema, usually with thickened, pachydermatous, darker skin and an often extensive, dermographism with bullous reactions. The clinical presentation may be dramatic with severe blistering and hypotensive episodes, requiring hospitalization; however, the overall prognosis is good. Even though serum tryptase levels are often increased in DCM at presentation, evidence of systemic involvement is usually not found and clinical improvement or resolution over time is the rule.[11,26,27]

Cosmetic complaints may be a major issue in adolescents and younger adults and also an important aspect to address in children—and their worried parents. The challenge of treating the skin lesions is, as discussed previously, that the reduction of skin lesions demands reduction of the MC infiltration. The use of potentially toxic drugs in pediatric CM, however, is not warranted for cosmetic indication. The most important aspect in a majority of younger children and their parents is, therefore, reassurance of the benign nature of the disease and providing tools for the child to cope with their disease and accept their skin lesions. In younger adults, treatment options targeting the cosmetic burden of skin lesions are currently limited to UV therapy and short-term high-potency topical steroid. These treatments should be used cautiously due to potential cutaneous side effects but can make skin lesions less visible in addition to reducing pruritus and whealing.

Anaphylaxis

In adult SM, there is a 7-fold to 8-fold increased risk of anaphylaxis compared with the background population,[28] with a reported cumulative prevalence from specialized

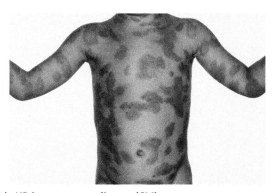

Fig. 3. Polymorphic UP in cutaneous disease (CM).

centers of 35% to 50%.[29–31] In comparison, the reported prevalence of anaphylaxis in pediatric mastocytosis is in the range of 1% to 9%, including mild episodes without cardiovascular compromise,[30,32] which seem higher than rates reported in the general pediatric population,[33] however, much lower than in adult SM, and overall severe anaphylaxis in pediatric mastocytosis is uncommon.

Patterns of elicitors of anaphylaxis in pediatric mastocytosis differ somewhat from those in adult SM. Here, cases of idiopathic anaphylaxis or unknown triggers are the most frequently reported, followed by foods and drugs, whereas Hymenoptera stings are not a frequent trigger of anaphylaxis in pediatric mastocytosis as opposed to in adult disease, where this is the most frequently reported trigger.[29,30,32]

In general, the incidence of IgE-mediated allergic rhinitis, asthma, and food allergies is not more frequent in mastocytosis,[30] but symptoms may be more difficult to control when the conditions coexist.

Currently, no clear predictors or surrogate markers have been identified to allow for an individual risk assessment for anaphylaxis in mastocytosis and further studies on this are needed. Suggested predictors for increased risk of anaphylaxis in pediatric mastocytosis include proved systemic disease, very extensive skin involvement, bullous skin reactions, persistently high serum tryptase levels, and previous anaphylaxis (**Box 1**).[32,34,35] In pediatric mastocytosis, the risk thus seems to correlate with the severity and character of skin lesions as well as MC burden/level of serum tryptase. By contrast, the risk of anaphylaxis in adult SM does not correlate to MC burden or may even correlate inversely—and adult patients without skin lesions (bone marrow mastocytosis [BMM]) may even be more prone to anaphylaxis than patients with typical ISM, which is an apparent paradox. Currently, even though firm evidence is lacking, most centers recommend that all adults patients are equipped with an adrenaline autoinjector for use in case of anaphylaxis, whereas this in general only is provided to pediatric patients in the presence of risk factors, as described previously (see **Box 1**). In addition, patients/families should be informed about potential MC triggers and risk situations individually, as described previously, and a thorough evaluation and allergological work-up is recommended in case of anaphylaxis.

Other Symptoms and Disease Manifestations

In general, extracutaneous symptoms occur less often in pediatric mastocytosis compared with adult SM. GI symptoms, such as reflux, abdominal cramping, and loose stools, may be encountered in pediatric patients, especially with flushing events. This may be caused by an increase in intestinal MCs and/or MC mediator effects in the GI tract; however, in children with such GI symptoms, a thorough evaluation for differential diagnoses is mandatory. Similarly, other symptoms that are frequent in adult

---

Box 1
Suggested risk factors for anaphylaxis in pediatric mastocytosis

Very extensive skin involvement

Severe blistering disease

Significantly elevated basal serum tryptase

Systemic disease

KIT D816V mutation

Previous anaphylaxis

SM, such as fatigue, moods, lack of concentration, depression, and musculoskeletal pain, are rare in pediatric mastocytosis—and should prompt a search for other causes when present. At present, little is known about the bone metabolism in pediatric mastocytosis compared with adult SM, where osteoporosis is prevalent; however, from clinical experience, this does not constitute a problem in children.

MAST CELL ACTIVATION SYNDROME

MCA syndrome (*MCAS*) is a term proposed to describe a severe constellation of episodic multisystem symptoms resulting from MCA.[1,36] MCAS and its diagnostic criteria were primarily introduced in the adult population, and little has been published about MCAS in children.

To meet criteria for MCAS a patient must fulfill all of the following 3 criteria:

1. Episodic symptoms consistent with MCA involving 2 or more organ systems (skin [flushing, urticaria, and angioedema], GI tract [diarrhea, abdominal cramping, nausea, and vomiting], airways/naso-ocular [wheezing, conjunctival injection, and nasal stuffiness], or cardiovascular system [hypotensive syncope, and tachycardia])
2. Appropriate response to medications targeting MCA
3. A documented increase in a validated marker of MCA during a symptomatic episode compared with the patient's baseline value. The most commonly used marker is serum tryptase and an increase of 20% from baseline plus 2 ng/mL is suggested as a meaningful indicator of MCA[37]

By this definition, anaphylaxis is 1 category of MCAS, and, when clinical diagnostic criteria for anaphylaxis are met,[38] it is more appropriate to use this designation, whereas patients with chronic MCAS typically present with milder systemic symptoms from MCA.

Currently, MCAS is applied in patients with mastocytosis or with evidence of clonal MC disease not fulfilling WHO criteria for SM (MMAS), that is, clonal or primary MCAS, as well as in patients without identifiable cause for MCA, that is, idiopathic or nonclonal MCAS.[39]

The current literature on MCAS does not address the pediatric population and there is a need for studies to better understand and classify this in children.

In a child referred for suspected MCAS, it is currently advised to apply the criteria discussed previously, after ruling out mastocytosis (ie, presence of UP skin lesions) as well as other etiologies with similar clinical manifestations. A final diagnosis of nonclonal MCAS should not be assigned unless all these 3 criteria are fulfilled.

In clinical practice, an increasing number of referrals for investigation of MCAS are seen—also in the pediatric population—due to more diffuse, nonspecific symptoms without an identifiable cause. These symptoms often present on a chronic basis without well-defined episodes of MCA and include intolerance to environmental factors, foods, and drugs; chronic fatigue; headaches; and memory problems. Currently, there is no evidence to suggest that an abnormal MC phenotype or a continuous state of MCA with chronic MC mediator release is the cause for these symptoms.[36] In some of these patients, a slightly elevated baseline serum tryptase level might have led to the suspicion of MCAS. Familial alpha-tryptasemia resulting from duplication or triplication of the alpha-tryptase gene (TPSAB1) may be the cause and is reported in 4% to 6% of the general population.[40] Alpha-tryptase is enzymatically inactive (as opposed to beta-tryptase) and there are currently no data to suggest that patients with an elevated tryptase level caused by familial alpha-tryptasemia have an activated MC phenotype.

DIAGNOSIS

In children, a diagnosis of mastocytosis is largely clinical and based on the typical appearance of skin lesions associated with the Darier sign, which is also accepted as the major diagnostic criterion for cutaneous involvement in mastocytosis in general. Minor diagnostic criteria are increased numbers of MCs in biopsy sections of lesional skin and/or the detection of a *KIT* mutation in lesional skin tissue.[26]

In contrast to adult SM, children with mastocytosis always present with skin lesions, that is, so far no cases of pediatric BMM or clonal MCAD without skin lesions have been reported.

Baseline serum tryptase is most often in the normal range or only slightly elevated in pediatric mastocytosis, except for in children with DCM or ISM who in a majority of cases have a value greater than 20 ng/mL.[11,41]

Typically serum tryptase values decrease over time in all children with mastocytosis in conjunction with improvement of clinical symptoms.[11,41]

The application of sensitive, allele-specific quantitative polymerase chain reaction *KIT* D816V mutation analysis in peripheral blood has become a standard diagnostic screening tool in adult mastocytosis; however, experiences in pediatric patients are limited.[42] For diagnostic purposes, this approach may be less valuable in pediatric mastocytosis for 3 reasons; first, children present with UP skin lesions on objective examination; second, only approximately one-third of children carry this specific mutation; and, finally, the mutation analysis may be negative in blood even though the *KIT* D816V mutation is detected in lesional skin (personal communication, Broesby-Olsen S, 2017). Therefore, a negative result of a *KIT* D816V mutation analysis in peripheral blood should be interpreted cautiously in pediatric mastocytosis and further studies are needed on this topic.

A recent study has shown that the most reliable predictor for systemic disease in children with mastocytosis is organomegaly and even in children with serum tryptase greater than 20 ng/mL and severe MC mediator symptoms, but no organomegaly, evidence of SM was not detected on bone marrow examination.[11] When making a decision whether to perform a bone marrow examination in pediatric mastocytosis, it must be considered whether bone marrow findings will alter disease management in the child. In general, a bone marrow examination is only warranted in severely affected children with a failure to thrive and where there is a significant concern for the health of the child, in combination with organomegaly and a persistently elevated serum tryptase indicating systemic disease.[11] On the other hand, CM is usually accepted as the final diagnosis for polymorphic lesions without the other variables.

DIFFERENTIAL DIAGNOSIS

Usually UP skin lesions have distinct features, as described previously, including the Darier sign, which is close to pathognomonic for mastocytosis. Localized smooth muscle hamartoma, an uncommon benign skin tumor in children, appearing typically as a slightly hyperpigmented 1-cm to 2-cm skin lesion, may also feature redness and a slight swelling (ie, pseudo–Darier sign) after rubbing and thus be taken for a solitary mastocytoma.

Other differential diagnoses in cases of multiple pigmented skin lesions include melanocytic nevi, café au lait spots and neurofibromatosis, tuberous sclerosis, postinflammatory pigmentation, juvenile xanthogranulomas, and lentigines among others. Bullous eruptions in mastocytosis may be taken for bullous impetigo, phytophotodermatitis, or autoimmune bullous skin diseases.

TREATMENT AND MANAGEMENT

Children with mastocytosis are generally best handled by comprehensive care centers with experience in managing the disease, using a coordinated, multidisciplinary approach. Treatment and follow-up should focus on the individual child and be tailored to symptoms, disease manifestations, and clinical course.

Treatment options in mastocytosis is divided into antimediator therapy, aiming at reducing release or effects of MC mediators, and cytoreductive therapies, aiming to reduce the MC burden. Due to potential side effects, currently available cytoreductive drugs are not relevant in the vast majority of pediatric patients and reserved for very rare cases of advanced SM.

Antimediator treatment should be symptom-directed and is not mandatory in all pediatric patients. Information on common triggers for MCA, such as friction, heat, and cold, should be given but should be individualized and, apart from physical stimuli to the skin most other theoretic triggers, do not have clinical relevance in childhood mastocytosis. It must be stressed that it is not helpful to provide a long list of potential MC triggers to avoid in pediatric mastocytosis. To that end, counseling and thorough information for often worried parents are often helpful, because information found on the Internet on this heterogeneous disease may vary greatly in quality and lead to unnecessary concerns and misinformation.

Antihistamines are most often sufficient to control skin symptoms. Second-generation, nonsedating H_1-antihistamines are generally recommended and may be updosed,[43] whereas sedating H_1-receptor blockers should be used cautiously and only for short periods for sleep-disturbing symptoms but should not be applied for long-term use. Emollients may be helpful to decrease the sensitivity to physical stimuli. Topical corticosteroids may relieve skin symptoms and increase threshold for MCA but should only be prescribed for short-term use due to potential side effects in the skin.[12]

Risk of anaphylaxis in pediatric mastocytosis is much lower than in adult mastocytosis, as discussed previously, and most expert mastocytosis centers only prescribe an adrenaline pen as emergency medication to selected children (see **Box 1**).[32,34,35]

PROGNOSIS

A yet unsolved enigma is the spontaneous resolution observed in a majority of children, as discussed previously.[7] This is in contrast to the increasing evidence that pediatric mastocytosis is a clonal disease in the great majority of children. One possible explanation is differences in mutational profiles compared with adults, with the KIT D816V mutation only detectable in approximately 25% to 35% of children as opposed to 80% to 95% of adult patients. In addition, children have more mutations in the transmembrane and extracellular domains of KIT.[21] Mechanisms involved in the resolution of an apparent clonal disease, however, are yet to be elucidated. From a clinical perspective, recent data have suggested that children presenting with monomorphic small-sized lesions similar to adult patients may have a higher risk of having persistent mastocytosis, whereas in those with polymorphic larger lesions, the disease more often resolves before or at puberty.[26,44] Similarly a late onset in childhood, evidence of systemic disease at diagnosis, and persistently elevated levels of serum tryptase have been proposed to predict persistency (**Box 2**); however, further studies, including long-term studies, are needed for clarification.

CURRENT CONTROVERSIES

In general, knowledge about pediatric mastocytosis is limited, because invasive tests, such as bone marrow biopsies, are not routinely performed in children and, thus, the

Box 2
Suggested predictors for persistent disease

Small, monomorphic skin lesions (adult-type UP)

Systemic disease (often related to monomorphic UP)

KIT D816V mutation

Persistently elevated basal serum tryptase

Onset after 3 years of age

Skin lesions present after 12 years of age

true prevalence of systemic disease in pediatric patients is not known. Given that systemic involvement most likely is equal to persistent disease as well as associated with an increased risk for anaphylaxis, osteoporosis, and other comorbidities in adulthood, this lack of knowledge limits the possibility of properly counseling and treating the pediatric patients. It is possible that development of improved diagnostic methods, such as highly sensitive methods for detection of non-*KIT* D816V mutations and highly sensitive flow cytometry, may in the future provide a better understanding and guide a personalized approach to affected children.

So far, no children with mastocytosis without skin lesions, that is, BMM/monoclonal MCAD, have been reported. This is, however, a frequently encountered entity in the adult population, often only recognized by diagnostic screening using a highly sensitive *KIT* D816V mutation analysis in peripheral blood[45] or by performing a bone marrow examination in, for example, anaphylaxis patients based on proposed scoring systems.[46–48] Although evidence of a similar high prevalence of underlying mastocytosis in pediatric venom anaphylaxis patients is lacking,[49] further research is needed to understand to what extent clonal MC disease without skin lesions may be found in the pediatric population when systematically applying diagnostic screening methods with very high analytical sensitivity, which in the future may be able to detect even lower levels of mutated cells and non-*KIT* D816V mutations.

Similarly, future studies on idiopathic MCAS are of paramount importance to better classify this newly introduced entity in the pediatric population and to understand to what extent the current knowledge from adult patients can be transferred to children. To that end, there is a need for further studies to clarify if a chronic, nonepisodic form of MCAS may exist with multiple symptoms caused by but not specific to MC mediators and if a continuous state of MCA is possible in such patients, which for now remains speculative.

SUMMARY AND FUTURE CONSIDERATIONS

This article focuses on pediatric mastocytosis, which in a broader perspective may be grouped among MCADs. Although symptoms in pediatric mastocytosis are typically mild and often limited to the skin,[6,12,50] several aspects of the disease are in need of further research, such as the pathogenesis, disease course and prognostication, risk of persistent disease, and extracutaneous manifestations. It is, therefore, generally recommended that children with mastocytosis are offered an evaluation by specialized multidisciplinary mastocytosis centers.

REFERENCES

1. Akin C, Valent P, Metcalfe DD. Mast cell activation syndrome: proposed diagnostic criteria. J Allergy Clin Immunol 2010;126(6):1099–104.e4.

2. Metcalfe DD. Mast cells and mastocytosis. Blood 2008;112(4):946–56.
3. Valent P, Akin C, Escribano L, et al. Standards and standardization in mastocytosis: consensus statements on diagnostics, treatment recommendations and response criteria. Eur J Clin Invest 2007;37(6):435–53.
4. Valent P, Horny HP, Escribano L, et al. Diagnostic criteria and classification of mastocytosis: a consensus proposal. Leuk Res 2001;25(7):603–25.
5. Horny HP, Akin C, Metcalfe DD, et al. Mastocytosis (mast cell disease). In: Swerdlow CD, Campo E, Harris NL, et al, editors. World Health Organization (WHO) classification of tumours of the haematopoietic and lymphoid tissues, vol. 2. Lyon (France): IARC Press; 2008. p. 54–63.
6. Carter MC, Metcalfe DD. Paediatric mastocytosis. Arch Dis Child 2002;86(5):315–9.
7. Uzzaman A, Maric I, Noel P, et al. Pediatric-onset mastocytosis: a long term clinical follow-up and correlation with bone marrow histopathology. Pediatr Blood Cancer 2009;53(4):629–34.
8. Meni C, Bruneau J, Georgin-Lavialle S, et al. Paediatric mastocytosis: a systematic review of 1747 cases. Br J Dermatol 2015;172(3):642–51.
9. Cohen SS, Skovbo S, Vestergaard H, et al. Epidemiology of systemic mastocytosis in Denmark. Br J Haematol 2014;166(4):521–8.
10. Brockow K. Epidemiology, prognosis, and risk factors in mastocytosis. Immunol Allergy Clin North Am 2014;34(2):283–95.
11. Carter MC, Clayton ST, Komarow HD, et al. Assessment of clinical findings, tryptase levels, and bone marrow histopathology in the management of pediatric mastocytosis. J Allergy Clin Immunol 2015;136(6):1673–9.e3.
12. Hartmann K, Metcalfe DD. Pediatric mastocytosis. Hematol Oncol Clin North Am 2000;14(3):625–40.
13. Lange M, Niedoszytko M, Renke J, et al. Clinical aspects of paediatric mastocytosis: a review of 101 cases. J Eur Acad Dermatol Venereol 2013;27(1):97–102.
14. Bibi S, Langenfeld F, Jeanningros S, et al. Molecular defects in mastocytosis: KIT and beyond KIT. Immunol Allergy Clin North Am 2014;34(2):239–62.
15. Broesby-Olsen S, Kristensen TK, Moller MB, et al. Adult-onset systemic mastocytosis in monozygotic twins with KIT D816V and JAK2 V617F mutations. J Allergy Clin Immunol 2012;130(3):806–8.
16. Zanotti R, Simioni L, Garcia-Montero AC, et al. Somatic D816V KIT mutation in a case of adult-onset familial mastocytosis. J Allergy Clin Immunol 2013;131(2):605–7.
17. Kristensen T, Broesby-Olsen S, Vestergaard H, et al. KIT D816V mutation-positive cell fractions in lesional skin biopsies from adults with systemic mastocytosis. Dermatology 2013;226(3):233–7.
18. Kristensen T, Broesby-Olsen S, Vestergaard H, et al, Mastocytosis Centre Odense University Hospital (MastOUH). Circulating KIT D816V mutation-positive non-mast cells in peripheral blood are characteristic of indolent systemic mastocytosis. Eur J Haematol 2012;89(1):42–6.
19. Kristensen T, Vestergaard H, Bindslev-Jensen C, et al, Mastocytosis Centre, Odense University Hospital (MastOUH). Sensitive KIT D816V mutation analysis of blood as a diagnostic test in mastocytosis. Am J Hematol 2014;89(5):493–8.
20. Kristensen T, Vestergaard H, Moller MB. Improved detection of the KIT D816V mutation in patients with systemic mastocytosis using a quantitative and highly sensitive real-time qPCR assay. J Mol Diagn 2011;13(2):180–8.
21. Bodemer C, Hermine O, Palmerini F, et al. Pediatric mastocytosis is a clonal disease associated with D816V and other activating c-KIT mutations. J Invest Dermatol 2010;130(3):804–15.

22. Theoharides TC, Valent P, Akin C. Mast cells, mastocytosis, and related disorders. N Engl J Med 2015;373(19):1885–6.

23. Pec M, Plank L, Szepe P, et al. A case of systemic mastocytosis–an ultrastructural and immunohistochemical study of the dermal mast cells in relation to activation of the epidermal melanin unit. J Eur Acad Dermatol Venereol 1998;11(3):258–61.

24. Tomita Y, Maeda K, Tagami H. Histamine stimulates normal human melanocytes in vitro: one of the possible inducers of hyperpigmentation in urticaria pigmentosa. J Dermatol Sci 1993;6(2):146–54.

25. Hartmann K, Henz BM. Cutaneous mastocytosis – clinical heterogeneity. Int Arch Allergy Immunol 2002;127(2):143–6.

26. Hartmann K, Escribano L, Grattan C, et al. Cutaneous manifestations in patients with mastocytosis: consensus report of the European Competence Network on Mastocytosis; the American Academy of Allergy, Asthma & Immunology; and the European Academy of Allergology and Clinical Immunology. J Allergy Clin Immunol 2016;137(1):35–45.

27. Carter MC, Metcalfe DD, Clark AS, et al. Abnormal bone marrow histopathology in paediatric mastocytosis. Br J Haematol 2015;168(6):865–73.

28. Broesby-Olsen S, Farkas DK, Vestergaard H, et al. Risk of solid cancer, cardiovascular disease, anaphylaxis, osteoporosis and fractures in patients with systemic mastocytosis: a nationwide population-based study. Am J Hematol 2016; 91(11):1069–75.

29. Gulen T, Hagglund H, Dahlen B, et al. High prevalence of anaphylaxis in patients with systemic mastocytosis - a single-centre experience. Clin Exp Allergy 2014; 44(1):121–9.

30. Gonzalez de Olano D, de la Hoz Caballer B, Nunez Lopez R, et al. Prevalence of allergy and anaphylactic symptoms in 210 adult and pediatric patients with mastocytosis in Spain: a study of the Spanish network on mastocytosis (REMA). Clin Exp Allergy 2007;37(10):1547–55.

31. Broesby-Olsen S, Kristensen T, Vestergaard H, et al. KIT D816V mutation burden does not correlate to clinical manifestations of indolent systemic mastocytosis. J Allergy Clin Immunol 2013;132(3):723–8.

32. Brockow K, Jofer C, Behrendt H, et al. Anaphylaxis in patients with mastocytosis: a study on history, clinical features and risk factors in 120 patients. Allergy 2008; 63(2):226–32.

33. Huang F, Chawla K, Jarvinen KM, et al. Anaphylaxis in a New York City pediatric emergency department: triggers, treatments, and outcomes. J Allergy Clin Immunol 2012;129(1):162–8.e1-e3.

34. Alvarez-Twose I, Vano-Galvan S, Sanchez-Munoz L, et al. Increased serum baseline tryptase levels and extensive skin involvement are predictors for the severity of mast cell activation episodes in children with mastocytosis. Allergy 2012;67(6): 813–21.

35. Brockow K, Ring J, Alvarez-Twose I, et al. Extensive blistering is a predictor for severe complications in children with mastocytosis. Allergy 2012;67(10):1323–4.

36. Akin C. Mast cell activation syndromes. J Allergy Clin Immunol 2017;140(2):349–55.

37. Schwartz LB. Diagnostic value of tryptase in anaphylaxis and mastocytosis. Immunol Allergy Clin North Am 2006;26(3):451–63.

38. Sampson HA, Munoz-Furlong A, Bock SA, et al. Symposium on the definition and management of anaphylaxis: summary report. J Allergy Clin Immunol 2005; 115(3):584–91.

39. Valent P, Akin C, Arock M, et al. Definitions, criteria and global classification of mast cell disorders with special reference to mast cell activation syndromes: a consensus proposal. Int Arch Allergy Immunol 2012;157(3):215–25.
40. Lyons JJ, Yu X, Hughes JD, et al. Elevated basal serum tryptase identifies a multisystem disorder associated with increased TPSAB1 copy number. Nat Genet 2016;48(12):1564–9.
41. Lange M, Zawadzka A, Schrors S, et al. The role of serum tryptase in the diagnosis and monitoring of pediatric mastocytosis: a single-center experience. Postepy Dermatol Alergol 2017;34(4):306–12.
42. Kristensen T, Vestergaard H, Bindslev-Jensen C, et al. Prospective evaluation of the diagnostic value of sensitive KIT D816V mutation analysis of blood in adults with suspected systemic mastocytosis. Allergy 2017;72(11):1737–43.
43. Zuberbier T, Aberer W, Asero R, et al. The EAACI/GA(2) LEN/EDF/WAO guideline for the definition, classification, diagnosis, and management of urticaria: the 2013 revision and update. Allergy 2014;69(7):868–87.
44. Wiechers T, Rabenhorst A, Schick T, et al. Large maculopapular cutaneous lesions are associated with favorable outcome in childhood-onset mastocytosis. J Allergy Clin Immunol 2015;136(6):1581–90.e3.
45. Broesby-Olsen S, Oropeza AR, Bindslev-Jensen C, et al. Recognizing mastocytosis in patients with anaphylaxis: value of KIT D816V mutation analysis of peripheral blood. J Allergy Clin Immunol 2015;135(1):262–4.
46. Carter MC, Desai A, Komarow HD, et al. A distinct biomolecular profile identifies monoclonal mast cell disorders in patients with idiopathic anaphylaxis. J Allergy Clin Immunol 2018;141(1):180–8.e3.
47. Alvarez-Twose I, Gonzalez-de-Olano D, Sanchez-Munoz L, et al. Validation of the REMA score for predicting mast cell clonality and systemic mastocytosis in patients with systemic mast cell activation symptoms. Int Arch Allergy Immunol 2012;157(3):275–80.
48. Zanotti R, Lombardo C, Passalacqua G, et al. Clonal mast cell disorders in patients with severe hymenoptera venom allergy and normal serum tryptase levels. J Allergy Clin Immunol 2015;136(1):135–9.
49. Yavuz ST, Sackesen C, Sahiner UM, et al. Importance of serum basal tryptase levels in children with insect venom allergy. Allergy 2013;68(3):386–91.
50. Torrelo A, Alvarez-Twose I, Escribano L. Childhood mastocytosis. Curr Opin Pediatr 2012;24(4):480–6.

Bone Marrow Expression of Mast Cell Disorders

Laura Sánchez-Muñoz, MD, PhD[a,b,*], Ana Filipa Henriques, BSc, PhD[a,b],
Iván Alvarez-Twose, MD, PhD[a,b], Almudena Matito, MD, PhD[a,b]

KEYWORDS

- Mast cells • Mastocytosis • Flow cytometry • Bone marrow • Cell purification
- Diagnosis • KIT mutation • Prognosis

KEY POINTS

- Mast cell disorders constitute a group of heterogeneous diseases that should be managed in specialized reference centers, in order to increase patient access to high-quality diagnostic tests and treatment.
- To establish the correct diagnosis and prognosis of the disease, highly specialized laboratory diagnostic tests should be applied in the diagnostic workup in suspected systemic mastocytosis.
- Multiparameter flow cytometry stands as the most sensitive technique to determine the grade of involvement of the bone marrow, together with the exact diagnosis, subtype, and prognosis of mastocytosis.
- Sensitive approaches for detecting KIT mutation in highly purified bone marrow mast cells are mandatory to avoid false negative results, moreover when a pathologic low bone marrow mast cell burden is suspected.

INTRODUCTION

The World Health Organization (WHO) recently updated the classification of mastocytosis[1–3] in the following categories:

I. Cutaneous mastocytosis (CM) when it is limited to the skin;
II. Systemic mastocytosis (SM) when abnormal mast cells (MCs) are located in extracutaneous organs, including the bone marrow (BM); it is divided into indolent

Disclosure Statement: The authors declare no competing financial interest.

Funding: This work was supported by grants from the Asociación Española de Mastocitosis y enfermedades relacionadas (AEDM 2017); Fondos de Investigación para Enfermedades Raras del Ministerio de Sanidad, Servicios sociales e Igualdad; Ensayo clínico independiente del Ministerio de Salud y Política Social (EC11-287); Hospital Virgen de la Salud Biobank (BioB-HVS) is supported by grant PT13/0010/0007 from the Instituto de Salud Carlos III (Spain).

[a] Instituto de Estudios de Mastocitosis de Castilla La Mancha, Hospital Virgen del Valle, Ctra. Cobisa s/n, Toledo 45071, Spain; [b] Spanish Network on Mastocytosis (REMA), Toledo, Spain
* Corresponding author. Instituto de Estudios de Mastocitosis de Castilla La Mancha, Hospital Virgen del Valle, Ctra. Cobisa s/n, Toledo 45071, Spain.
E-mail address: lsmunoz@sescam.jccm.es

SM (ISM), smoldering SM, SM with an associated hematologic (non-MC lineage) neoplasm (SM-AHN), aggressive SM (ASM), and mast cell leukemia (MCL);

III. MC sarcoma. Furthermore, 2 other subvariants of mastocytosis have been recognized:

1. Well-differentiated forms with cutaneous and systemic (WDSM) involvement[4]; these forms show unique features that require specific diagnostic criteria;
2. ISM in the absence of skin lesions (ISMs−).[5–7]

According to the WHO criteria,[2,3] the diagnosis of SM is based on the coexistence of one major criterion (presence of multifocal dense aggregates of $\geq$15 MCs in BM biopsies and/or in sections of other extracutaneous organs) plus one minor criterion or simultaneous detection of 4 minor criteria:

A. Identification of greater than 25% of atypical MCs on BM smears or infiltrates of spindle-shaped MCs on sections of visceral organs,
B. KIT point mutation at codon 816 in the BM or another extracutaneous organ,
C. MCs in BM or blood or another extracutaneous organ exhibit CD2 and/or CD25,
D. Baseline serum tryptase levels greater than 20 ng/mL.

In clinical practice, the suspicion of an underlying MC disorder is based on the presence of the typical skin lesions of mastocytosis or in patients without skin lesions presenting with systemic symptoms of MC activation (MCA) (eg, anaphylaxis).[8]

Despite the great relevance and efficiency of the WHO criteria in the diagnosis of SM, frequently in nonaggressive categories of SM, MCs represent a very small proportion of all nucleated BM cells ($<10^{-3}$ BM MCs, as assessed by flow cytometry).[9,10] Along this line, BM MC aggregates are not found in 30% to 54% of the ISMs− patients and serum tryptase levels are frequently less than 20 ng/mL in 31% to 38% of the ISMs− cases (anaphylaxis elicited by other triggers vs insects, respectively).[11] Therefore, it is mandatory to apply highly sensitive and specific methodological approaches to the study of BM MCs, including detailed cytologic analysis of BM smears, flow cytometry immunophenotyping using specific strategies for detecting MCs present at low frequencies,[12,13] detection of KIT mutations in highly purified BM MCs,[14] as well as the rational combination of the SM criteria in the routine diagnosis of SM,[10,15] in order to improve the diagnostic efficiency and quality as previously reported.[16]

Of note, the sensitivity and specificity of the methodological approaches used in the diagnosis of ISMs− contribute to explain the differences in the percentage of SM among adults presenting with systemic symptoms of MCA in the absence of skin lesions described in different reports.[7,17–19] In addition, different terms such as (mono) clonal MC activation syndrome (MMAS)[8,18,19] or primary MC activation syndrome[20] or clonal MC activation disorder (c-MCAD)[7] emerged to name those cases who do not meet the WHO criteria for SM, despite KIT mutated clonal MCs that usually express CD25 are found (Fig. 1).

The mast cell activation syndrome (MCAS) includes a heterogeneous group of diseases that are characterized by systemic symptoms secondary to the release of MC mediators that may or may not have a known trigger, may or may not present specific immunoglobulin E (IgE) antibodies in response to that trigger, and are associated with normal or elevated baseline tryptase levels in the absence of skin lesions of mastocytosis.[8,21] The diagnosis and classification of MCAS are based on previous described clinical and laboratory criteria.[8] The Spanish Network of Mastocytosis (REMA) supports that the most relevant fact to classify the MCAS is the presence versus absence of clonal MCs (based on the expression of CD25$^+$ and/or KIT mutation).[21] When

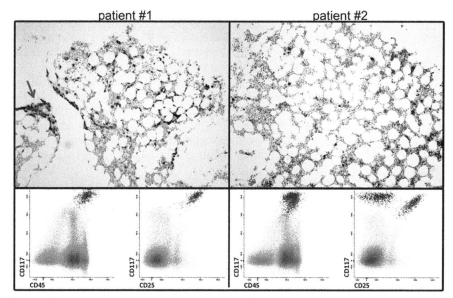

Fig. 1. BM sections showed increased numbers of interstitial MCs and MC aggregates (*red arrow*) in patient 1 (ISMs−), but scattered MCs in the absence of aggregates in patient 2 (c-MCAS/MMAS); (*upper panels*) tryptase stain, ×400. BM aspirate analysis by flow cytometry showed 0.09%/0.002% of BMMCs (*red dots*) in patients 1 and 2, respectively. Expression of CD25 was detected in all BMMCs in patient 1, whereas only 53% in patient 2.

MCAS diagnostic criteria are fulfilled but there is no evidence of clonality, nonclonal MCAS should be considered. Along this line, the European Competence Network on Mastocytosis recommends using the REMA score[7] to predict the presence of clonal MCs in the BM of patients diagnosed of MCAS, in order to select those cases that should undergo a complete BM study.

The clonal nature of MCs in mastocytosis or clonal MC disorders can be established through demonstration of KIT mutations in lesional skin and/or BM cells,[14,22–25] resulting the KIT D816V as the most frequently mutation found in SM.

BM is the most appropriate site for screening systemic involvement in mastocytosis because it is the most frequently documented site of extracutaneous involvement, resulting in the expansion and accumulation of aberrant MCs in distinct tissues.[2,26]

Because diagnosis of mastocytosis may be a challenge because of the wide variety of clinical presentation, abnormal morphology of MC, and variation in histologic features, a thorough histologic, immunohistochemical, and morphologic BM examination remains an important feature in the diagnostic workup in suspected SM.[27]

Bone Marrow Histopathologic Features of Mast Cell Disorders

The presence of multifocal, dense aggregates of ≥15 MCs in tissue sections from biopsy specimens from BM and/or other extracutaneous organs is highly specific of mastocytosis. In addition, mastocytosis may also present with a predominantly diffuse or a mixed (diffuse and focal) infiltration pattern.[28,29] Depending on the number and distribution of MCs in the BM, different histologic patterns can be observed.[28] Accordingly, whereas ASM and MCL cases systematically show a dense, diffuse MC infiltration, ISM may have different patterns of BM involvement ranging from an increase of interstitial MCs without evidence of compact MC aggregates, to focal, dense MC aggregates with or without a diffuse component.[30]

Bone Marrow Immunohistochemistry

Immunohistochemical staining of BM biopsy sections with tryptase is recommended for MC-detection and evaluation of BM MC infiltration,[28] resulting more informative than using only conventional stains (eg, hematoxylin and eosin or Giemsa).[31]

c-Kit staining is routinely used to identify both normal and abnormal MCs, whereas CD25 is a reliable and specific marker for SM MCs.[30] Despite this, its utility is limited in cases lacking MC aggregates (resulting difficult to differentiate between abnormal MCs and CD25-positive T lymphocytes), and in CD25-negative WDSM. In addition, expression of CD30 has been reported to be a potentially useful prognostic marker because it is strongly expressed by MCs from poor-prognosis categories of mastocytosis, ASM and MCL.[32,33]

Morphologic Expression of Mast Cell Disorders

MCs can be easily identified in toluidine blue–stained BM smears as red-purple elements over a blue background (**Fig. 2**). On the other hand, May-Grünwald-Giemsa stain allows a better cytomorphologic characterization of MCs (mainly outside the BM particles), as well as the identification of other morphologic features suspicious of a coexisting hematological malignancy. Wright and Giemsa stains of BM MCs of patients with clonal MCD show morphologic features such as the following:

I. Metachromatic granulated blast and immature atypical MCs with bilobed or multilobed nuclei: promastocyte or atypical MC type II,
II. More mature cells, which show an atypical morphology with prominent surface projections, frequently spindle-shaped, with a hypogranulated cytoplasm and/or an oval eccentric nucleus, atypical MC type I, and
III. Typical mature (tissue) MC features, consisting of round or oval-shaped cells with a round central nucleus and a well-granulated cytoplasm.[34]

Along this line, ASM and MCL typically show immature cytologic features such as a wide-sized heterogeneity, multilobed nuclei (promastocytes), or a poorly differentiated morphology (metachromatic blasts)[10,34]; round or polygonal BM MCs may coexist with fusiform shapes in some SM cases,[10] and WDSM BM MCs typically exhibit mature, increased size, round shaped with round nucleus, and fully granulated cytoplasm with relatively frequent degranulation phenomena, vacuoles.[35]

Origin, Identification, and Enumeration of Bone Marrow Mast Cells by Flow Cytometry

MCs derive from BM hematopoietic progenitors and circulate through the vascular system as immature progenitors, before they migrate into peripheral tissues, where they complete the final stages of their maturation under the influence of a tissue-specific local microenvironment.[36]

As stated previously, MCs represent an infrequent cell population in normal BM-aspirated samples (0.008% $\pm$ 0.0082% of all nucleated cells in adult human BM).[13,37] Although reactive BM samples and BM samples from patients with non-MC–related hematologic disorders may show slightly increased mean BM MC numbers (0.027% $\pm$ 0.17%), in most instances, these cells represent less than 0.1% the whole BM cellularity.[38] Interestingly, despite the increased frequency of BM MCs found in reactive samples versus normal BM, few immunophenotypic differences have been described between normal and reactive MCs.[13,37,39]

MCs strongly express CD117, CD203c, and the high-affinity receptor for IgE, FcεRI[38,40] (**Fig. 3**); nevertheless, none of them is a specific marker for MC.[41–43] In early

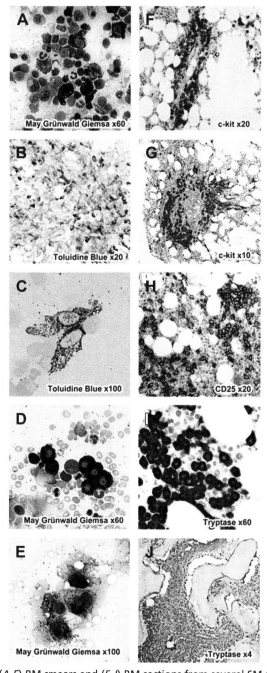

Fig. 2. Images of (A-E) BM smears and (F-J) BM sections from several SM patients. (A) High-power view showing fusiform MC together with round and oval MCs from a case of ISM. (B) Low-power view showing a marked increase of atypical MCs from a case of ASM. (C) High-power view showing 2 spindle-shaped MC. (D) High-power view showing round, fully granulated MCs from a case of WDSM. (E) High-power view showing morphologically poor-differentiated MC, some of which display 2 nuclei (promastocytes) from a case of

studies, the identification of MCs was based on their strong reactivity for CD117 in the absence of expression for CD38, CD34, and CD138, to discriminate MCs from CD34 HPC and CD117[+] plasma cells; in turn, the coexpression of FcεRI and CD33 together with strong positivity for CD117 allows the discrimination between MCs and basophils.[12] More recently, it has been suggested that using a CD117high/CD45low combination could accurately identify BM MC[12,13] (see **Fig. 3**).

Immunophenotypic Characteristics of Bone Marrow Mast Cells in Systemic Mastocytosis

Early studies on the immunophenotypic features of BM MCs in SM reported several aberrant phenotypes with a clear discrimination from normal and pathologic MCs.[44–47] These early studies reported aberrant expression for CD2 and CD25 as a hallmark for SM, because both of these proteins were absent in normal/reactive BM MC, but expressed in most SM patients.[9,48] From these 2 markers, CD25 has been described to be the most sensitive, specific, and stable, whereas positivity for CD2 may vary depending on the sensitivity of the fluorochrome-conjugated monoclonal antibody used in the study.[12] Also, in a recent publication,[49] it was shown that CD2 expression does not contribute to improve the diagnosis of SM when compared with aberrant CD25 expression alone.

Apart from the aberrant expression of CD2 and CD25, BM MCs from SM patients also display abnormally high expression of CD33[44] and of the CD2 ligand CD58.[45] Increased expression for activation markers such as CD69[50] or CD63[51] and complement-associated molecules, such as CD11c, CD35,[52] CD59, and/or CD88,[52,53] are also commonly found in BM MCs from SM. In contrast, expression of CD117,[45] the CD71 transferrin receptor, and CD29 integrin is abnormally downregulated on BM MCs from these patients[48] (**Table 1**).

Aberrant expression of other molecules, such as CD30 (TNFR superfamily 8), seems not to be associated with the D816V KIT mutation itself. This receptor has been described recently to be widely expressed on BM MCs from SM patients and allows for the identification of a minor group of patients who typically lack expression of CD25/CD2 and activating exon 17 KIT mutations, WDSM patients, ultimately improving the overall diagnosis of the disease.[4,54]

Coexistence of Normal and Pathologic Bone Marrow Mast Cells

Although the BM MC burden in ISM patients can be extremely low, the coexistence of normal and pathologic MCs in the same patient is frequent in specific disease categories (33% of ISMs− and 18% of ISM patients).[7] Furthermore, the coexistence of normal and aberrant BM MC populations is usually restricted to SM patients with KIT mutation limited to the BM MC compartment,[55] and it should be considered a good prognosis factor because of its association with indolent forms of the disease.

ASM. (F) Low-power view showing a perivascular infiltrate of MCs from a case of ISM. (G) Low-power view showing a large lymphoid aggregate admixed with MCs from a case of ISM. (H) Low-power view showing CD25-positive MCs from a case of ISM. (I) High-power view showing round, fully granulated, tryptase-positive MCs from a case of WDSM. (J) Low-power view showing a dense, diffuse MC infiltration from a case of ASM. (From Alvarez-Twose I, Morgado JM, Sánchez-Muñoz L, et al. Current state of biology and diagnosis of clonal mast cell diseases in adults. Int J Lab Hematol 2012;34(5):452; with permission.)

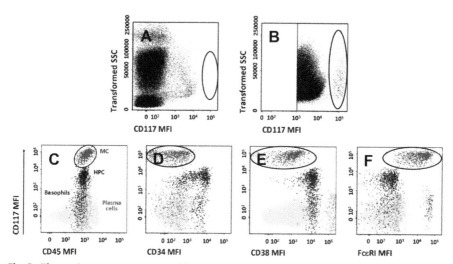

Fig. 3. The gating strategy proposed by REMA for the immunophenotypic identification and characterization of BM MCs by use of MFC. Whole BM cellularity (*A*) live gated to enrich on CD117⁺-nucleated cells corresponding to 3×10^6 total events (*B*) from an individual with a BM MC load of 0.009% is shown. (*C–F*) The gating strategy used for the identification of the BM MC population (*red events*) within the CD117⁺ cells gated in (*B*) and its phenotypic discrimination from CD34⁺ HPC (*blue dots*), plasma cells (*green dots*), and basophils (*violet dots*) coexisting in the same BM sample. (*Adapted from* Teodosio C, Mayado A, Sánchez-Muñoz L, et al. The immunophenotype of mast cells and its utility in the diagnostic work-up of systemic mastocytosis. J Leukoc Biol 2015;97(1):51; with permission.)

Mast Cell Immunophenotypical Expression of Different Types of Systemic Mastocytosis

Considering that SM is a group of heterogeneous diseases regarding both their clinical behavior and their prognosis,[7,19,27,56–59] the differences in the immunophenotypic profiles of the distinct subtypes of SM were studied individually[13,55]; in such an analysis, 3 different patterns were identified[13] (**Fig. 4**).

Overall, the most frequently detected immunophenotypic pattern of BM MCs corresponds to a good-prognosis group of SM patients (ISM). These patients typically show a mature immunophenotype associated with aberrant expression of CD2 and CD25 and increased expression of MC activation-associated molecules.[13] In line with this activation-related pattern, upregulation of molecules associated with MC degranulation (eg, the lysosomal glycoprotein CD63 and CD203c) is also observed in this subgroup of SM patients. Overall, these findings indicate that MCs from patients with ISM display an activated mature phenotype in the BM, associated with aberrant CD25 and CD2 expression (see **Fig. 4**).[13] This activation-associated MC phenotype might result from the presence of the D816V KIT mutation, because this KIT mutation is shared by most (>95%) of these patients.[14]

In contrast to ISM, most BM MCs from WDSM patients typically do not carry the D816V KIT mutation in the absence of CD2 and CD25 expression, although approximately -third of cases are partially positive for CD25 or show dim expression of CD2 on its BM MC.[13,49] BM MCs from WDSM patients display an overall phenotype similar to that observed for mature-resting, normal BM MCs (strong expression for CD117 and FcεRI).[38] Aberrant MC phenotypes from WDSM in most patients are

Table 1
Qualitative and semiquantitative patterns of expression of individual markers on normal, reactive, and systemic mastocytosis bone marrow mast cells

Functional Group of Proteins	Surface Antigen	CD Code	Normal BM (% of Positive Cases)	Reactive BM (% of Positive Cases)	Overall SM (% of Positive Cases)
Cytokine receptor	IL-2Rα	CD25	—	—	-/+ (93)
	IL-3Rα	CD123	—	NR	-/+ (72)
	c-Kit	CD117	+++ (100)	+++ (100)	++/+++ (100)
Adhesion-related molecules	LFA-2	CD2	—	—	-/+ (72)
	Integrin alpha-L	CD11a	-/+ (20)	NR	—
	Integrin alpha-M	CD11 b	-/+ (50)	-/+ (50)	-/+ (50)
	Integrin alpha-X	CD11c	-/+ (71)	NR	+/++ (100)
	Integrin beta-2	CD18	+ (65)	NR	-/+ (44)
	Siglec-2	CD22	-/+ (60)	-/+ (50)	-/+ (96)
	Integrin beta-1	CD29	++ (100)	++ (100)	+ (100)
	Siglec-3	CD33	++/+++ (100)	++/+++ (100)	+++ (100)
	HPCA-1	CD34	—	—	—
	Pgp-1	CD44	++ (100)	++ (100)	++ (100)
	Integrin alpha-4	CD49 d	+/++ (100)	NR	-/+ (80)
	Integrin alpha-5	CD49e	+ (100)	NR	-/+ (30)
	Integrin alpha-V	CD51	+ (100)	+	-/+ (45)
	ICAM-1	CD54	-/+ (75)	NR	++ (100)
Complement-related molecules	CR1	CD35	—	+	+ (100)
	Complement decay-accelerating factor	CD55	+ (100)	+ (100)	+/++ (100)
	Membrane attack complex inhibition factor	CD59	+ (100)	+ (100)	+/++ (100)
	C5aR	CD88	-/+ (18)	NR	-/+ (54)
Immunoglobulin receptors	FcεRI	NA	++/+++ (100)	++/+++ (100)	++/+++ (100)
	FcγRIIIB	CD16	-/+ (13)	-/+ (13)	-/+ (69)
	FcγRII	CD32	+ (100)	+ (100)	+/++ (100)
	FcγRI	CD64	-/+ (4)	-/+ (4)	-/+ (84)

Category	Marker	Antigen			
MHC-related molecules	HLA-I	NA	++ (100)	++ (100)	+/+++ (100)
	HLA-DR	NA	-/+ (25)	-/+ (25)	-/+ (85)
Tetraspanins	CD9 antigen	CD9	+++ (100)	+++ (100)	++/+++ (100)
	LAMP3	CD63	++ (100)	++/+++[a] (100)	++/+++ (100)
TNF receptor family proteins	CD30 L receptor	CD30	—	NR	-/+ (80)
	CD40 L receptor	CD40	-/+ (65)	-/+ (65)	-/+ (65)
Mast cell proteases	Tryptase	NA	++ (100)	++ (100)	+/+++ (100)
	Carboxypeptidase A	NA	++ (100)	++ (100)	+/+++ (100)
Activation markers	Early activation antigen CD69	CD69	+ (100)	+ (100)	+/++ (100)
	E-NPP 3	CD203c	+ (100)	NR	+/++ (100)
Other	LCA	CD45	+ (100)	+ (100)	+/++ (100)
	Transferrin receptor protein 1	CD71	+ (100)	NR	-/+ (38)
	Bcl-2	NA	-/+ (94)	-/+ (94)	-/+ (87)

Abbreviations: NA, not applicable; NR, not reported; -/+, expressed in a subset of patients (percentage of positive cases); −, absent expression; +dim, dim positive expression; +, moderate positive expression; ++, positive expression; +++, strong positive expression. Mixed symbols indicate variable reactivity, either among cases or among cells from the same individual.

[a] Expression of CD63 is increased in BM MCs from myelodysplastic syndromes.

Data from Refs. [13,44–46,48,50–53,59,86]

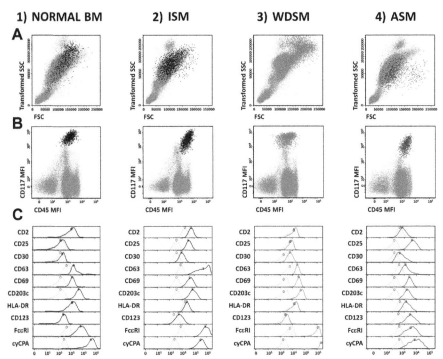

Fig. 4. (*A, B*) Representative bivariate dot plots and (*C*) histograms, illustrating the (*A*) light-scatter features and (*C*) immunophenotypical profiles of BM MCs from healthy donors (highlighted in black in *A1*, *B1*, and *C1*), ISM (highlighted in blue in *A2*, *B2*, and *C2*), WDSM (highlighted in green in *A3*, *B3*, and *C3*), and ASM (highlighted in red in *A4*, *B4*, and *C4*), identified on the basis of their reactivity for (*B*) CD45 and CD117. Baseline MC autofluorescence for each protein is indicated in the histograms in gray in *C1–C4*. cyCPA, cytoplasmic carboxypeptidase A. (*From* Teodosio C, Mayado A, Sánchez-Muñoz L, et al. The immunophenotype of mast cells and its utility in the diagnostic work-up of systemic mastocytosis. J Leukoc Biol 2015;97(1):55; with permission.)

restricted to expression of CD30 in the absence of CD25 high[54] and increased cytoplasmic contents in MC enzymes (eg, tryptase and CPA), which probably contribute to the typical hypergranulated, morphologic appearance of BM MCs in WDSM cases,[4,15] and their abnormally increased size and internal complexity[13] (see **Fig. 4**).

Oppositely, the poor-prognosis subvariants of the disease (ASM and MCL) typically display bright expression of CD25, frequently in the absence of CD2.[13,49] This aberrant phenotype is commonly associated with increased expression of the CD123 and HLA-DR antigens, which are typically expressed by immature BM MC,[38,60,61] together with abnormally low levels of cytoplasmic tryptase and CPA and decreased light-scatter (SSC and FSC) features (see **Fig. 4**).[13] Overall, BM MCs from poor-prognosis variants of SM (ASM and MCL) display a relatively immature phenotype, potentially associated with an early blockade of MC maturation.

KIT Mutation Analysis in Mastocytosis

Most adults with mastocytosis carry the activating somatic KIT D816V mutation, whereas most cases of childhood-onset and familial mastocytosis would lack these mutations. Nevertheless, the frequency of the D816V KIT mutation is highly variable in the literature, which could be due to several reasons:

I. The relatively low number of cases included in some studies;
II. The patient selection with predominance of aggressive versus indolent forms of the disease;
III. The sensitivity of the methods used to assess the presence/absence of KIT mutations, particularly in cases with low MC burden;
IV. The type of samples used for the identification of KIT mutations (eg, total BM samples versus highly purified BM MC).[14]

Standard Molecular Assays for Detection of KIT D816V

Mutation analysis based on genomic DNA (gDNA) or the expressed messenger RNA should be performed with caution, especially to avoid false-negative results in those BM samples with low MC numbers when low sensitive assays for detection of the KIT D816V mutation are used.[14] Overall, in 6% of ISMs— other mutations involving exon 17 are described,[14] such as D815K,[62] D816F, E839K,[24] R815K,[62] I817V,[14] N819Y,[63] N822I,[64] D816Y,[14,24] D816H,[65] insV815_I81618, and D820G mutations.[66] In addition, other mutations of KIT out of exon 17 should be ruled out (eg, F522C, A533D, K509I, R634W, V560G, among others),[67–74] as well as the pattern of inactivation of chromosome X by using HUMARA in BM MC,[4] moreover in familial and WD mastocytosis.

Multiple molecular methods can be used to specifically detect the D816V KIT mutation in patients suspected of mastocytosis:

I. Reverse transcriptase (RT)-polymerase chain reaction (PCR) assays plus restriction fragment length polymorphism,
II. Nested RT-PCR followed by denaturing high-performance liquid chromatography of PCR amplicons,
III. Peptide nucleic acid (PNA)-mediated PCR,
IV. Allele specific PCR (ASO-PCR) and the quantitative variant of the method (ASO-qPCR) on DNA or RNA/complementary DNA (cDNA).[75]

Other techniques include enrichment of MCs and other cell lineage from BM samples via laser microdissection, and both immunomagnetic[76,77] and fluorescence-activated cell sorting[12,14,76] of MCs followed by PNA-mediated PCR-clamping technique.[55,62] These approaches showed the KIT mutation not only in BM MCs but also in other highly purified hematopoietic lineages in SM patients; 27% of ISM and almost all poor-prognosis SM patients carry the KIT mutation in other non-MC hematopoietic lineage, multilineal KIT mutation involvement,[14] resulting the most powerful independent prognostic factor for progression of ISM to more aggressive forms of the disease.[57,78] Multilineal KIT D816V mutation in SM can be detected in gDNA from CD34+ hematopoietic stem and precursor cells, eosinophils, monocytes, and maturing neutrophils, and, to a less extent also in T lymphocytes, in addition to BM MC.[14,79] In order to evaluate the multilineal KIT pattern in SM, the REMA recommends performing the KIT mutation assays in at least one highly purified population (>97%) of myeloid cells (eg, BM monocytes and/or maturing neutrophils) and a population of lymphoid cells, apart from MC.[10,57]

The D816V mutation in a peripheral blood (PB) sample from a patient with SM in the absence of detectable circulating MCs was described in 1995.[22] Recently, several groups[80–84] have confirmed the feasibility of detecting the KIT mutation in PB leukocytes using highly sensitive assays (eg, ASO-qPCR-assays). These approaches also show that the mutation burden differs significantly among patients with different categories of the disease, but can be detected in PB leukocytes in nearly all adult patients with mastocytosis, including ISM and CM. In addition, the KIT D816V allele burden is of prognostic significance concerning survival and can be followed quantitatively during the natural course or during therapy and may be rapidly adopted as a valuable follow-up parameter in untreated and drug-treated patients with advanced SM.[75,81]

Despite all the above, discrepant results regarding both the frequency of SM cases carrying the KIT D816V[+] in PB and the prognostic impact of the KIT D816V allele burden have been published.[81,83,85] These discrepant findings might be related to the different approaches and sensitivity of the techniques used to assess KIT mutation involvement in PB (analysis on gDNA vs cDNA), and also to SM cases with a very low KIT mutated MC burden. For these reasons, BM samples are still the preferred specimen to rule out the mutation of KIT, moreover when a very low BM MC burden is suspected.[80,81,83]

REFERENCES

1. Arber DA, Orazi A, Hasserjian R, et al. The 2016 revision to the World Health Organization classification of myeloid neoplasms and acute leukemia. Blood 2016; 127(20):2391–405.

2. Horny HP, Akin C, Arber D, et al. Mastocytosis. World Health Organization (WHO) Classification of Tumours. In: Swerdlow SH, Campo E, Harris NL, et al, editors. Pathology & genetics. Tumours of haematopoietic and lymphoid tissues. Lyon (France): IARC Press; 2016.

3. Valent P, Akin C, Metcalfe DD. Mastocytosis: 2016 updated WHO classification and novel emerging treatment concepts. Blood 2017;129(11):1420–7.

4. Alvarez-Twose I, Jara-Acevedo M, Morgado JM, et al. Clinical, immunophenotypic, and molecular characteristics of well-differentiated systemic mastocytosis. J Allergy Clin Immunol 2016;137:168–78.

5. Metcalfe DD. Clinical advances in mastocytosis: an interdisciplinary roundtable discussion. J Invest Dermatol 1991;96(suppl):1S–65S.

6. Florian S, Krauth MT, Simonitsch-Klupp I, et al. Indolent systemic mastocytosis with elevated serum tryptase, absence of skin lesions, and recurrent severe anaphylactoid episodes. Int Arch Allergy Immunol 2005;136(3):273–80.

7. Alvarez-Twose I, Gonzalez de Olano D, Sánchez-Muñoz L, et al. Clinical, biological and molecular characteristics of systemic mast cell disorders presenting with severe mediator-related symptoms. J Allergy Clin Immunol 2010;125(6):1269–78.

8. Valent P, Akin C, Arock M, et al. Definitions, criteria and global classification of mast cell disorders with special reference to mast cell activation syndromes: a consensus proposal. Int Arch Allergy Immunol 2012;157(3):215–25.

9. Escribano L, Orfao A, Villarrubia J, et al. Sequential immunophenotypic analysis of mast cells in a case of systemic mast cell disease evolving to a mast cell leukemia. Cytometry 1997;30:98–102.

10. Sánchez-Muñoz L, Alvarez-Twose I, Garcia-Montero AC, et al. Evaluation of the WHO criteria for the classification of patients with mastocytosis. Mod Pathol 2011;24(9):1157–68.

11. Alvarez-Twose I, Zanotti R, Gonzalez-de-Olano D, et al. Nonaggressive systemic mastocytosis (SM) without skin lesions associated with insect-induced anaphylaxis shows unique features versus other indolent SM. J Allergy Clin Immunol 2014;133:520–8.

12. Escribano L, Diaz-Agustin B, López A, et al. Immunophenotypic analysis of mast cells in mastocytosis: when and how to do it. Proposals of the Spanish Network on Mastocytosis (REMA). Cytometry B Clin Cytom 2004;58B(1):1–8.

13. Teodosio C, Garcia-Montero AC, Jara-Acevedo M, et al. Mast cells from different molecular and prognostic subtypes of systemic mastocytosis display distinct immunophenotypes. J Allergy Clin Immunol 2010;125(3):719–26.

14. Garcia-Montero AC, Jara-Acevedo M, Teodosio C, et al. KIT mutation in mast cells and other bone marrow haematopoietic cell lineages in systemic mast cell disorders. A prospective study of the Spanish Network on Mastocytosis (REMA) in a series of 113 patients. Blood 2006;108(7):2366–72.

15. Escribano L, Garcia-Montero A, Sánchez-Muñoz L, et al. Diagnosis of adult mastocytosis: role for bone marrow analysis. In: Kottke-Marchant K, Davis B, editors. Laboratory hematology practice. London: Wiley-Blackwell; 2012. p. 388–98.

16. Sánchez-Muñoz L, Morgado JM, varez-Twose I, et al. Diagnosis and classification of mastocytosis in non-specialized versus reference centres: a Spanish Network on Mastocytosis (REMA) study on 122 patients. Br J Haematol 2016; 172(1):56–63.

17. Akin C, Scott LM, Kocabas CN, et al. Demonstration of an aberrant mast cell population with clonal markers in a subset of patients with "idiopathic" anaphylaxis. Blood 2007;110:2331–3.

18. Sonneck K, Florian S, Mullauer L, et al. Diagnostic and subdiagnostic accumulation of mast cells in the bone marrow of patients with anaphylaxis: monoclonal mast cell activation syndrome. Int Arch Allergy Immunol 2006;142(2):158–64.

19. Bonadonna P, Perbellini O, Passalacqua G, et al. Clonal mast cell disorders in patients with systemic reactions to Hymenoptera stings and increased serum tryptase levels. J Allergy Clin Immunol 2009;123(3):680–6.

20. Valent P. Mast cell activation syndromes: definition and classification. Allergy 2013;68(4):417–24.

21. Gonzalez de Olano D, Matito A, Orfao A, et al. Advances in the understanding and clinical management of mastocytosis and clonal mast cell activation syndromes. F1000Res 2016;5:2666.

22. Nagata H, Worobec AS, Oh CK, et al. Identification of a point mutation in the catalytic domain of the protooncogene c-kit in peripheral blood mononuclear cells of patients who have mastocytosis with an associated hematologic disorder. Proc Natl Acad Sci U S A 1995;92(23):10560–4.

23. Longley BJ, Tyrrell L, Lu SZ, et al. Somatic c-KIT activating mutation in urticaria pigmentosa and aggressive mastocytosis: establishment of clonality in a human mast cell neoplasm. Nat Genet 1996;12(3):312–4.

24. Longley BJ Jr, Metcalfe DD, Tharp M, et al. Activating and dominant inactivating c-KIT catalytic domain mutations in distinct clinical forms of human mastocytosis. Proc Natl Acad Sci USA 1999;96(4):1609–14.

25. Yavuz AS, Lipsky PE, Yavuz S, et al. Evidence for the involvement of a hematopoietic progenitor cell in systemic mastocytosis from single-cell analysis of mutations in the c-kit gene. Blood 2002;100(2):661–5.

26. Orfao A, Garcia-Montero AC, Sanchez L, et al. Recent advances in the understanding of mastocytosis: the role of KIT mutations. Br J Haematol 2007;138(1): 12–30.

27. Valent P, Akin C, Escribano L, et al. Standards and standardization in mastocytosis: consensus statements on diagnostics, treatment recommendations and response criteria. Eur J Clin Invest 2007;37(6):435–53.

28. Horny HP, Valent P. Diagnosis of mastocytosis: general histopathological aspects, morphological criteria, and immunohistochemical findings. Leuk Res 2001;25(7):543–51.

29. Sandes AF, Medeiros RS, Rizzatti EG. Diagnosis and treatment of mast cell disorders: practical recommendations. Sao Paulo Med J 2013;131(4):264–74.

30. Alvarez-Twose I, Morgado JM, Sánchez-Muñoz L, et al. Current state of biology and diagnosis of clonal mast cell diseases in adults. Int J Lab Hematol 2012; 34:446–60.

31. Horny HP, Sotlar K, Valent P. Mastocytosis: immunophenotypical features of the transformed mast cells are unique among hematopoietic cells. Immunol Allergy Clin North Am 2014;34(2):315–21.

32. Maric I, Calvo KR. Mastocytosis: the new differential diagnosis of CD30-positive neoplasms. Leuk Lymphoma 2011;52(5):732–3.

33. Sotlar K, Cerny-Reiterer S, Petat-Dutter K, et al. Aberrant expression of CD30 in neoplastic mast cells in high-grade mastocytosis. Mod Pathol 2011;24(4):585–95.

34. Sperr W, Escribano L, Jordan JH, et al. Morphologic properties of neoplastic mast cells: delineation of stages of maturation and implication for cytological grading of mastocytosis. Leuk Res 2001;25:529–36.

35. Alvarez-Twose I, Gonzalez P, Morgado JM, et al. Complete response after imatinib mesylate therapy in a patient with well-differentiated systemic mastocytosis. J Clin Oncol 2012;30(12):e126–9.

36. Moon TC, St Laurent CD, Morris KE, et al. Advances in mast cell biology: new understanding of heterogeneity and function. Mucosal Immunol 2010;3(2):111–28.

37. Sánchez-Muñoz L, Teodosio C, Morgado JM, et al. Immunophenotypic characterization of bone marrow mast cells in mastocytosis and other mast cell disorders. Methods Cell Biol 2011;103:333–59.

38. Escribano L, Garcia Montero AC, Nunez R, et al. Flow cytometric analysis of normal and neoplastic mast cells: role in diagnosis and follow-up of mast cell disease. Immunol Allergy Clin North Am 2006;26(3):535–47.

39. Sánchez-Muñoz L, Teodosio C, Morgado JM, et al. Flow cytometry in mastocytosis: utility as a diagnostic and prognostic tool. Immunol Allergy Clin North Am 2014;34(2):297–313.

40. Hauswirth AW, Escribano L, Prados A, et al. CD203c is overexpressed on neoplastic mast cells in systemic mastocytosis and is upregulated upon IgE receptor cross-linking. Int J Immunopathol Pharmacol 2008;21(4):797–806.

41. Escribano L, Ocqueteau M, Almeida J, et al. Expression of the c-kit (CD117) molecule in normal and malignant hematopoiesis. Leuk Lymphoma 1998;30: 459–66.

42. Valent P, Majdic O, Maurer D, et al. Further characterization of surface membrane structures expressed on human basophils and mast cells. Int Arch Allergy Appl Immunol 1990;91:198–203.

43. Valent P, Bettelheim P. Cell surface structures on human basophils and mast cells: biochemical and functional characterization. Adv Immunol 1992;52: 333–423.

44. Escribano L, Díaz Agustín B, Bellas C, et al. Utility of flow cytometric analysis of mast cells in the diagnosis and classification of adult mastocytosis. Leuk Res 2001;25:563–70.

45. Escribano L, Diaz-Agustin B, Nunez R, et al. Abnormal expression of CD antigens in mastocytosis. Int Arch Allergy Immunol 2002;127(2):127–32.

46. Bodni RA, Sapia S, Galeano A, et al. Indolent systemic mast cell disease: immunophenotypic characterization of bone marrow mast cells by flow cytometry. J Eur Acad Dermatol Venereol 2003;17(2):160–6.
47. Pardanani A, Kimlinger T, Reeder T, et al. Bone marrow mast cell immunophenotyping in adults with mast cell disease: a prospective study of 33 patients. Leuk Res 2004;28(8):777–83.
48. Escribano L, Orfao A, Diaz-Agustin B, et al. Indolent systemic mast cell disease in adults: immunophenotypic characterization of bone marrow mast cells and its diagnostic implications. Blood 1998;91(8):2731–6.
49. Morgado JM, Sánchez-Muñoz L, Teodosio CG, et al. Immunophenotyping in systemic mastocytosis diagnosis: 'CD25 positive' alone is more informative than the 'CD25 and/or CD2' WHO criterion. Mod Pathol 2012;25(4):516–21.
50. Diaz-Agustin B, Escribano L, Bravo P, et al. The CD69 early activation molecule is overexpressed in human bone marrow mast cells from adults with indolent systemic mast cell disease. Br J Haematol 1999;106(2):400–5.
51. Escribano L, Orfao A, Díaz Agustín B, et al. Human bone marrow mast cells from indolent systemic mast cell disease constitutively express increased amounts of the CD63 protein on their surface. Cytometry 1998;34:223–8.
52. Escribano L, Orfao A, Villarrubia J, et al. Immunophenotypic characterization of human bone marrow mast cells. A flow cytometric study of normal and pathological bone marrow samples. Annal Cell Pathol 1998;16:151–9.
53. Nuñez R, Escribano L, Schernthaner G, et al. Overexpression of complement receptors and related antigens on the surface of bone marrow mast cells in patients with systemic mastocytosis. Br J Haematol 2002;120:257–65.
54. Morgado JM, Perbellini O, Johnson RC, et al. CD30 expression by bone marrow mast cells from different diagnostic variants of systemic mastocytosis. Histopathology 2013;63(6):780–7.
55. Teodosio C, Garcia-Montero AC, Jara-Acevedo M, et al. An immature immunophenotype of bone marrow mast cells predicts for multilineage D816V KIT mutation in systemic mastocytosis. Leukemia 2012;26(5):951–8.
56. Akin C, Escribano L, Núñez R, et al. Well-differentiated systemic mastocytosis: a new disease variant with mature mast cell phenotype and lack of codon 816 c-Kit mutations. J Allergy Clin Immunol 2004;113(2):S327.
57. Escribano L, Alvarez-Twose I, Sánchez-Muñoz L, et al. Prognosis in adult indolent systemic mastocytosis: a long-term study of the Spanish Network on Mastocytosis in a series of 145 patients. J Allergy Clin Immunol 2009;124:514–21.
58. Lim KH, Tefferi A, Lasho TL, et al. Systemic mastocytosis in 342 consecutive adults: survival studies and prognostic factors. Blood 2009;113(23):5727–36.
59. Valent P, Horny HP, Escribano L, et al. Diagnostic criteria and classification of mastocytosis: a consensus proposal. Leuk Res 2001;25:603–25.
60. Matarraz S, Lopez A, Barrena S, et al. The immunophenotype of different immature, myeloid and B-cell lineage-committed CD34+ hematopoietic cells allows discrimination between normal/reactive and myelodysplastic syndrome precursors. Leukemia 2008;22(6):1175–83.
61. Schernthaner GH, Hauswirth AW, Baghestanian M, et al. Detection of differentiation- and activation-linked cell surface antigens on cultured mast cell progenitors. Allergy 2005;60(10):1248–55.
62. Sotlar K, Escribano L, Landt O, et al. One-step detection of c-kit point mutations using PNA-mediated PCR-clamping and hybridization probes. Am J Pathol 2003; 162(3):737–46.

63. Jara-Acevedo M, Garcia-Montero A, Teodosio C, et al. Well-differentiated systemic mastocytosis (WDSM): a novel form of mastocytosis. Haematologica 2008;93(supplement 1):91.

64. Wasag B, Niedoszytko M, Piskorz A, et al. Novel, activating KIT-N822I mutation in familial cutaneous mastocytosis. Exp Hematol 2011;39(8):859–65.

65. Pullarkat VA, Bueso-Ramos C, Lai R, et al. Systemic mastocytosis with associated clonal Hematological non-mast-cell lineage disease: analysis of clinicopathologic features and activating c-kit mutations. Am J Hematol 2003;73(1):12–7.

66. Pignon JM, Giraudier S, Duquesnoy P, et al. A new c-kit mutation in a case of aggressive mast cell disease. Br J Haematol 1997;96(2):374–6.

67. Akin C, Fumo G, Yavuz AS, et al. A novel form of mastocytosis associated with a transmembrane c-kit mutation and response to imatinib. Blood 2004;103(8): 3222–5.

68. Astle JM, Rose MG, Racke FK, et al. R634W KIT mutation in an adult with systemic mastocytosis. Lab Med 2017;48(3):253–7.

69. Conde-Fernandes I, Sampaio R, Moreno F, et al. Systemic mastocytosis with KIT V560G mutation presenting as recurrent episodes of vascular collapse: response to disodium cromoglycate and disease outcome. Allergy Asthma Clin Immunol 2017;13:21.

70. Pollard WL, Beachkofsky TM, Kobayashi TT. Novel R634W c-kit mutation identified in familial mastocytosis. Pediatr Dermatol 2015;32(2):267–70.

71. Tang X, Boxer M, Drummond A, et al. A germline mutation in KIT in familial diffuse cutaneous mastocytosis. J Med Genet 2004;41(6):e88.

72. Wang HJ, Lin ZM, Zhang J, et al. A new germline mutation in KIT associated with diffuse cutaneous mastocytosis in a Chinese family. Clin Exp Dermatol 2014; 39(2):146–9.

73. Wohrl S, Moritz KB, Bracher A, et al. A c-kit mutation in exon 18 in familial mastocytosis. J Invest Dermatol 2013;133(3):839–41.

74. Zhang LY, Smith ML, Schultheis B, et al. A novel K509I mutation of KIT identified in familial mastocytosis - in vitro and in vivo responsiveness to imatinib therapy. Leuk Res 2006;30(4):373–8.

75. Arock M, Sotlar K, Akin C, et al. KIT mutation analysis in mast cell neoplasms: recommendations of the European Competence Network on Mastocytosis. Leukemia 2015;29(6):1223–32.

76. Kocabas CN, Yavuz AS, Lipsky PE, et al. Analysis of the lineage relationship between mast cells and basophils using the c-kit D816V mutation as a biologic signature. J Allergy Clin Immunol 2005;115(6):1155–61.

77. Molderings GJ, Meis K, Kolck UW, et al. Comparative analysis of mutation of tyrosine kinase kit in mast cells from patients with systemic mast cell activation syndrome and healthy subjects. Immunogenetics 2010;62(11–12):721–7.

78. Matito A, Morgado JM, varez-Twose I, et al. Serum tryptase monitoring in indolent systemic mastocytosis: association with disease features and patient outcome. PLoS One 2013;8(10):e76116.

79. Akin C, Kirshenbaum AS, Semere T, et al. Analysis of the surface expression of c-kit and occurrence of the c-kit Asp816Val activating mutation in T cells, B cells, and myelomonocytic cells in patients with mastocytosis. Exp Hematol 2000;28(2): 140–7.

80. Jara-Acevedo M, Teodosio C, Sánchez-Muñoz L, et al. Detection of the KIT D816V mutation in peripheral blood of systemic mastocytosis: diagnostic implications. Mod Pathol 2015;28(8):1138–49.

81. Hoermann G, Gleixner KV, Dinu GE, et al. The KIT D816V allele burden predicts survival in patients with mastocytosis and correlates with the WHO type of the disease. Allergy 2014;69(6):810–3.

82. Kristensen T, Vestergaard H, Moller MB. Improved detection of the KIT D816V mutation in patients with systemic mastocytosis using a quantitative and highly sensitive real-time qPCR assay. J Mol Diagn 2011;13(2):180–8.

83. Kristensen T, Vestergaard H, Bindslev-Jensen C, et al. Sensitive KIT D816V mutation analysis of blood as a diagnostic test in mastocytosis. Am J Hematol 2014; 89(5):493–8.

84. Valent P, Escribano L, Broesby-Olsen S, et al. Proposed diagnostic algorithm for patients with suspected mastocytosis: a proposal of the European Competence Network on Mastocytosis. Allergy 2014;69:1267–74.

85. Erben P, Schwaab J, Metzgeroth G, et al. The KIT D816V expressed allele burden for diagnosis and disease monitoring of systemic mastocytosis. Ann Hematol 2014;93(1):81–8.

86. Escribano L, Díaz Agustín B, Bravo P, et al. Immunophenotype of bone marrow mast cells in indolent systemic mast cell disease in adults. Leuk Lymphoma 1999;35:227–35.

Mast Cell Mediators of Significance in Clinical Practice in Mastocytosis

Joseph H. Butterfield, MD[a,*], Anupama Ravi, MD[b],
Thanai Pongdee, MD[a]

KEYWORDS

- N-methylhistamine • 2,3,dinor-11βProstaglandin(PG) F2α • Leukotriene(LT) E4
- Tryptase • Histamine • Neuropeptide

KEY POINTS

- Mast cells are known to store and secrete a variety of mediators; however, it is not possible for clinical laboratories to measure most of them.
- Although several mast cell mediator metabolites are measured in the urine, aside from serum tryptase measurement no other mast cell mediator is included in diagnostic criteria for systemic mastocytosis.
- By quantitating an increase in one or more mast cell mediators coincident with acute symptoms and comparison with baseline values, evidence of mast cell participation in clinical syndromes is verified.
- Emerging evidence suggests that various cytokines and neuropeptides may have clinical relevance in systemic mastocytosis.

INTRODUCTION

The local and/or remote symptoms that result from mast cell (MC) mediator release are common reasons that patients with systemic mastocytosis (SM) seek medical care. Documentation of an increase in the level of one or more MC mediators, obtained at baseline or during acute symptom flares, serves to confirm the participation of these cells in the pathogenesis of a clinical condition. However, the clinical laboratory's ability to routinely measure MC mediators day-to-day is severely limited.

MCs and their mediators have been hypothesized to participate in a great number of disorders and to contribute to the pathogenesis of clinical conditions outside that of SM.[1]

Disclosure Statement: None to disclose.
[a] Division of Allergic Diseases, Mayo Clinic, 200 Southwest 1st Street, Rochester, MN 55902, USA; [b] Division of Pediatric Allergy and Immunology, Mayo Clinic, 200 1st Street Southwest, Rochester, MN 55905, USA
* Corresponding author.
E-mail address: butterfield.joseph@mayo.edu

Immunol Allergy Clin N Am 38 (2018) 397–410
https://doi.org/10.1016/j.iac.2018.04.011
0889-8561/18/© 2018 Elsevier Inc. All rights reserved.

immunology.theclinics.com

MCs are induced to activate by IgE-triggered stimuli and non-IgE causes including hormones, complement fragments, physical factors, immunoglobulins, toll-like receptor ligands, pathogens and their components, antimicrobial peptides, neuropeptides, toxins, cytokines and other inflammatory mediators, chemokines, other chemoattractants, and exogenous molecules and drugs.[2,3] However, aside from the physical presence of increased numbers of MC infiltrating tissue it is difficult to substantiate a primary contribution of MCs in a legion of disorders ranging from chronic bronchitis to chronic fatigue syndrome[4] using currently available tests to quantify MC mediators.

Hardly a month goes by in which new factors or pathways affecting MC degranulation are not reported. Many of these reports come from studies in nonhuman species or from in vitro studies that may use nonhuman MCs. The applicability of these reports to the clinical practice of diagnosing and managing patients with SM is frequently unproven.

MCs are factories for the production of mediators that are released immediately or in a delayed fashion. These products have proinflammatory, immunomodulatory, or chemokine effects that in turn can impact other immune cells in the body and stimulate the production of inflammatory mediators by these cells. In SM, the greatly increased number of MCs has the potential to magnify the results from mediator release. Furthermore, production of mediators by MCs themselves is affected by exposure to other inflammatory products.[5] These observations suggest a complex web of interacting systems affecting MC mediator secretion.

Rather than being a compendium of MC products, this article is focused on those MC mediators with current or potential relevance to the management of patients with SM. It is hoped that this serves as a useful resource to clinicians for evaluation and management of these patients.

PREFORMED MEDIATORS
Biologic Amines

Histamine
Histamine (2-[4-imidazolyl]-ethylamine) is an endogenous amine that is synthesized by histidine decarboxylase, which removes a carboxylic acid residue from the semiessential amino acid L-histidine. Histamine may be produced by a wide variety of cell types that express histidine decarboxylase including MCs, basophils, gastric enterochromaffin-like cells, histaminergic neurons, platelets, dendritic cells, and lymphocytes. MCs and basophils store large quantities of histamine in secretory granules, whereas other cell types, such as lymphocytes, secrete histamine after synthesis and do not store it intracellularly. MCs and basophils release histamine on degranulation in response to immunologic and nonimmunologic stimuli.[6,7]

Once released, histamine is metabolized rapidly (half-life of 1 minute) via two enzymatic pathways. Most histamine is metabolized by histamine N-methyltransferase (HNMT), which is an S-adenosyl-methionine-dependent enzyme responsible for 70% to 80% of histamine biotransformation. HNMT acts as a catalyst for the transfer of a methyl group from S-adenosyl-L-methionine to histamine, resulting in the formation of N-methylhistamine. N-Methylhistamine is then metabolized further by monoamine oxidase to N-methylimidazole acetic acid, which is then excreted in the urine.[7,8] HNMT is found in tissues throughout the body and is particularly important in the central nervous system and bronchial epithelium, where it is the only known metabolic process to inactivate histamine.[7]

The second enzymatic pathway metabolizing the remaining 20% to 30% of histamine occurs through the activities of diamine oxidase. Diamine oxidase is a membrane glycoprotein that is mainly found in the kidney and colon. Diamine oxidase is stored in plasma membrane vesicles and is released on stimulation to oxidatively deaminate histamine and other substrates. Diamine oxidase converts histamine to imidazole acetaldehyde, which is then subsequently converted to imidazole acetic acid and conjugated with ribose phosphate.[7,8]

Histamine induces widespread responses and plays important physiologic roles in human health.[7,9] Histamine exerts its diverse effects via binding to four subtypes of histamine receptors (HRs), which are named chronologically in order of their discovery (H1R to H4R).[6]

H1R-mediated effects include itching, swelling, rhinorrhea, conjunctivitis, urticaria, bronchoconstriction, and anaphylaxis. In addition, H1R may have centrally mediated effects affecting attention, sleep regulation, and regulation of food and water intake.[6]

H2R activation results in relaxation of smooth muscle in the airway and vasculature. H2R-mediated effects are most discussed in relation to gastric acid secretion, because occupation of parietal cell H2R results in hydrogen ion production. H2R activation may also be involved in regulation of gastric motility, and in the cardiovascular system, may induce negative chronotropic and ionotropic effects.[7]

H3R inhibits histamine release from histaminergic neurons in the human brain and also seems to be involved in the regulation of the release of neurotransmitters, such as dopamine, serotonin, noradrenaline, γ-aminobutyric acid, and acetylcholine in the human brain.[7] Thereby, H3R is shown to be important in the sleep-wake cycle, cognition, homeostatic regulation of energy levels, and inflammation.[6] H4R is emerging as an important receptor for chemotaxis and modulation of inflammatory responses.[6]

Overproduction of histamine in SM has been reported for more than 30 years, but histamine levels in blood or urine are not used in current diagnostic criteria. In patients with SM, plasma histamine levels demonstrate a diurnal variation with highest levels observed in the early morning. Although patients with SM have elevated plasma histamine levels on average, the determination of such levels has not proven to be reliable to screen patients for mastocytosis.[10] However, measurement of the urinary histamine metabolites N-methylhistamine and N-methylimidazole acetic acid, rather than measurement of urinary histamine, has been shown to correlate with serum tryptase levels and bone marrow biopsy findings in multiple studies.[11–14] In addition, urinary histamine metabolite measurements have been included in diagnostic algorithms proposed by the European Competency Network on Mastocytosis and other groups to select patients for bone marrow examination to establish a diagnosis of SM.[12]

In one study involving 37 patients with elevated levels of urinary N-methylhistamine, the optimal predictive value for detecting MC aggregates in the bone marrow biopsy was an N-methylhistamine level of 297 μmol/mol creatinine (Cr) at which the sensitivity was 67% with a specificity of 84%. Another study involving 161 different patients demonstrated a significant correlation between serum tryptase and urinary N-methylhistamine levels. Of these 161 patients, 13 patients had retrievable bone marrow biopsies, and significant differences were found for serum tryptase and urinary N-methylhistamine levels between bone marrow biopsies with an increased number of MC aggregates and those without such increases. It was noted, however, that serum tryptase discriminated better than urinary N-methylhistamine between patients with and without increased MC aggregates in bone marrow biopsies.[13]

A more recent study[12] involving 142 patients undergoing evaluation for mastocytosis included 53 patients without urticaria pigmentosa who were diagnosed with indolent SM (ISM) and 89 patients who ultimately were not diagnosed with mastocytosis. In this study, when tryptase levels were greater than 10 μg/L, the highest combination of sensitivity and specificity for a diagnosis of SM was 2.0 mmol/mol Cr for methylimidazole acetic acid (sensitivity, 0.85; specificity, 0.86) and 176 μmol/mol Cr for methylhistamine (sensitivity, 0.81; specificity, 0.93).[12] One final study[14] involving 90 patients found that urinary N-methylhistamine levels positively correlated with serum tryptase levels and the percentage of MCs on bone marrow biopsy. There was also a significant difference of urinary N-methylhistamine levels between subjects found to have atypical MCs on bone marrow biopsy and those who did not. Furthermore, urinary N-methylhistamine levels were statistically different between the patient group positive for c-kit mutation versus the group that lacked the mutation. It was also noted that as urinary N-methylhistamine levels increased, greater proportions of patients demonstrated the aforementioned associated correlations. Thereby, this study found that a urinary N-methylhistamine level that is twice the upper limit of normal (400 μg/g Cr), corresponds to 95% MC atypia and 85% MC aggregates on bone marrow biopsy, and thus may be clinically useful to predict bone marrow findings in SM.[14] In summary, several investigations of urinary histamine metabolites have demonstrated clear utility to aid SM evaluation and diagnosis, and evolving diagnostic criteria for SM may reflect the measurement of urinary N-methylhistamine levels in the future.

Chemokines

Chemokines are low-molecular-weight chemotactic cytokines divided into four main families depending on the position of conserved cysteine residues near the N terminus. Cultured MCs produce the chemokines monocyte chemotactic protein-1[15] and interleukin (IL)-8.[16]

Interleukin-8

IL-8 (CXCL8) is produced by many cell types including MCs. Clinically, significant elevations of IL-8 serum levels are found in patients with interstitial cystitis/bladder pain syndrome.[17] Among a cohort of 46 patients with ISM, aggressive SM (ASM), and SM with associated clonal hematopoietic disorder (SM-AHN) a panel of assayed cytokines showed only IL-8 levels to be significantly different in SM-AHN versus ISM/ASM patients (P<.0002).[18] A clinical study of patients with SM demonstrated that serum IL-8 and monocyte chemotactic protein-1 were significantly elevated in patients with anaphylaxis versus patients without anaphylaxis.[19]

Enzymes

Tryptase

Tryptase is the most specific marker of MC activation and burden. Tryptase is a serine protease concentrated in the secretory granules of all MCs. Basophils also have a negligible amount of tryptase, about 0.4% of that of MCs.[20]

Tryptase has multiple biologic activities. Tryptase promotes tissue repair and generates bradykinin from kininogen leading to increased vascular permeability and facilitating cellular migration. Tryptase has chemotactic effects on neutrophils and eosinophils via release of IL-8. It upregulates ICAM-1 expression on epithelial cells. Tryptase is a growth factor for epithelial cells, respiratory smooth muscle cells, and fibroblasts.[21] Tryptase-mediated degradation of bronchodilators vasoactive intestinal peptide and peptide histidine-methionine seems to contribute to bronchial hyperresponsiveness and the decrease in immunoreactive vasoactive intestinal peptide in airway nerves associated with asthma.[22]

Tryptase cleaves α and β chains of fibrinogen. Thrombin-initiated clot formation is thereby inhibited.[23] The anticoagulant activity of β tryptase can partially explain the bleeding episodes in patients with SM and anaphylaxis.

α-Pro-tryptase is the predominant form of tryptase in serum at baseline in normal subjects and in those with SM. β-tryptase is the predominant form from MCs in skin and lung and in the blood during systemic anaphylaxis. Release of β-tryptase parallels histamine but diffuses more slowly because it is associated with protease-proteoglycan complex. β-tryptase peaks at 30 to 90 minutes following MC activation or an anaphylactic event, with a half-life of 2 hours, whereas histamine peaks at 5 minutes and returns to baseline within 15 to 30 minutes. Thus, optimal time to obtain tryptase is 1 to 2 hours after precipitating event.[24]

Total MC tryptase (α- and β-tryptases) reflect the total MC burden. The normal tryptase level in adults is 1 to 15 ng/mL, with average of 5 ng/mL. A serum level greater than 11.5 ng/mL, the 95th percentile, is considered increased. The median tryptase level in children is 3.30 ng/mL (range, 2.38–4.36) and is inversely related to age.[25] There is one currently available blood tryptase assay (Phadia Laboratory Systems, Uppsala, Sweden), performed via fluorescence enzyme immunoassay. This assay does not distinguish between α- and β-tryptases.

Higher tryptase levels increase the likelihood of SM. Serum tryptase greater than 20 ng/mL is one of the minor criteria of SM. Tryptase levels vary among forms of SM. Highest levels are detected in MC leukemia and smoldering SM, compared to isolated bone marrow (no cutaneous or multi organ involvement).[26] Also, in ISM-suspected patients greater than 50 years with a body mass index greater than 25 kg/m^2, there is diminished reliability of tryptase as risk indicator for mastocytosis.[27]

Elevation of tryptase is not specific to SM. Elevation of tryptase has also been seen in systemic anaphylaxis, acute myelocytic leukemia, various myelodysplastic syndromes, hypereosinophilic syndrome associated with the FLP1L1-PDGFRA mutation, end-stage renal failure, treatment of onchocerciasis, and familial hypertryptasemia. Among patients with myeloid neoplasm, blood tryptase greater than 15 ng/mL was found in greater than 90% of SM cases, 38% of acute myelocytic leukemia, 34% of patients with chronic myelogenous leukemia, and 25% of patients with myelodysplastic syndrome. A corollary of these observations is that serum tryptase levels cannot be used as a minor criterion when diagnosing SM in those patients with an associated hematologic neoplasm. Serum tryptase levels do not correlate with therapy-induced bone marrow complete response at a given single time point.[28] Also, non-SM obese individuals were found to have elevated tryptase. Detecting elevated baseline serum tryptase levels in individuals who experienced anaphylaxis to a stinging insect can indicate underlying SM.

In contrast to ASM, patients with ISM usually present with urticaria pigmentosa-like skin lesions. Lack of these lesions does not exclude ISM even if the serum tryptase is elevated. Increasing tryptase levels in patients with ISM is associated with poor prognosis and increased progression. Patients with SM have increased risk for decreased bone density and pathologic fractures; however, elevated tryptase levels are actually associated with greater bone density in a cohort of patients with SM. Patients with SM with less severe disease and lower serum tryptase levels should particularly have bone density evaluated.

Children Increased tryptase levels were also found in children with systemic disease and correlated to skin lesion density and bone marrow pathology. In children with extensive cutaneous involvement, increased serum baseline tryptase identifies patients at risk for severe MC activation events in pediatric mastocytosis. In cutaneous mastocytosis organomegaly was the strongest predictor of SM, whereas serum tryptase values alone were not predictive in the determination of systemic involvement. Sequential tryptase measurements, however, were helpful in supplementing clinical judgment as to disease course.[29] **Table 1** lists a selection of preformed MC mediators whose contribution to acute and/or chronic symptoms in SM remains to be fully validated.

Table 1
Mast cell enzymes of possible, but unproven, clinical significance in mastocytosis

Mast Cell Mediator	Action	Reference
Carboxypeptidase A	• Skin MCs have greater content than lung MCs • Selectively localized to tryptase-positive, chymase-positive MCs • Increased in children with allergic disease	Pan et al,[30] 2011
Chymase	• Indolent mastocytosis patient revealed tryptase-positive, chymase-positive MCs in skin and bone marrow	Weidner et al,[31] 1992
Kininogenase	• Released via IgE-mediated mechanism • Kinin formation	Proud et al,[32] 1985
Metalloproteinase-9	• Mast cell migration into tissues	Tanaka et al,[33] 1999
Peroxidase	• Found in mast cells in urticaria pigmentosa • Appearance associated with cells' ability to synthesize PGD_2 • Marker of in vitro maturation of bone marrow–derived mast cells	Akiyama et al,[34] 1989
Arylsulfatase, nitric oxide synthase, nitric oxide, phospholipase, β-hexosaminidase	• Limited animal studies	

Proteoglycans

Chondroitin sulfate

Mast cell granules contain the proteoglycan serglycin, which has glycosaminoglycan side chains of negatively charged heparin, chondroitin, or dermatan sulfate.[35] These proteoglycans are responsible for the metachromatic staining of MCs and serve as storage sites for positively charged proteases.[36] Although chondroitin sulfate when preincubated with LAD2 human MCs inhibits substance P–induced IL-8 and tumor necrosis factor release, there are no studies implicating chondroitin sulfate in the pathophysiology or clinical symptoms of SM.

Heparin

Human MC granules contain the highly sulfated proteoglycan heparin (5 pg/10^6 cells).[37] Heparin and chondroitin sulfate diB/E containing serglycin proteoglycans are located within the electron dense MC secretory granules. By binding to antithrombin heparin induces a conformational change in antithrombin that greatly enhances its anticoagulant activity through inactivation of thrombin and factor Xa.[38]

Serglycin proteoglycans also bind and stabilize tetramer-forming tryptases in MC secretory granules and are essential in maintaining activity of human tryptase-β to cleave the α and β chains of human fibrinogen thereby inhibiting clot formation.[39] An elevation of the plasma heparin level, particularly after stimulation of MC degranulation by obstruction of venous flow for 10 minutes, has been proposed as a marker for MC activation disorder,[40] but has not been evaluated in SM. In one series clinical signs of bleeding including hematoma formation, bruising, prolonged bleeding after biopsies, gingival bleeding, epistaxis, gastrointestinal, and other were reported in patients with MC activation disorder.[41] In SM bleeding is not a commonly reported problem. There are only occasional reports of clotting abnormalities related to MC degranulation[42] and/or organ infiltration by MCs in patients with SM-AHN[43] or MC leukemia.[44]

DE NOVO MEDIATORS
Phospholipid Metabolites

Prostaglandins
Prostaglandin (PG) D_2 is a lipid-derived MC mediator that is rapidly degraded into D-, F-, and J-ring metabolites, which are excreted as more stable urinary metabolites (**Fig. 1**). Mast cells, not basophils, remain the predominant source of PGD_2. patients with SM excrete four times more PG-F-ring compared with PG-D-ring metabolites. The predominant clinically measured urinary metabolite is 2,3-dinor-11βprostaglandin F2α (2,3-BPG) (**Fig. 2**).

Multiple studies have shown elevated urinary excretion of PGD_2 in SM. A patient treated with antihistamines and aspirin, 975 mg orally four times a day, for 8 months had reduced excretion of PGD_2 metabolite by 80% to 85% and symptom reduction.

PGD-M is a downstream metabolite of PGD_2. Measurement of urine PGD-M was increased greater than normal by 300% in patients with SM.[45] PGD-M is measured

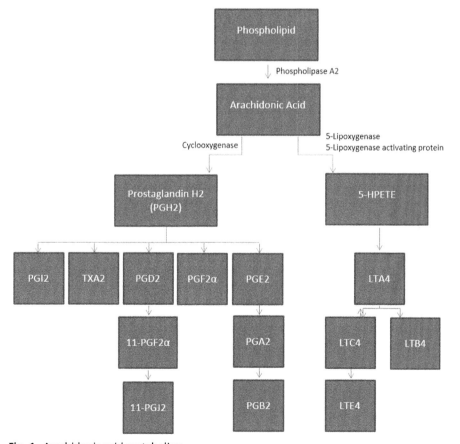

Fig. 1. Arachidonic acid metabolism.

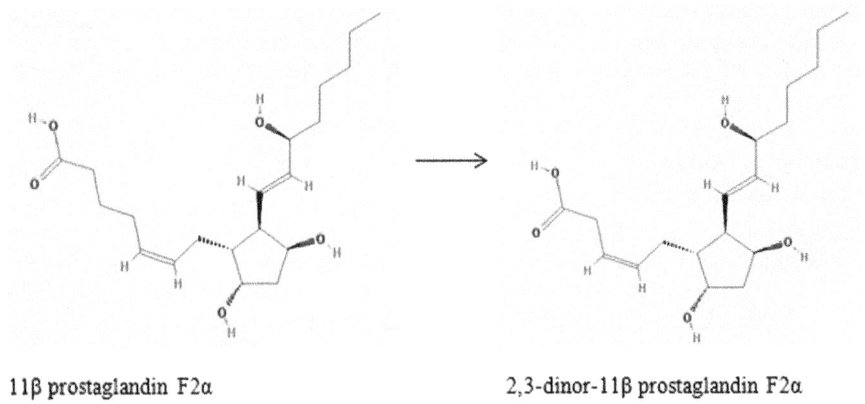

11β prostaglandin F2α   2,3-dinor-11β prostaglandin F2α

Fig. 2. Prostaglandin F-ring. (*From* National Center for Biotechnology Information. Pub-Chem Compound Database; CID = 5280886. Available at: https://pubchem.ncbi.nlm.nih.gov/compound/5280886. Accessed November 17, 2017; and National Center for Biotechnology Information. PubChem Compound Database; CID = 5283032. Available at: https://pubchem.ncbi.nlm.nih.gov/compound/5283032. Accessed November 17, 2017.)

by gas chromatography compared with the measurement of 2,3-BPG, which uses liquid chromatography and tandem mass spectrometry. Mean urinary excretion of PGD-M was significantly higher ($P<.01$) in patients with SM compared with control subjects (37.2 vs 11.5 ng/mg Cr) with 65% of 17 patients with SM showing elevated levels.[46]

The clinical sensitivity of 11β-PGF2α (>1000 ng/mL) alone for diagnosis of SM was determined to be 53%.[47] In a Mayo Clinic study of 22 patients with SM, elevated urinary excretion levels of 11β-PGF2α greater than 3494 ng/24 hours correlated with the presence of bone marrow MC aggregates (89%) and atypical MC (100%) but not with c-kit positivity.[14]

Cysteinyl leukotrienes: leukotriene E4

Cysteinyl leukotrienes are mediators produced by activated MCs, neutrophils, eosinophils, and macrophages. Leukotriene C4 is a lipid mediator that is metabolized into leukotriene D4 and subsequently into leukotriene E4 (LTE4) (see **Fig. 1**). LTE4 is the primary stable metabolite of cysteinyl leukotrienes.

LTE4 is excreted in the urine, where it is assayed by liquid chromatography followed by tandem mass spectroscopy. Patients with SM have significantly increased excretion of LTE4 pg/mg Cr (median, 30 ng/g Cr; range, 3.0–188 ng/g Cr) compared with the control group (median, 7.0 ng/g Cr; range, 1.0–128 ng/g Cr; $P = .01$).[48]

Median urine LTE4 among patients with SM was 97 pg/mg Cr, significantly higher than patients without SM 50 pg/mg Cr ($P<.01$). The 95th percentile of the reference interval population was less than 104 pg/mg Cr. The reference interval cutoff of 104 pg/mg Cr for LTE4 was 48% sensitive and 84% specific for a diagnosis of SM.[47]

Platelet activating factor

Platelet activating factor (PAF) is produced by MCs, endothelial cells, polymorphonuclear leukocytes, eosinophils, macrophages, monocytes, and platelets. In allergic disorders, the source of PAF is antigen-stimulated basophils and MCs. PAF activates eosinophils and Polymorphonuclear leukocytes. PAF has been detected in blister fluid in a patient with bullous mastocytosis. In 1988, treatment of adult SM with a PAF-acether antagonist BN52063 resulted in resolution of symptoms.[49] The role of PAF in the day-to-day symptoms of SM has yet to be elucidated. **Table 2** summarizes the symptoms caused by mast cell mediators that can be measured in clinical laboratories.

Cytokines

Human MCs have demonstrated the capability to synthesize and release several multifunctional cytokines including IL-1, IL-3, IL-5, IL-6, IL-13, IL-16, IL-18, IL-31, tumor necrosis factor-α, transforming growth factor-β, and macrophage inflammatory protein-1α. These cytokines have physiologic effects primarily with inflammation and leukocyte migration and proliferation. Cytokines are typically synthesized de novo and are released several hours after MC activation. MCs may be activated via IgE- or IgG-dependent mechanisms or also in response to bacterial products through Toll-like receptors.[50–54] Much of the data associating these cytokines with MCs were obtained from studies with human MC lines and primary MC cultures. Cytokine expression and regulation by resident tissue MCs in those with mastocytosis remain largely undetermined.[55] The limited number of cytokines that have been studied in SM include IL-6 and IL-31.

Table 2
Symptoms from mast cell–derived mediators routinely measured in clinical laboratories

Mast Cell Mediator	Collection Method	Symptom
Histamine N-Methylhistamine	Urine	Headache
		Nasal obstruction/rhinorrhea/sneezing
		Hypotension
		Urticaria $\pm$ angioedema
		Pruritus
		Flushing
		Nausea/vomiting
		Diarrhea
		Abdominal pain
PGD$_2$	Urine	Mucus secretion
		Bronchoconstriction
		Vascular instability/vasodilator
		Coronary and pulmonary vasoconstrictor
		Inhibition of platelet aggregation
		Eosinophil and neutrophil chemoattractant
		Dendritic cell activation
		Augmentation of basophil histamine release
2,3Dinor 11β-PGF2α PGD$_2$ metabolite	Urine	Bronchoconstriction
		Peripheral vasodilation
		Coronary vasoconstriction
		Inhibition of platelet aggregation
LTE4	Urine	Bronchoconstriction
		Enhanced bronchial responsiveness
		Increased vascular permeability
		Mucus secretion
		Edema formation
Tryptase	Serum	Bleeding
		Bronchospasm
		Increased fibroblast proliferation and collagen synthesis
Heparin	Plasma	Bleeding

Interleukin-6

Of the cytokines studied in SM, IL-6 potentially has the most clinical relevance to date. IL-6 has been shown to be increased in SM with plasma levels correlating with disease severity and progression.[55–58] Specifically, increased plasma IL-6 levels of patients with SM correlated with serum tryptase levels, symptom severity, aggressive disease category, severity of bone marrow pathology, organomegaly, hematologic abnormalities, presence of osteoporosis, and extent of skin involvement.[55–57] Furthermore, plasma IL-6 levels greater than 2.5 pg/mL identified all patients with severe disease, aggressive disease categories, and all with organomegalies. Increased plasma IL-6 levels of this magnitude also identified more than 90% of patients with diffuse infiltrates found on bone marrow biopsy. These increased IL-6 levels were not found in control subjects or in patients with cutaneous mastocytosis.[56] Not only do IL-6 levels seem to be a useful surrogate marker for disease, IL-6 levels also have demonstrated prognostic significance. In patients with ISM, high levels of IL-6 were associated with disease severity, organomegalies, and disease progression to more aggressive disease.[58] These findings suggest that IL-6 blockade may be beneficial to lessen MC-related symptoms and pathology in patients with mastocytosis and increased IL-6 levels.

Interleukin-31

IL-31 seems to be a cytokine playing a key role in the induction of chronic skin inflammation. Increased serum IL-31 levels and increased IL-31 mRNA levels in the skin have been demonstrated in patients with atopic dermatitis, chronic urticaria, allergic contact dermatitis, prurigo nodularis, and primary cutaneous lymphomas.[59–63] Sources of IL-31 include $CD4^+$ T cells, CD45R0 CLA^+ T cells, and MCs.[59] In one study, serum IL-31 levels were found to be significantly increased in patients with mastocytosis compared with that found in healthy control subjects.[59] Moreover, patients with more advanced disease categories, such as ASM, demonstrated significantly increased IL-31 levels compared with those with nonadvanced disease, such as cutaneous mastocytosis or ISM. All IL-31 levels exceeding 313.9 pg/mL were measured in patients with advanced disease categories, and none of the patients with advanced disease had IL-31 levels less than 81.9 pg/mL. In addition, IL-31 levels also correlated with serum tryptase levels and with the percentage of MC infiltrates in the bone marrow. In contrast, IL-31 levels did not correlate with other clinical parameters including disease duration; presence of a KitD816 V mutation; skin lesion involvement; or presence of MC activation symptoms, such as pruritus, flushing, or anaphylaxis. Through immunohistochemistry, MCs in skin and bone marrow were shown to be able to produce IL-31.[59] Thus, IL -31 levels may be another potential diagnostic biomarker for mastocytosis.

Growth Factors

Stem cell factor

The most important cytokine that contributes to MC differentiation and maturation is the ligand stem cell factor (SCF),[64] which binds to its specific tyrosine kinase receptor, *kit*, encoded by the *kit* proto-oncogene. Cardiac MCs from patients with idiopathic dilated cardiomyopathy were first shown to contain SCF in their secretory granules by immunogold staining. Subsequent studies using skin MCs and human lung MCs also demonstrated the presence of immunoreactive SCF.[65] Chymase, present in MC secretory granules, cleaves recombinant human SCF (SCF^{1-166}). The larger cleaved fragment, SCF^{1-159}, but not the minor cleavage product $SCF^{159-166}$ activates human lung MCs, potentiates anti-IgE-induced activation of these cells, and stimulates human lung MCs chemotaxis.[66] Specific clinical symptoms attributable to SCF apart from these effects on MCs have not been identified.

Nerve growth factor

Mast cells respond to and produce nerve growth factor (NGF), a unique neurotrophic factor with a wide range of biologic effects.[67] Patients with SM show elevated serum levels of NGF, neurotrophin (NT)-3, and NT4. Levels of NGF-β and NT4 also correlate with serum tryptase levels and expression of receptors for NT have been demonstrated on intestinal and skin MCs of patients with SM.[68] Although the release of NGF can contribute to the accumulation of MCs in inflammatory and autoimmune states, the specific contribution of this trophic factor to symptoms of patients with SM awaits further study.

SUMMARY

For diagnosing and treating SM the utility of quantitating levels of released MC mediators remains to be fully explored. Aside from tryptase, other MC products are not current criteria for diagnosing SM. Mediator levels are used to document excessive levels of released MC products present chronically or contemporaneously during MC activation events. By blocking the synthesis of these mediators or their receptors, relief of MC-induced symptoms is achieved (**Table 2**).

REFERENCES

1. Shi GP, Bot I, Kovanen PT. Mast cells in human and experimental cardiometabolic diseases. Nat Rev Cardiol 2015;12:643–58.
2. Hilderbrand SC, Murrell RN, Gibson JE, et al. Marine brevetoxin induces IgE-independent mast cell activation. Arch Toxicol 2011;85:135–41.
3. Yu Y, Blokhuis BR, Garssen J, et al. Non-IgE mediated mast cell activation. Eur J Pharmacol 2016;778:33–43.
4. Singh J, Shah R, Singh D. Targeting mast cells: uncovering prolific therapeutic role in myriad diseases. Int Immunopharmacol 2016;40:362–84.
5. Lorentz A, Wilke M, Sellge G, et al. IL-4-induced priming of human intestinal mast cells for enhanced survival and Th2 cytokine generation is reversible and associated with increased activity or ERK1/2 and c-Fos. J Immunol 2005;174:6751–6.
6. O'Mahony L, Akdis M, Akdis CA. Regulation of the immune response and inflammation by histamine and histamine receptors. J Allergy Clin Immunol 2011;128:1153–62.
7. Jones BL, Kearns GL. Histamine: new thoughts about a familiar mediator. Clin Pharmacol Ther 2011;89(2):189–97.
8. Lieberman P. The basics of histamine biology. Ann Allergy Asthma Immunol 2011; 106:S2–5.
9. Simons FER, Simons KJ. Histamine and H_1-antihistamines: celebrating a century of progress. J Allergy Clin Immunol 2011;128:1139–50.
10. Friedman BS, Steinberg SC, Meggs WJ, et al. Analysis of plasma histamine levels in patients with mast cell disorders. Am J Med 1989;87:649–54.
11. Oranje AP, Mulder PG, Heide R, et al. Urinary N-methylhistamine as an indicator of bone marrow involvement in mastocytosis. Clin Exp Dermatol 2002;27:502–6.
12. van Doormaal JJ, van der Veer E, van Voorst Vader PC, et al. Tryptase and histamine metabolites as diagnostic indicators of indolent systemic mastocytosis without skin lesions. Allergy 2012;67:683–90.
13. van Toorenenbergen AW, Oranje AP. Comparison of serum tryptase and urine N-methylhistamine in patients with suspected mastocytosis. Clin Chim Acta 2005; 359:72–7.

14. Divekar R, Butterfield J. Urinary 11β-PGF2α and N-methyl histamine correlate with bone marrow biopsy findings in mast cell disorders. Allergy 2015;70:1230–8.

15. Lappalainen J, Lindstedt KA, Oksjoki R, et al. OxLDL-IgG immune complexes induce expression and secretion of proatherogenic cytokines by cultured human mast cells. Atherosclerosis 2011;214:357–63.

16. Möller A, Lippert U, Lessmann D, et al. Human mast cells produce IL-8. J Immunol 1993;151:3261–6.

17. Jiang YH, Peng CH, Liu HT, et al. Increased pro-inflammatory cytokines, C-reactive protein and nerve growth factor expressions in serum of patients with interstitial cystitis/bladder pain syndrome. PLoS One 2013;8:e76779.

18. Pardanani A, Finke C, Lasho TL, et al. Comprehensive cytokine profiling in systemic mastocytosis: prognostic relevance of increased plasma IL-2R levels. Blood 2012;120:2836. Conference: 54th Annual Meeting of the American Society of Hematology.

19. Niedoszytko M, Nedoszytko B, Lange M, et al. Serum markers which could predict the risk of anaphylaxis in mastocytosis patients [abstract]. Allergy: European Journal of Allergy and Clinical Immunology 2013;68:575.

20. Castells MC, Irani AM, Schwartz LB. Evaluation of human peripheral leukocytes for mast cell tryptase. J Immunol 1987;138:2184–9.

21. Vitte J. Human mast cell tryptase in biology and medicine. Mol Immunol 2015; 63(1):18–24.

22. Tam EK, Caughey GH. Degradation of airway neuropeptides by human lung tryptase. Am J Respir Cell Mol Biol 1990;3(1):27–32.

23. Prieto-García A, Castells MC, Hansbro PM, et al. Mast cell-restricted tetramer-forming tryptases and their beneficial roles in hemostasis and blood coagulation. Immunol Allergy Clin North Am 2014;34(2):263–81.

24. Schwartz LB. Clinical utility of tryptase levels in systemic mastocytosis and associated hematologic disorders. Leuk Res 2001;25(7):553–62.

25. Sahiner UM, Yavuz ST, Buyuktiryaki B, et al. Serum basal tryptase levels in healthy children: correlation between age and gender. Allergy Asthma Proc 2014;35(5):404–8.

26. Sperr WR, Jordan JH, Fiegl M, et al. Serum tryptase levels in patients with mastocytosis: correlation with mast cell burden and implication for defining the category of disease. Int Arch Allergy Immunol 2002;128(2):136–41.

27. Vos BJ, van der Veer E, van Voorst Vader PC. Diminished reliability of tryptase as risk indicator of mastocytosis in older overweight subjects. J Allergy Clin Immunol 2015;135(3):792–8.

28. Quintás-Cardama A, Sever M, Cortes J. Bone marrow mast cell burden and serum tryptase level as markers of response in patients with systemic mastocytosis. Leuk Lymphoma 2013;54(9):1959–64.

29. Carter MC, Clayton ST. Komarow HDAssessment of clinical findings, tryptase levels, and bone marrow histopathology in the management of pediatric mastocytosis. J Allergy Clin Immunol 2015;136(6):1673–9.

30. Pan Q, Ding MF, Zhang S, et al. Measurement of plasma mast cell carboxypeptidase and chymase levels in children with allergic diseases. Zhongguo Dang Dai Er Ke Za Zhi 2011;13(10):814–6 [in Chinese].

31. Weidner N, Horan RF, Austen KF. Mast-cell phenotype in indolent forms of mastocytosis. Ultrastructural features, fluorescence detection of avidin binding, and immunofluorescent determination of chymase, tryptase, and carboxypeptidase. Am J Pathol 1992;140(4):847–57.

32. Proud D, MacGlashan DW, Newball HH. Immunoglobulin E-mediated release of a kininogenase from purified human lung mast cells. Am Rev Respir Dis 1985; 132(2):405–8.

33. Tanaka A, Arai K, Kitamura Y. Matrix metalloproteinase-9 production, a newly identified function of mast cell progenitors, is downregulated by c-kit receptor activation. Blood 1999;94(7):2390–5.

34. Akiyama M, Watanabe Y, Nishikawa T. Peroxidase activity in mast cell granules in urticaria pigmentosa. Dermatologica 1989;178(3):145–50.

35. Mulloy B, Lever R, Page CP. Mast cell glycosaminoglycans. Glycoconj J 2017;34: 351–61.

36. Ronnberg E, Melo FR, Pejler G. Mast cell proteoglycans. J Histochem Cytochem 2012;60:950–62.

37. Metcalfe DD, Lewis RA, Silbert JE, et al. Isolation and characterization of heparin from human lung. J Clin Invest 1979;64:1537–43.

38. Rosenberg RD. Role of heparin and heparinlike molecules in thrombosis and atherosclerosis. Fed Proc 1985;44:404–9.

39. Prieto-Garcia A, Zheng D, Adachi R, et al. Mast cell restricted mouse and human tryptase-heparin complexes hinder thrombin-induced coagulation of plasma and the generation of fibrin by proteolytically destroying fibrinogen. J Biol Chem 2012; 287:7834–44.

40. Vysniauskaite M, Hertfelder HJ, Oldenburg J, et al. Determination of plasma heparin level improves identification of systemic mast cell activation disease. PLoS One 2015;10:e0124912.

41. Seidel H, Molderings GJ, Oldenburg J, et al. Bleeding diathesis in patients with mast cell activation disease. Thromb Haemost 2011;106:987–9.

42. Sucker C, Mansmann G, Steiner S, et al. Fatal bleeding due to a heparin-like anticoagulant in a 37 year old woman suffering from systemic mastocytosis. Clin Appl Thromb Hemost 2008;14:360–4.

43. Carvalhosa AB, Aouba A, Damaj G, et al. A French national survey on clotting disorders in mastocytosis. Medicine 2015;94:e1414.

44. Travis WD, Li C-Y, Hoagland HC, et al. Mast cell leukemia: report of a case and review of the literature. Mayo Clin Proc 1986;61:957–66.

45. Morrow JD, Guzzo C, Lazarus G. Improved diagnosis of mastocytosis by measurement of the major urinary metabolite of prostaglandin D2. J Invest Dermatol 1995;104(6):937–40.

46. Cho C, Nguyen A, Bryant KJ. Prostaglandin D2 metabolites as a biomarker of in vivo mast cell activation in systemic mastocytosis and rheumatoid arthritis. Immun Inflamm Dis 2015;4(1):64–9.

47. Lueke AJ, Meeusen JW, Donato LJ. Analytical and clinical validation of an LC-MS/MS method for urine leukotriene E4: a marker of systemic mastocytosis. Clin Biochem 2016;49(13–14):979–82.

48. Butterfield JH. Increased leukotriene E4 excretion in systemic mastocytosis. Prostaglandins Other Lipid Mediat 2010;92(1–4):73–6.

49. Guinot P, Summerhayes C, Berdah L. Treatment of adult systemic mastocytosis with a PAF-acether antagonist BN52063. Lancet 1988;2(8602):114.

50. Metcalfe DD. Mast cells and mastocytosis. Blood 2008;112:946–56.

51. Sayed BA, Christy A, Quirion MR, et al. The master switch: the role of mast cells in autoimmunity and tolerance. Annu Rev Immunol 2008;26:705–39.

52. Theoharides TC, Alysandratos KD, Angelidou A, et al. Mast cells and inflammation. Biochim Biophys Acta 2012;1822:21–33.

53. Hoermann G, Greiner G, Valent P. Cytokine regulation of microenvironmental cells in myeloproliferative neoplasms. Mediators Inflamm 2015;2015:869242.

54. Brockow K, Akin C, Huber M, et al. Levels of mast-cell growth factors in plasma and in suction skin blister fluid in adults with mastocytosis: correlation with dermal mast-cell numbers and mast-cell tryptase. J Allergy Clin Immunol 2002;109:82–8.

55. Theoharides TC, Boucher W, Spear K. Serum interleukin-6 reflects disease severity and osteoporosis in mastocytosis patients. Int Arch Allergy Immunol 2002;128(4):344–50.

56. Brockow K, Akin C, Huber M, et al. IL-6 levels predict disease variant and extent of organ involvement in patients with mastocytosis. Clin Immunol 2005;115:216–23.

57. Rabenhorst A, Christopeit B, Leja S, et al. Serum levels of bone cytokines are increased in indolent systemic mastocytosis associated with osteopenia or osteoporosis. J Allergy Clin Immunol 2013;132:1234–7.

58. Mayado A, Teodosio C, Garcia-Montero AC, et al. Increased IL6 plasma levels in indolent systemic mastocytosis are associated with high risk of disease progression. Leukemia 2016;30:124–30.

59. Hartmann K, Wagner N, Rabenhorst A, et al. Serum IL-31 levels are increased in a subset of patients with mastocytosis and correlate with disease severity in adult patients. J Allergy Clin Immunol 2013;132:233–5.

60. Dillon SR, Sprecher C, Hammond A, et al. Interleukin 31, a cytokine produced by activated T cells, induces dermatitis in mice. Nat Immunol 2004;5:752–60.

61. Cornelissen C, Luscher-Firzlaff J, Baron JM, et al. Signaling by IL-31 and functional consequences. Eur J Cell Biol 2012;91:552–66.

62. Raap U, Wichmann K, Bruder M, et al. Correlation of IL-31 serum levels with severity of atopic dermatitis. J Allergy Clin Immunol 2008;122:421–3.

63. Niyonsaba F, Ushio H, Hara M, et al. Antimicrobial peptides human β-defensins and cathelicidin LL-37 induce the secretion of a pruritogenic cytokine IL-31 by human mast cells. J Immunol 2010;184:3526–34.

64. Valent P, Spanblochl E, Sperr WR, et al. Induction of differentiation of human mast cells from bone marrow and peripheral blood mononuclear cells by recombinant human stem cell factor (SCF) kit ligand (KL) in long term culture. Blood 1992;80:2237–45.

65. dePaulis A, Minopoli G, Arbustini E, et al. Stem cell factor is localized in, released from and cleaved by human mast cells. J Immunol 1999;163:2799–808.

66. Longley BJ, Tyrrel L, Ma Y, et al. Chymase cleavage of stem cell factor yields a bioactive, soluble product. Proc Natl Acad Sci U S A 1997;94:9017–21.

67. Skaper SD. Nerve growth factor: a neuroimmune crosstalk mediator for all seasons. Immunology 2017;151:1–15.

68. Peng WM, Maintz L, Allam JP, et al. Increased circulating levels of neurotrophins and elevated expression of their high-affinity receptors on skin and gut mast cells in mastocytosis. Blood 2013;122:1779–88.

Kit Mutations
New Insights and Diagnostic Value

Lorenzo Falchi, MD[a], Srdan Verstovsek, MD, PhD[b],*

KEYWORDS

- KIT mutations • *KIT* D816V • Cutaneous mastocytosis • Systemic mastocytosis
- Imatinib • Midostaurin • Avapritinib

KEY POINTS

- KIT mutations are the molecular hallmark of mastocytosis and are present in the vast majority of patients, despite the clinical heterogeneity of the disease.
- *KIT* D816V is the most common KIT mutation, particularly in patients with more advanced forms, and it is believed to represent a driver lesion of the disease.
- Testing for *KIT* D816V is part of the diagnostic criteria for mastocytosis. The mutation can be detected through allele-specific–oligonucleotide quantitative polymerase chain reaction in peripheral blood in most patients.
- Mutated KIT inhibition with imatinib mesylate has represented the first advancement in the targeted therapy of systemic mastocytosis, but it is ineffective in patients with *KIT* D816V.
- Novel agents capable of overcoming *KIT* D816V–mediated tyrosine kinase inhibitor resistance include the multikinase inhibitor midostaurin, the selective *KIT* D816V inhibitor avapritinib, and the so-called switch-pocket inhibitors.

INTRODUCTION

Mastocytosis is a neoplastic disorder originating from the malignant transformation and clonal proliferation of mast cells (MCs), which accumulate in one or multiple organs. The true incidence of the disease is difficult to ascertain due to potential underdiagnosis. It is estimated, however, at 0.89 per 100,000 per year, according to a recent European study.[1] The prevalence of mastocytosis was hypothesized to be approximately 1 in 10,000 people.[2]

The clinical spectrum of mastocytosis ranges from isolated cutaneous forms (cutaneous mastocytosis [CM]) that is more frequent in younger patients, with tendency to

Disclosure Statement: The authors have nothing to declare.
[a] Division of Hematology/Oncology, Columbia University Medical Center, 177 Fort Washington Avenue, MHB 6GN-435, New York, NY 10032, USA; [b] Leukemia Department, The University of Texas MD Anderson Cancer Center, 1515 Holcombe Boulevard, Unit 428, Houston, TX 77030, USA
* Corresponding author.
E-mail address: sverstov@mdanderson.org

Immunol Allergy Clin N Am 38 (2018) 411–428
https://doi.org/10.1016/j.iac.2018.04.005   immunology.theclinics.com
0889-8561/18/© 2018 Elsevier Inc. All rights reserved.

spontaneously resolve,[3] to aggressive diffuse variants (systemic mastocytosis [SM]) typically seen in adult patients and associated with poorer outcome.[4] In addition, because SM is a hematopoietic stem cell disorder, it can coexist with other World Health Organization (WHO)-defined myeloid (or, more rarely, lymphoid) neoplasms.[5]

Once comprised within the group of myeloproliferative neoplasms (MPNs), mastocytosis is now recognized as a distinct clinicopathologic entity in the 2016 revision of the WHO classification of myeloid tumors (**Box 1**).[6]

The symptoms of mastocytosis are largely due to the release of MC products. Histamine (acting through receptors H_1–H_4) mediates vasodilation, brochoconstriction, gastrointestinal hypermotility, and increased gastric acid production, which account for rapid-onset symptoms like headache, hypotension, pruritus, urticaria, angioedema, cramping, diarrhea, and anaphylaxis.[7] Chymase is responsible for cardiovascular symptoms like arrhythmias, myocardial ischemia, and hypotension. Other mediators of mastocytosis symptoms include platelet-activating factor, prostaglandin D2,[8] serotonin, and substance P.[9] Rare manifestations of mastocytosis include tissue eosinophilia (due to interleukin [IL]-5 production) and bone remodeling (due to space-occupying MC burden, as well as to IL-1β and IL-6 secreted by MCs).[10]

CM, the most common form of mastocytosis, can present as urticaria pigmentosa, particularly on the torso and extremities; diffuse CM; or solitary skin mastocytoma. SM is defined by MC involvement of end organs other than the skin (most commonly the bone marrow [BM]). Indolent SM primarily causes gastrointestinal, skin, and cognitive symptoms, but does not affect organ function (e.g., BM, although involved with mastocytosis, functions well and patients have normal blood cell counts). Smoldering SM is a subtype of indolent SM, with organ enlargement (B findings) but preserved organ function, and possibly with more variable course.[11] Although indolent SM is a rather benign condition, end-organ damage is the

---

Box 1
World Health Organization classification of mastocytosis (2016)

1. Cutaneous mastocytosis
   a. Urticaria pigmentosa/maculopapular cutaneous mastocytosis
   b. Diffuse cutaneous mastocytosis
   c. Solitary mastocytoma of skin

2. SM
   a. ISM: meets criteria for SM; no C findings; no evidence of associated clonal hematologic non–MC lineage disease[a]
   b. Smoldering SM: as above (ISM) but with 2 or more B findings and no C findings[a]
   c. SM-AHN[b]: meets criteria for SM and criteria for an associated hematologic neoplasm as a distinct entity per the WHO classification
   d. ASM: meets criteria for SM; 1 or more C findings; no evidence of MCL[a]
   e. MCL

3. MC sarcoma
   a. Unifocal MC tumor; no evidence of SM; destructive growth pattern; high-grade cytology

[a] These subtypes require information regarding B findings and C findings for complete diagnosis (see **Box 2**), all of which may not be available at the time of initial tissue diagnosis.

[b] The terms, systemic mastocytosis with an associated clonal hematologic non-MC lineage disease (SM-AHNMD) and SM-AHN, can be used synonymously.

Adapted from Swerdlow SH, Campo E, Harris N, et al. WHO classification of tumours of haematopoietic and lymphoid tissues. 4th edition. Lyon (France): International Agency for Research on Cancer (IARC); 2017; with permission.

hallmark of aggressive SM (C findings). SM with associated hematologic neoplasms (SM-AHN) exhibits a yet more aggressive behavior and can associate with chronic myelomonocytic leukemia, myelodysplastic syndrome, B-cell lymphoma/leukemia, plasma cell neoplasms, MPNs, and acute myeloid leukemia.[12] MC leukemia (MCL) is a form of acute nonlymphoid leukemia and it is associated with dismal outcomes.

Characteristics of mastocytosis differ in children and adults. In the former, the disease is usually cutaneous and self-limited, anaphylaxis is rare, and the basal tryptase level is less than 20 μg/L [70]. Tryptase levels greater than 20 μg/L usually portend diffuse skin involvement and possible underlying systemic disease.[13] Cutaneous manifestations of adulthood-onset mastocytosis exhibit a more chronic course, typically presenting with diffuse maculopapular lesions, anaphylaxis that is more common, and tryptase levels frequently greater than 20 μg/L.[14] In general, serum tryptase levels tend to increase in more aggressive forms.[4] This test, however, is nonspecific because tryptase can be increased in other conditions, such as acute myeloid leukemia, chronic myeloid leukemia, and myelodysplastic syndrome.[15]

In adults with suspected SM, a BM biopsy is always performed because it allows confirming the diagnosis and ruling out an associated hematologic neoplasm.[5] BM histopathology reveals dense perivascular and/or paratrabecular aggregates of spindle-shaped MCs with hypogranulation or abnormal nuclei. Tryptase staining is extremely sensitive for the detection of MCs,[16] but it is also found in normal MCs[17] and other myeloid neoplasms.[5] In contrast, expressions of CD2 and CD25[6] are more specific markers.[18] WHO criteria for the diagnosis of SM are outlined in **Box 2**. Additional descriptors of the severity of the disease, the so-called B finding and C findings, are also reported.

THE ROLE OF KIT IN THE PATHOBIOLOGY OF MASTOCYTOSIS

Over the past few years significant progress has been made in the understanding of the pathobiology of mastocytosis. This has led to the discovery, development, and, in some cases, regulatory approval of targeted therapies. Other agents specifically interfering with the pathogenetic mechanisms of mastocytosis are under preclinical or clinical development.

Physiology

KIT (or CD117) is a type III receptor tyrosine kinase found on various cell types, including hematopoietic progenitor cells, MCs, germ cells, melanocytes, and interstitial cells of Cajal. It plays an important role in organogenesis, development, and physiologic regulation of several organs/systems.[19] In the hematopoietic system, KIT expression is lost in all mature cells, but it remains high in MCs. The 145-kDa KIT molecule is encoded by a 21-exon gene on chromosome 4q12 and is composed of 5 extracellular immunoglobulin-like domains (ECD), a juxtamembrane domain (JMD), and a tyrosine-kinase domain (TKD). The first 3 Ig-like domains bind to stem cell factor (SCF), the KIT ligand. Domains 4 and 5 initiate intracellular signaling in cooperation with the JMD. The TKD contains 2 subdomains: a phosphotransferase domain (PTD) and an ATP binding site.[20–22]

SCF is expressed by fibroblasts and endothelial cells[23,24] and subsequently cleaved to be released in soluble form.[25] Binding to KIT triggers conformational changes[22] that cause activation of multiple downstream kinases, and signaling through the mitogen-activated protein kinase pathway, which is required for MC activation,[26] or JAK-STAT pathway, required for MC development, survival, and proliferation (**Fig. 1**).[27]

Box 2
World Health Organization criteria for the diagnosis of systemic mastocytosis

Major criterion

Multifocal, dense infiltrates of MCs (≥15 MCs in aggregates) detected in sections of BM and/or other extracutaneous organs

Minor criteria
a. In biopsy sections of bone marrow or other extracutaneous organs, greater than 25% of the MCs in the infiltrate are spindle-shaped or have atypical morphology or, of all MCs in BM aspirate smears, greater than 25% are immature or atypical.
b. Detection of an activating point mutation at codon 816 of *KIT* in BM, blood, or other extracutaneous organ.
c. MCs in BM, blood, or other extracutaneous organ express CD2 and/or CD25 in addition to normal MC markers.
d. Serum total tryptase persistently exceeds 20 ng/mL (unless there is an associated clonal myeloid disorder, in which case this parameter is not valid).

Diagnosis of SM requires major criterion + 1 minor criterion or greater than or equal to 3 minor criteria

B findings
1. Greater than 30% BM infiltration by MCs in focal, dense aggregates and/or serum total tryptase level greater than 20 ng/mL
2. Signs of dysplasia or myeloproliferation, in non-MC lineage(s), not meeting criteria for a hematopoietic neoplasm, with normal or slightly abnormal blood counts
3. Hepatomegaly and/or splenomegaly without functional impairment, and/or lymphadenopathy

C findings
1. One or more cytopenia(s) without obvious non-MC hematopoietic malignancy
2. Palpable hepatomegaly with impairment of liver function, ascites, and/or portal hypertension
3. Osteolytic lesions and/or pathologic fractures
4. Palpable splenomegaly with hypersplenism
5. Malabsorption with weight loss due to gastrointestinal MC infiltrates

Adapted from Swerdlow SH, Campo E, Harris N, et al. WHO classification of tumours of haematopoietic and lymphoid tissues, 4th edition. Lyon (France): International Agency for Research on Cancer (IARC); 2017; with permission.

Molecular Epidemiology of KIT Mutations

A point mutation resulting in the replacement of aspartate with valine in codon 816 of the *KIT* sequence (D816V) was originally identified in the peripheral blood (PB) of both patients with CM and SM.[28] Later it became clear that an activating mutation of *KIT*, primarily affecting the TKD, could be found in most SM patients across disease subtypes.[4] At a cellular level, this point mutation results in enhanced survival and autonomous growth of neoplastic MCs.[29]

In adult patients, D816V is the most common *KIT* mutation (>90% of cases). Other mutations, such as V560G,[30,31] D815K,[32] D816Y,[32–35] insVI815-816,[33] D816F,[32,35] D816H,[36] and D820G,[37] have been identified. In children, mastocytosis is also associated with activating *KIT* mutations, but the frequency of *KIT* D816V is lower (25%–36%)[19,38–40] and the type and location of alterations in the remaining cases are varied (often in the ECD), potentially accounting for the different characteristics and clinical course of the disease in the two age groups. Mutations in exons 8 and 9 have been found in rare familial mastocytosis, alone or as part of clinical syndromes.[41–44] A synopsis of the most common *KIT* mutations and their distribution is illustrated in **Fig. 2**.

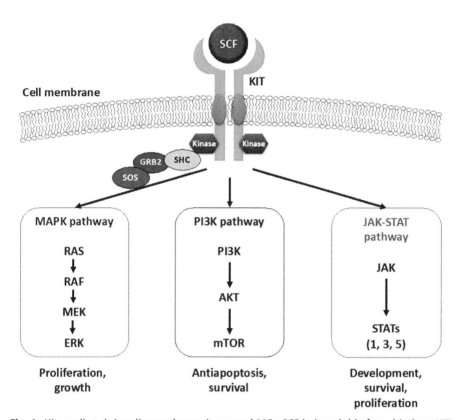

Fig. 1. Kit-mediated signaling pathways in normal MCs. SCF in its soluble form binds to KIT and promotes its dimerization and autophosphorilation. The latter causes activation of multiple downstream signaling pathways, including the mitogen-activated protein kinase pathway (through the recruitment of intermediary molecules, such as SHC and GRB2, required for MC activation), the PI3K pathways, important in MC survival, and the JAK-STAT pathway, required for MC development, survival, and proliferation). ERK, extracellular signal-regulated kinases; GRB2, growth-factor-receptor-bound protein 2; JAK-STAT, Janus kinase-signal transducer and activator of transcription; MAPK, mitogen-activated protein kinase; MEK, MAP/extracellular signal-regulated kinase; mTOR, mammalian target of rapamycin; PI3K, phosphoinositide 3-kinase; RAF, rapidly accelerated fibrosarcoma; RAS, rat sarcomaSHC, SRC homology 2 (SH2)-domain-containing transforming protein C; SOS, son of sevenless homologue.

The type and frequency of *KIT* mutations vary to some degree in different subtypes of mastocytosis. For example, some patients with indolent SM (ISM) may carry a non-*KIT* D816V (or no *KIT* mutation), whereas those with smoldering SM, aggressive SM (ASM), and SM-AHN are nearly always *KIT* D816V–positive in MC[17,37,45] and sometimes in non-MC populations.[33] A significant proportion of the latter also carries the mutation in the myeloid (virtually never lymphoid) AHN component,[4] consistent with the hypothesis that transformation affects early progenitors capable of generating cells of different lineages that undergo further, distinct transformation events.[12] In patients with MCL, there is a relatively higher prevalence of non-D816V mutations or wild-type *KIT*. Finally, in MC sarcoma no *KIT* D816V mutations have been reported.[46]

Several single-nucleotide polymorphisms have been described in the *KIT* gene although their clinical impact remains unclear.[47]

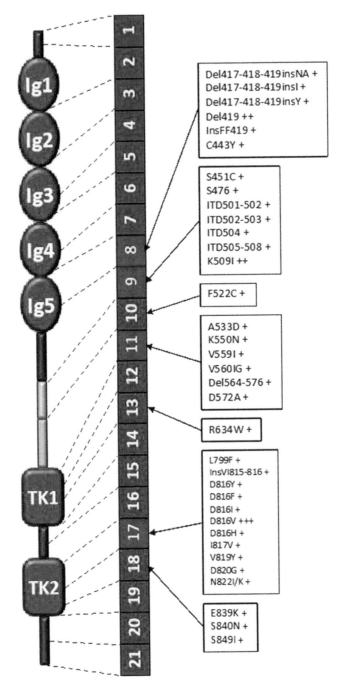

Fig. 2. Distribution of mutations of KIT (depicted in its monomeric form) in pediatric and adult patients with mastocytosis. In the former, *KIT* D816V PTD mutation (exon 17) is found in nearly 30% of the cases and in greater than 80% in the latter. A list of mutations described at each hotspot is represented. The approximate frequency of each mutation is also described: +, less than 10% of the patients; ++, 5% to 20%; +++ and approximately 30% (pediatric) or greater than 80% (adult). Del, deletion; Ig, immunoglobulin; Ins, insertion; ITD, internal tandem duplication. (*Modified from* Arock M, Sotlar K, Akin C, et al. KIT mutation analysis in mast cell neoplasms: recommendations of the European Competence Network on Mastocytosis. Leukemia 2015;29(6):1224–5; with permission.)

Oncogenicity

The *KIT* D816V is believed to induce conformational changes in the PTD of the receptor causing constitutive, ligand-independent activation.[48] Activating *KIT* mutations can affect regulation of the kinase domain or change the sequence of the enzymatic site itself, causing its stabilization in an activated state and/or a decreased affinity for type I tyrosine kinase inhibitors (TKIs), such as imatinib mesylate (IM), that recognize the active conformation of a kinase.[49] Rarely, more than 1 *KIT* mutation is present in the same patient.[50]

In one set of experiments, transgenic mice expressed *KIT* D816V under the control of the chymase promoter. Upon sacrifice of the animals and a group of control mice, researchers noticed abnormal accumulation of MCs in spleen, heart, and lymph nodes (the chymase promoter would not be functional in hematopoietic progenitors, hence the lack of BM involvement). Only transgenic MCs could be maintained in continuous cultures. These, however, became growth factor–independent only after several months. Moreover, transgenic mice only developed clinical signs of mastocytosis after 12 months to 18 months and with a penetrance of only 30% (**Fig. 3**).[51] These observations suggest that, despite the oncogenic potential of *KIT* D816V, additional genetic events are likely necessary for the development of overt mastocytosis in a majority of cases.

In another experience, transgenic mice expressing *KIT* D814V (the murine homolog of *KIT* D816V) under the *KIT* promoter, developed severe mastocytosis in 100% of cases early in life. In approximately 50% of them, an associated non-MC hematologic neoplasm was also found. Again, when the expression of KIT was restricted to more differentiated MCs, the phenotype was milder and developed later in life.[52] Both experiments suggest that the severity of the disease might at least in part depend on the timing of acquisition of the *KIT* mutation along the differentiation chain of MCs.

Mutations of Genes other than KIT

The discrepancy between a unique defining mutation (*KIT* D816V) and a heterogeneous clinical course and prognosis may be explained in part by the presence of additional mutations in the MC clone. These additional alterations may also be responsible for the variable response to KIT-targeted therapy and are correlated with poorer outcomes.

For instance, a *TET2* mutation was detected in 20% to 29% of mastocytosis cases across subtypes, albeit more frequently in patients with aggressive forms, including SM-AHN.[53–57] In half of these patients KIT D816V and *TET2* mutations coexisted. *ASXL1* is mutated in 12% to 20% of patients with mastocytosis and it seems to confer poorer prognosis.[56–58] Other recurrent mutations involve genes of the spliceosome machinery (*SF3B1*, *SRSF2*, and *U2AF1*), *CBL*, *DNMT3A*, *KRAS*, *NRAS*, *JAK2*, *EZH2*, and *ETV6*.[57,59,60] Some patients with SM, particularly in its later stage, harbor multiple mutations in the same MC clone,[57] often before acquiring the *KIT* D816V.[55] These individuals have a poorer prognosis. Although some mutations may contribute more strongly to the negative prognosis[61] the precise contribution of each of these alterations and/or their order is presently unknown.

KIT TESTING IN THE DIAGNOSIS OF MASTOCYTOSIS

The presence of *KIT* D816V represents a minor criterion for the diagnosis of mastocytosis according to the WHO.[6] In general, in children with CM, *KIT* mutation is screened for only if the diagnosis in not unequivocal,[38] or an underlying ASM is suspected.[62] The likelihood of detecting *KIT* mutations depends on the amount of MCs in the sample and

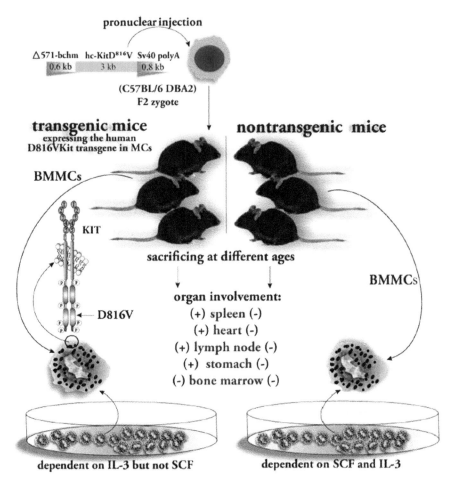

pronuclear injection

Δ571-bchm hc-KitD⁸¹⁶V Sv40 polyA
0.6 kb   3 kb   0.8 kb

(C57BL/6 DBA2)
F2 zygote

transgenic mice
expressing the human
D816VKit transgene in MCs

nontransgenic mice

BMMCs

KIT

sacrificing at different ages

D816V

BMMCs

organ involvement:
(+) spleen (-)
(+) heart (-)
(+) lymph node (-)
(+) stomach (-)
(-) bone marrow (-)

dependent on IL-3 but not SCF   dependent on SCF and IL-3

Fig. 3. Transgenic mice expressing the human D816VKit transgene in MCs were assessed at different ages for developing SM symptoms and compared with normal nontransgenic mice. They were found to have organ involvement in the spleen, heart, lymph nodes, and stomach but not in the BM. Comparing BM-derived cultured MCs (BMMCs) of these 2 groups of mice revealed that BMMCs from the transgenic ones became independent to SCF for proliferation and activation. (*From* Komi DEA, Rambasek T, Wöhrl S. Mastocytosis: from a molecular point of view. Clinic Rev Allerg Immunol 2017; with permission.)

the sensitivity of the diagnostic technique.[63] In most SM patients, the *KIT* D816V allele burden is less than 1% by allele-specific oligonucleotide quantitative polymerase chain reaction (ASO-qPCR).[64–66] Moreover, routine testing only detects *KIT* D816V. Therefore, for those SM patients who have *KIT* mutations other than D816V, dedicated assays, such as restriction fragment length polymorphism (RFLP) or high-performance liquid chromatography (HPLC) of PCR products, should be performed.[64,67]

Historically, *KIT* testing has been performed by conventional sequencing of PCR products from BM-derived MCs.[68] Given the low diagnostic yield of this technique,[69] assays such as PCR plus RFLP,[70] peptide nucleic acid (PNA)-mediated PCR clamping,[32] nested reverse transcriptase–PCR (RT-PCR) followed by denaturing HPLC (D-HPLC)[64] and ASO-qPCR assays[64,71–73] were developed.

Several studies have consistently shown that PB ASO-qPCR allows detection of the *KIT* D816V in almost all adults with SM, regardless of the presence of MCs in the circulation.[64–66,71] This test is currently recommended for the initial screening of individuals with suspected SM by the European Competence Network on Mastocytosis (ECNM).[74] ASO-qPCR presents other advantages. It can be performed both on fresh samples and stored material, such as on fresh-frozen paraffin-embedded tissue, including biopsy samples of the skin[75] and other affected organs.[76,77] Moreover, because it is a quantitative method, it allows measurement of *KIT* D816V allele burden at the time of diagnosis and/or during the course of disease.[65,71,73]

The technique has limitations. For instance, when the MC burden is very low, PB testing may be not sensitive enough and the BM by ASO-qPCR,[64,71] or (less frequently) MC enrichment by laser microdissection or flow cytometry may need to be examined.[33,78] In addition, ASO-qPCR cannot detect non-D816V *KIT* mutations. Therefore, in *KIT* D816V–negative patients with strong clinical suspicion for, but no formal diagnosis of, SM other techniques, such as PC plus RFLP or D-HPLC, should be considered, followed, if negative, by next-generation sequencing of the entire *KIT* coding region. This is especially important for patients with ASM or MCL who may have non–D816V *KIT* mutations sensitive to imatinib therapy. Finally, ASO-qPCR has not yet undergone rigorous standardization and harmonization among centers.

In this regard, digital droplet PCR (which allows a more accurate quantitative measurement of the target DNA without the need for calibration material)[79] was recently shown to be more sensitive than PNA-mediated PCR clamping and comparable to ASO-qPCR for the detection and quantitation of *KIT* D816V in PB and BM, with the appealing advantage of being suitable for readily interlaboratory standardization.[79] A comparison of standard assays for the detection of *KIT* mutations is outlined in **Table 1**.

Table 1
Advantages and disadvantages of standard techniques for the detection of *KIT* mutations

Technique	Advantages	Disadvantages
RT-PCR and RFLP	• Easy to perform • Rapid • Reliable • Cost effective • Sensitivity: 0.05%	• Does not detect mutations other than in codon 816 • Not quantitative
Nested RT-PCR followed by D-HPLC of PCR products	• Detects all mutations in the amplified region	• Sensitivity: 0.5%–1% • Not quantitative • Time consuming • HPLC requires dedicated infrastructure
PNA-mediated PCR	• Detects other mutations in codon 816 or in adjacent codons • Method of choice for testing of formalin-fixed, paraffin-embedded tissue	• Not quantitative • Sensitivity: 0.1%
ASO-qPCR (performed on DNA or RNA-cDNA)	• Simple • Rapid • Inexpensive • Sensitivity: 0.01% • Quantitative	• Detects only *KIT* D816V mutation • Requires, validation and interlaboratory standardization and harmonization

Abbreviations: cDNA, complementary DNA.

OTHER USES OF KIT MUTATION TESTING

In retrospective series of patients with mastocytosis, the *KIT* D816V allele burden was found to gradually increase in advanced disease stages, from CM to ASM. Moreover, an increase in the allele burden over time correlated with disease progression. Conversely, a response to cytoreductive therapy was accompanied by a decrease of it.[64,66] Based on these observations, the ECNM recommends measuring the *KIT* D816V allele burden in patients with previously stable ISM who display signs of disease progression and in patients with aggressive forms treated with cytoreductive therapies to monitor the response to treatment.[80]

KIT testing can be helpful in certain diagnostically challenging situations. For instance, patients who do not meet criteria for a formal diagnosis of mastocytosis, but present with symptoms of MC activation and have clonal MCs by *KIT* mutation testing or CD25 staining, are assigned a provisional diagnosis of "monoclonal mast cell activation syndrome." Its course and tendency to evolve into a more aggressive form are undefined.[81] On the other hand, some patients with SM may have a relatively uninformative BM picture, but are found to have non–D816V *KIT* mutations and may be sensitive to IM therapy.[33,43]

A recent prospective study confirmed the concordance of PB and BM *KIT* D816V mutation analysis (of 44 patients who tested positive in PB, 43 did so in BM as well). Moreover, among 13 patients with SM who had presented with Hymenoptera venom–induced anaphylaxis as the only manifestation of disease, 12 tested D816V-positive. Without molecular testing, an SM diagnosis could have been easily missed in these individuals. Among the 14 patients who tested negative, 5 were subsequently found to have SM, indicating that BM biopsy cannot be avoided in adults with strong suspicion for SM.[82]

Finally, an important diagnostic distinction is made between *KIT*-mutated SM and Philadelphia chromosome–negative MPN with features of chronic eosinophilic leukemia associated with splenomegaly, marked elevation of vitamin B_{12}, elevation of tryptase, and increased BM MCs. In the latter, MCs are usually scattered rather than clustered and rearrangements of platelet derived growth factor A (PDGFRA) or PDGFRB are commonly found, conferring sensitivity to IM treatment.[6]

THERAPEUTIC RELEVANCE OF KIT MUTATIONS

In contrast to other hematologic malignancies, where the knowledge of specific genetic lesions has been critical to direct the therapeutic strategy, in SM, such knowledge has been less consequential, partly because of the limited efficacy of KIT-targeted approaches in this patient population and partly because of the significant genetic complexity of the disease.

Nonetheless, understanding the structural changes of KIT has helped explain how certain mutations determine sensitivity or resistance to targeted drugs.[83,84]

Two drugs are currently approved by the US Food and Drug Administration (FDA) for the treatment of patients with SM. IM is approved for use in adult patients with ASM without the *KIT* D816V mutation as determined with an FDA-approved test or with *KIT* mutational status unknown. Midostaurin is approved for the treatment of patients with ASM, SM-AHN, or MCL, regardless of their *KIT* D816V mutational status.

Early small studies showed variable responses to IM in all-comer SM patients. Among those with *KIT* D816V responses were also variable (0%–36%).[85–88] Because it is an ATP-competitive TKI, IM can only inhibit mutations that modulate the receptor's conformational change. Thus, patients with KIT mutations outside the PTD (ie, JMD or ECD) exhibit response to imatinib.[42,89–91] In contrast, in *KIT* D816V mutants, the receptor is found in a permanently active conformation that cannot be inhibited by imatinib.[48,87,92] Other instances in which IM has shown remarkable efficacy include patients with transmembrane domain *KIT* mutations (F522C or K509I),[42,43] individuals with familial syndromes associated with mastocytosis,[42] and patients with wild-type *KIT*.[93]

Midostaurin (PKC412) is a pleiotropic kinase inhibitor with activity against KIT mutants, including D816V.[94,95] After encouraging preliminary results from small studies,[96] midostaurin was tested, at a dose of 100 mg twice daily, in a multinational phase 2 study that included 116 patients with advanced SM, 87% of whom were D816V-positive. Among 89 patients evaluable for efficacy, the overall response rate was 60%, consistently across ASM, SM-AHN, and MCL subtypes and regardless of the presence of *KIT* D816V. Remarkably, progression-free survival lasted approximately 1 year for patients in the latter 2 groups.[97] Based on these results, the FDA approved midostaurin for the treatment of aggressive SM on April 28, 2017.

In an effort to identify biomarkers of response, a recent study sought to evaluate the impact of mutations in *SRSF2*, *ASXL1*, and/or *RUNX1* [S/A/R] in 38 midostaurin-treated ASM patients. Responses and survival were significantly lower in S/A/R-positive compared with non-S/A/R patients. In multivariate analysis, however, only a reduction of *KIT* D816V allele burden greater than or equal to 25% was independently associated with improved survival. Patients with progression of disease had acquired additional mutations (*K/NRAS*, *RUNX1*, *IDH2*, or *NPM1*).[98]

Other TKIs have been tested and/or are in development for SM. Dasatinib and nilotinib showed good preclinical activity against KIT mutants, including D816V, but modest clinical efficacy in patients with ASM.[99–101] Ponatinib, another multikinase inhibitor, showed activity against *KIT* V560G and *KIT* D816V cell lines[102] and may be synergistic with midostaurin.[103] Avapritinib (BLU-285) is a highly selective KIT D816V inhibitor, with activity in preclinical models, including those resistant to midostaurin.[61,104] A phase 1 trial of this drug in patients with ASM, most with 1 or more additional mutations, was recently presented. Significant clinical benefit was seen in the majority of patients. Responses occurred rapidly and were durable. Treatment was well tolerated.[105] Masatinib mesilate (AB1010) is a KIT and LYN inhibitor[106] with weak activity against *KIT* D816V. This agent is being developed for patients with ISM, where it showed promising activity and good tolerability in pilot experiences[107,108] and, more recently, proved superior to placebo in randomized phase 3 trial.[109] Finally, strategies have been developed to target the so-called switch-pocket region of KIT, which confers the receptor either an active or inactive conformation. DP-2976 and DP-4851 are non-ATP competitors that showed potent antineoplastic activity in primary malignant MCs.[110] DCC-2618 is a type II switch-pocket control inhibitor, which potently inhibits exon 17 KIT mutations resistant to conventional TKI and is being tested in an ongoing phase 1 trial (NCT02571036).[111]

SUMMARY

Mastocytosis is a rare WHO-defined distinct clonal disorder, according to the latest version of the WHO classification of myeloid tumors. Despite significant heterogeneity from clinical and prognostic points of view, at a molecular level mastocytosis is characterized by a mutation of the *KIT* gene sequence, most commonly the D816V, in almost all cases across disease subtypes. Thus, although *KIT* D816V can be considered a driver lesion based on experiments in animal models, other genetic events are likely responsible for the phenotypic diversity of the disease.

On the other hand, the discovery of *KIT* mutations as central to the pathobiology of mastocytosis, and the availability of KIT inhibitors, opened avenues for the development of targeted TKIs, including FDA-approved IM and midostaurin, as well as promising new agents (such as avapritinib).

Several other mutations involving genes other than *KIT*, such as *TET2, ASXL1*, and *DNMT3A*, among others, may preexist or accumulate in the neoplastic MC clone during the course of disease. These alterations likely contribute to the clinicopathologic diversity of mastocytosis, cause resistance to targeted (and conventional) therapy, and, ultimately, impart poorer prognosis. A deeper understanding of the complexity and dynamics of the genetic events occurring in mastocytosis is required to better identify patients who can most benefit from current therapies and to develop new agents capable of improving the outcome of patients with advanced SM.

REFERENCES

1. Cohen SS, Skovbo S, Vestergaard H, et al. Epidemiology of systemic mastocytosis in Denmark. Br J Haematol 2014;166(4):521–8.
2. Brockow K. Epidemiology, prognosis, and risk factors in mastocytosis. Immunol Allergy Clin North Am 2014;34(2):283–95.
3. Uzzaman A, Maric I, Noel P, et al. Pediatric-onset mastocytosis: a long term clinical follow-up and correlation with bone marrow histopathology. Pediatr Blood Cancer 2009;53(4):629–34.
4. Lim KH, Tefferi A, Lasho TL, et al. Systemic mastocytosis in 342 consecutive adults: survival studies and prognostic factors. Blood 2009;113(23):5727–36.
5. Horny HP, Sotlar K, Sperr WR, et al. Systemic mastocytosis with associated clonal haematological non-mast cell lineage diseases: a histopathological challenge. J Clin Pathol 2004;57(6):604–8.
6. Swerdlow SH, Campo E, Harris N, et al. WHO classification of tumours of haematopoietic and lymphoid tissues. 4th edition. Lyon (France): International Agency for research on Cancer (IARC); 2017.
7. Carter MC, Metcalfe DD, Komarow HD. Mastocytosis. Immunol Allergy Clin North Am 2014;34(1):181–96.
8. Picard M, Giavina-Bianchi P, Mezzano V, et al. Expanding spectrum of mast cell activation disorders: monoclonal and idiopathic mast cell activation syndromes. Clin Ther 2013;35(5):548–62.
9. Hannah-Shmouni F, Stratakis CA, Koch CA. Flushing in (neuro) endocrinology. Rev Endocr Metab Disord 2016;17(3):373–80.
10. Castells M, Austen KF. Mastocytosis: mediator-related signs and symptoms. Int Arch Allergy Immunol 2002;127(2):147–52.
11. Valent P, Akin C, Sperr WR, et al. Smouldering mastocytosis: a novel subtype of systemic mastocytosis with slow progression. Int Arch Allergy Immunol 2002;127(2):137–9.
12. Wang SA, Hutchinson L, Tang G, et al. Systemic mastocytosis with associated clonal hematological non-mast cell lineage disease: clinical significance and comparison of chomosomal abnormalities in SM and AHNMD components. Am J Hematol 2013;88(3):219–24.
13. Alvarez-Twose I, Vano-Galvan S, Sanchez-Munoz L, et al. Increased serum baseline tryptase levels and extensive skin involvement are predictors for the severity of mast cell activation episodes in children with mastocytosis. Allergy 2012;67(6):813–21.

14. Hartmann K, Escribano L, Grattan C, et al. Cutaneous manifestations in patients with mastocytosis: consensus report of the European competence network on mastocytosis; the American academy of allergy, asthma & immunology; and the European academy of allergology and clinical immunology. J Allergy Clin Immunol 2016;137(1):35–45.
15. Sperr WR, El-Samahi A, Kundi M, et al. Elevated tryptase levels selectively cluster in myeloid neoplasms: a novel diagnostic approach and screen marker in clinical haematology. Eur J Clin Invest 2009;39(10):914–23.
16. Horny HP, Sillaber C, Menke D, et al. Diagnostic value of immunostaining for tryptase in patients with mastocytosis. Am J Surg Pathol 1998;22(9):1132–40.
17. Jordan JH, Walchshofer S, Jurecka W, et al. Immunohistochemical properties of bone marrow mast cells in systemic mastocytosis: evidence for expression of CD2, CD117/Kit, and bcl-x(L). Hum Pathol 2001;32(5):545–52.
18. Sotlar K, Horny HP, Simonitsch I, et al. CD25 indicates the neoplastic phenotype of mast cells: a novel immunohistochemical marker for the diagnosis of systemic mastocytosis (SM) in routinely processed bone marrow biopsy specimens. Am J Surg Pathol 2004;28(10):1319–25.
19. Yanagihori H, Oyama N, Nakamura K, et al. c-kit Mutations in patients with childhood-onset mastocytosis and genotype-phenotype correlation. J Mol Diagn 2005;7(2):252–7.
20. Giebel LB, Strunk KM, Holmes SA, et al. Organization and nucleotide sequence of the human KIT (mast/stem cell growth factor receptor) proto-oncogene. Oncogene 1992;7(11):2207–17.
21. Chabot B, Stephenson DA, Chapman VM, et al. The proto-oncogene c-kit encoding a transmembrane tyrosine kinase receptor maps to the mouse W locus. Nature 1988;335(6185):88–9.
22. Lennartsson J, Ronnstrand L. Stem cell factor receptor/c-Kit: from basic science to clinical implications. Physiol Rev 2012;92(4):1619–49.
23. Bai CG, Hou XW, Wang F, et al. Stem cell factor-mediated wild-type KIT receptor activation is critical for gastrointestinal stromal tumor cell growth. World J Gastroenterol 2012;18(23):2929–37.
24. Cruse G, Metcalfe DD, Olivera A. Functional deregulation of KIT: link to mast cell proliferative diseases and other neoplasms. Immunol Allergy Clin North Am 2014;34(2):219–37.
25. Duttlinger R, Manova K, Chu TY, et al. W-sash affects positive and negative elements controlling c-kit expression: ectopic c-kit expression at sites of kit-ligand expression affects melanogenesis. Development 1993;118(3):705–17.
26. Metcalfe DD. Mast cells and mastocytosis. Blood 2008;112(4):946–56.
27. Morales JK, Falanga YT, Depcrynski A, et al. Mast cell homeostasis and the JAK-STAT pathway. Genes Immun 2010;11(8):599–608.
28. Akin C, Kirshenbaum AS, Semere T, et al. Analysis of the surface expression of c-kit and occurrence of the c-kit Asp816Val activating mutation in T cells, B cells, and myelomonocytic cells in patients with mastocytosis. Exp Hematol 2000;28(2):140–7.
29. Piao X, Bernstein A. A point mutation in the catalytic domain of c-kit induces growth factor independence, tumorigenicity, and differentiation of mast cells. Blood 1996;87(8):3117–23.
30. Buttner C, Henz BM, Welker P, et al. Identification of activating c-kit mutations in adult-, but not in childhood-onset indolent mastocytosis: a possible explanation for divergent clinical behavior. J Invest Dermatol 1998;111(6):1227–31.

31. Furitsu T, Tsujimura T, Tono T, et al. Identification of mutations in the coding sequence of the proto-oncogene c-kit in a human mast cell leukemia cell line causing ligand-independent activation of c-kit product. J Clin Invest 1993; 92(4):1736–44.

32. Sotlar K, Escribano L, Landt O, et al. One-step detection of c-kit point mutations using peptide nucleic acid-mediated polymerase chain reaction clamping and hybridization probes. Am J Pathol 2003;162(3):737–46.

33. Garcia-Montero AC, Jara-Acevedo M, Teodosio C, et al. KIT mutation in mast cells and other bone marrow hematopoietic cell lineages in systemic mast cell disorders: a prospective study of the Spanish Network on Mastocytosis (REMA) in a series of 113 patients. Blood 2006;108(7):2366–72.

34. Beghini A, Cairoli R, Morra E, et al. In vivo differentiation of mast cells from acute myeloid leukemia blasts carrying a novel activating ligand-independent C-kit mutation. Blood Cells Mol Dis 1998;24(2):262–70.

35. Longley BJ Jr, Metcalfe DD, Tharp M, et al. Activating and dominant inactivating c-KIT catalytic domain mutations in distinct clinical forms of human mastocytosis. Proc Natl Acad Sci U S A 1999;96(4):1609–14.

36. Pullarkat VA, Pullarkat ST, Calverley DC, et al. Mast cell disease associated with acute myeloid leukemia: detection of a new c-kit mutation Asp816His. Am J Hematol 2000;65(4):307–9.

37. Pignon JM, Giraudier S, Duquesnoy P, et al. A new c-kit mutation in a case of aggressive mast cell disease. Br J Haematol 1997;96(2):374–6.

38. Bodemer C, Hermine O, Palmerini F, et al. Pediatric mastocytosis is a clonal disease associated with D816V and other activating c-KIT mutations. J Invest Dermatol 2010;130(3):804–15.

39. Verzijl A, Heide R, Oranje AP, et al. C-kit Asp-816-Val mutation analysis in patients with mastocytosis. Dermatology 2007;214(1):15–20.

40. Bibi S, Langenfeld F, Jeanningros S, et al. Molecular defects in mastocytosis: KIT and beyond KIT. Immunol Allergy Clin North Am 2014;34(2):239–62.

41. Hartmann K, Wardelmann E, Ma Y, et al. Novel germline mutation of KIT associated with familial gastrointestinal stromal tumors and mastocytosis. Gastroenterology 2005;129(3):1042–6.

42. Zhang LY, Smith ML, Schultheis B, et al. A novel K509I mutation of KIT identified in familial mastocytosis-in vitro and in vivo responsiveness to imatinib therapy. Leuk Res 2006;30(4):373–8.

43. Akin C, Fumo G, Yavuz AS, et al. A novel form of mastocytosis associated with a transmembrane c-kit mutation and response to imatinib. Blood 2004;103(8): 3222–5.

44. Tang X, Boxer M, Drummond A, et al. A germline mutation in KIT in familial diffuse cutaneous mastocytosis. J Med Genet 2004;41(6):e88.

45. Sotlar K, Colak S, Bache A, et al. Variable presence of KITD816V in clonal haematological non-mast cell lineage diseases associated with systemic mastocytosis (SM-AHNMD). J Pathol 2010;220(5):586–95.

46. Georgin-Lavialle S, Aguilar C, Guieze R, et al. Mast cell sarcoma: a rare and aggressive entity–report of two cases and review of the literature. J Clin Oncol 2013;31(6):e90–7.

47. Nagata H, Worobec AS, Metcalfe DD. Identification of a polymorphism in the transmembrane domain of the protooncogene c-kit in healthy subjects. Exp Clin Immunogenet 1996;13(3–4):210–4.

48. Laine E, Chauvot de Beauchene I, Perahia D, et al. Mutation D816V alters the internal structure and dynamics of c-KIT receptor cytoplasmic region:

implications for dimerization and activation mechanisms. PLoS Comput Biol 2011;7(6):e1002068.

49. Longley BJ, Reguera MJ, Ma Y. Classes of c-KIT activating mutations: proposed mechanisms of action and implications for disease classification and therapy. Leuk Res 2001;25(7):571–6.

50. Lasho T, Finke C, Zblewski D, et al. Concurrent activating KIT mutations in systemic mastocytosis. Br J Haematol 2016;173(1):153–6.

51. Zappulla JP, Dubreuil P, Desbois S, et al. Mastocytosis in mice expressing human Kit receptor with the activating Asp816Val mutation. J Exp Med 2005; 202(12):1635–41.

52. Gerbaulet A, Wickenhauser C, Scholten J, et al. Mast cell hyperplasia, B-cell malignancy, and intestinal inflammation in mice with conditional expression of a constitutively active kit. Blood 2011;117(6):2012–21.

53. Tefferi A, Levine RL, Lim KH, et al. Frequent TET2 mutations in systemic mastocytosis: clinical, KITD816V and FIP1L1-PDGFRA correlates. Leukemia 2009; 23(5):900–4.

54. Soucie E, Hanssens K, Mercher T, et al. In aggressive forms of mastocytosis, TET2 loss cooperates with c-KITD816V to transform mast cells. Blood 2012; 120(24):4846–9.

55. Jawhar M, Schwaab J, Schnittger S, et al. Molecular profiling of myeloid progenitor cells in multi-mutated advanced systemic mastocytosis identifies KIT D816V as a distinct and late event. Leukemia 2015;29(5):1115–22.

56. Traina F, Visconte V, Jankowska AM, et al. Single nucleotide polymorphism array lesions, TET2, DNMT3A, ASXL1 and CBL mutations are present in systemic mastocytosis. PLoS One 2012;7(8):e43090.

57. Schwaab J, Schnittger S, Sotlar K, et al. Comprehensive mutational profiling in advanced systemic mastocytosis. Blood 2013;122(14):2460–6.

58. Damaj G, Joris M, Chandesris O, et al. ASXL1 but not TET2 mutations adversely impact overall survival of patients suffering systemic mastocytosis with associated clonal hematologic non-mast-cell diseases. PLoS One 2014;9(1):e85362.

59. Wilson TM, Maric I, Simakova O, et al. Clonal analysis of NRAS activating mutations in KIT-D816V systemic mastocytosis. Haematologica 2011;96(3):459–63.

60. Hanssens K, Brenet F, Agopian J, et al. SRSF2-p95 hotspot mutation is highly associated with advanced forms of mastocytosis and mutations in epigenetic regulator genes. Haematologica 2014;99(5):830–5.

61. Jawhar M, Schwaab J, Schnittger S, et al. Additional mutations in SRSF2, ASXL1 and/or RUNX1 identify a high-risk group of patients with KIT D816V(+) advanced systemic mastocytosis. Leukemia 2016;30(1):136–43.

62. Valent P, Akin C, Escribano L, et al. Standards and standardization in mastocytosis: consensus statements on diagnostics, treatment recommendations and response criteria. Eur J Clin Invest 2007;37(6):435–53.

63. Akin C. Molecular diagnosis of mast cell disorders: a paper from the 2005 William Beaumont Hospital Symposium on Molecular Pathology. J Mol Diagn 2006; 8(4):412–9.

64. Erben P, Schwaab J, Metzgeroth G, et al. The KIT D816V expressed allele burden for diagnosis and disease monitoring of systemic mastocytosis. Ann Hematol 2014;93(1):81–8.

65. Kristensen T, Broesby-Olsen S, Vestergaard H, et al, Mastocytosis Centre Odense University Hospital (MastOUH). Circulating KIT D816V mutation-positive non-mast cells in peripheral blood are characteristic of indolent systemic mastocytosis. Eur J Haematol 2012;89(1):42–6.

66. Hoermann G, Gleixner KV, Dinu GE, et al. The KIT D816V allele burden predicts survival in patients with mastocytosis and correlates with the WHO type of the disease. Allergy 2014;69(6):810–3.

67. Valent P, Akin C, Sperr WR, et al. Mastocytosis: pathology, genetics, and current options for therapy. Leuk Lymphoma 2005;46(1):35–48.

68. Sotlar K. c-kit mutational analysis in paraffin material. Methods Mol Biol 2013; 999:59–78.

69. Corless CL, Harrell P, Lacouture M, et al. Allele-specific polymerase chain reaction for the imatinib-resistant KIT D816V and D816F mutations in mastocytosis and acute myelogenous leukemia. J Mol Diagn 2006;8(5):604–12.

70. Tan A, Westerman D, McArthur GA, et al. Sensitive detection of KIT D816V in patients with mastocytosis. Clin Chem 2006;52(12):2250–7.

71. Kristensen T, Vestergaard H, Bindslev-Jensen C, et al. Mastocytosis Centre OUH. Sensitive KIT D816V mutation analysis of blood as a diagnostic test in mastocytosis. Am J Hematol 2014;89(5):493–8.

72. Schumacher JA, Elenitoba-Johnson KS, Lim MS. Detection of the c-kit D816V mutation in systemic mastocytosis by allele-specific PCR. J Clin Pathol 2008; 61(1):109–14.

73. Kristensen T, Vestergaard H, Moller MB. Improved detection of the KIT D816V mutation in patients with systemic mastocytosis using a quantitative and highly sensitive real-time qPCR assay. J Mol Diagn 2011;13(2):180–8.

74. Valent P, Escribano L, Broesby-Olsen S, et al. Proposed diagnostic algorithm for patients with suspected mastocytosis: a proposal of the European Competence Network on Mastocytosis. Allergy 2014;69(10):1267–74.

75. Kristensen T, Broesby-Olsen S, Vestergaard H, et al. KIT D816V mutation-positive cell fractions in lesional skin biopsies from adults with systemic mastocytosis. Dermatology 2013;226(3):233–7.

76. Jensen RT. Gastrointestinal abnormalities and involvement in systemic mastocytosis. Hematol Oncol Clin North Am 2000;14(3):579–623.

77. Wimazal F, Schwarzmeier J, Sotlar K, et al. Splenic mastocytosis: report of two cases and detection of the transforming somatic C-KIT mutation D816V. Leuk Lymphoma 2004;45(4):723–9.

78. Sotlar K, Marafioti T, Griesser H, et al. Detection of c-kit mutation Asp 816 to Val in microdissected bone marrow infiltrates in a case of systemic mastocytosis associated with chronic myelomonocytic leukaemia. Mol Pathol 2000;53(4): 188–93.

79. Greiner G, Gurbisz M, Ratzinger F, et al. Digital PCR: a sensitive and precise method for KIT D816V quantification in mastocytosis. Clin Chem 2017;64(3): 547–55.

80. Arock M, Sotlar K, Akin C, et al. KIT mutation analysis in mast cell neoplasms: recommendations of the European Competence Network on Mastocytosis. Leukemia 2015;29(6):1223–32.

81. Valent P, Akin C, Arock M, et al. Definitions, criteria and global classification of mast cell disorders with special reference to mast cell activation syndromes: a consensus proposal. Int Arch Allergy Immunol 2012;157(3):215–25.

82. Kristensen T, Vestergaard H, Bindslev-Jensen C, et al. Prospective evaluation of the diagnostic value of sensitive KIT D816V mutation analysis of blood in adults with suspected systemic mastocytosis. Allergy 2017;72(11):1737–43.

83. Frost MJ, Ferrao PT, Hughes TP, et al. Juxtamembrane mutant V560GKit is more sensitive to Imatinib (STI571) compared with wild-type c-kit whereas the kinase domain mutant D816VKit is resistant. Mol Cancer Ther 2002;1(12):1115–24.

84. Lasota J. Not all c-kit mutations can be corrected by imatinib. Lab Invest 2007; 87(4):317.

85. Lim KH, Pardanani A, Butterfield JH, et al. Cytoreductive therapy in 108 adults with systemic mastocytosis: outcome analysis and response prediction during treatment with interferon-alpha, hydroxyurea, imatinib mesylate or 2-chlorodeoxyadenosine. Am J Hematol 2009;84(12):790–4.

86. Droogendijk HJ, Kluin-Nelemans HJ, van Doormaal JJ, et al. Imatinib mesylate in the treatment of systemic mastocytosis: a phase II trial. Cancer 2006;107(2): 345–51.

87. Vega-Ruiz A, Cortes JE, Sever M, et al. Phase II study of imatinib mesylate as therapy for patients with systemic mastocytosis. Leuk Res 2009;33(11):1481–4.

88. Pagano L, Valentini CG, Caira M, et al. Advanced mast cell disease: an Italian Hematological Multicenter experience. Int J Hematol 2008;88(5):483–8.

89. Hoffmann KM, Moser A, Lohse P, et al. Successful treatment of progressive cutaneous mastocytosis with imatinib in a 2-year-old boy carrying a somatic KIT mutation. Blood 2008;112(5):1655–7.

90. Alvarez-Twose I, Gonzalez P, Morgado JM, et al. Complete response after imatinib mesylate therapy in a patient with well-differentiated systemic mastocytosis. J Clin Oncol 2012;30(12):e126–9.

91. Mital A, Piskorz A, Lewandowski K, et al. A case of mast cell leukaemia with exon 9 KIT mutation and good response to imatinib. Eur J Haematol 2011; 86(6):531–5.

92. Foster R, Griffith R, Ferrao P, et al. Molecular basis of the constitutive activity and STI571 resistance of Asp816Val mutant KIT receptor tyrosine kinase. J Mol Graph Model 2004;23(2):139–52.

93. Georgin-Lavialle S, Lhermitte L, Suarez F, et al. Mast cell leukemia: identification of a new c-Kit mutation, dup(501-502), and response to masitinib, a c-Kit tyrosine kinase inhibitor. Eur J Haematol 2012;89(1):47–52.

94. Fabbro D, Ruetz S, Bodis S, et al. PKC412–a protein kinase inhibitor with a broad therapeutic potential. Anticancer Drug Des 2000;15(1):17–28.

95. Growney JD, Clark JJ, Adelsperger J, et al. Activation mutations of human c-KIT resistant to imatinib mesylate are sensitive to the tyrosine kinase inhibitor PKC412. Blood 2005;106(2):721–4.

96. Gallogly MM, Lazarus HM. Midostaurin: an emerging treatment for acute myeloid leukemia patients. J Blood Med 2016;7:73–83.

97. Gotlib J, Kluin-Nelemans HC, George TI, et al. Efficacy and safety of midostaurin in advanced systemic mastocytosis. N Engl J Med 2016;374(26):2530–41.

98. Jawhar M, Schwaab J, Naumann N, et al. Response and progression on midostaurin in advanced systemic mastocytosis: KIT D816V and other molecular markers. Blood 2017;130(2):137–45.

99. Verstovsek S, Akin C, Manshouri T, et al. Effects of AMN107, a novel aminopyrimidine tyrosine kinase inhibitor, on human mast cells bearing wild-type or mutated codon 816 c-kit. Leuk Res 2006;30(11):1365–70.

100. Shah NP, Lee FY, Luo R, et al. Dasatinib (BMS-354825) inhibits KITD816V, an imatinib-resistant activating mutation that triggers neoplastic growth in most patients with systemic mastocytosis. Blood 2006;108(1):286–91.

101. Hochhaus A, Baccarani M, Giles FJ, et al. Nilotinib in patients with systemic mastocytosis: analysis of the phase 2, open-label, single-arm nilotinib registration study. J Cancer Res Clin Oncol 2015;141(11):2047–60.

102. Jin B, Ding K, Pan J. Ponatinib induces apoptosis in imatinib-resistant human mast cells by dephosphorylating mutant D816V KIT and silencing beta-catenin signaling. Mol Cancer Ther 2014;13(5):1217–30.
103. Gleixner KV, Peter B, Blatt K, et al. Synergistic growth-inhibitory effects of ponatinib and midostaurin (PKC412) on neoplastic mast cells carrying KIT D816V. Haematologica 2013;98(9):1450–7.
104. Evans EK, Gardino AK, Kim JL, et al. A precision therapy against cancers driven by KIT/PDGFRA mutations. Sci Transl Med 2017;9(414) [pii:eaao1690].
105. DeAngelo DJ, Quiery AT, Radia D, et al. Clinical activity in a phase 1 study of Blu-285, a potent, highly-selective inhibitor of KIT D816V in advanced systemic mastocytosis (AdvSM). Blood 2017;130:2.
106. Dubreuil P, Letard S, Ciufolini M, et al. Masitinib (AB1010), a potent and selective tyrosine kinase inhibitor targeting KIT. PLoS One 2009;4(9):e7258.
107. Paul C, Sans B, Suarez F, et al. Masitinib for the treatment of systemic and cutaneous mastocytosis with handicap: a phase 2a study. Am J Hematol 2010;85(12):921–5.
108. Hermine O, Lortholary O, Leventhal PS, et al. Case-control cohort study of patients' perceptions of disability in mastocytosis. PLoS One 2008;3(5):e2266.
109. Lortholary O, Chandesris MO, Bulai Livideanu C, et al. Masitinib for treatment of severely symptomatic indolent systemic mastocytosis: a randomised, placebo-controlled, phase 3 study. Lancet 2017;389(10069):612–20.
110. Bai Y, Bandara G, Ching Chan E, et al. Targeting the KIT activating switch control pocket: a novel mechanism to inhibit neoplastic mast cell proliferation and mast cell activation. Leukemia 2013;27(2):278–85.
111. Schneeweiss MA, Peter B, Blatt K, et al. The multi-kinase inhibitor DCC-2618 inhibits proliferation and survival of neoplastic mast cells and other cell types involved in systemic mastocytosis. Blood 2016;128:1965.

Gastrointestinal Involvement in Mast Cell Activation Disorders

Fred H. Hsieh, MD

KEYWORDS

- Systemic mastocytosis • Mast cell activation syndrome
- Mast cell activation disorder • Gastrointestinal symptoms • Mast cell disease
- Monoclonal mast cell activation syndrome • Monoclonal mast cell activation disorder

KEY POINTS

- Gastrointestinal involvement in systemic mastocytosis is considered common, and gastrointestinal symptoms may be more likely to be triggered by mast cell–derived mediators compared with pathologic mast cell infiltration of gastrointestinal tissues.
- Both the presence of gastrointestinal symptoms and a response of gastrointestinal symptoms to anti–mast cell mediator therapy is considered qualifying criteria in the current diagnostic schema of the idiopathic mast cell activation syndrome.
- A variety of anti–mast cell mediator therapies have been proposed to alleviate the gastrointestinal symptoms attributed to systemic mastocytosis and the idiopathic mast cell activation syndrome.

INTRODUCTION

Gastrointestinal (GI) symptoms have long been recognized in patients with systemic mastocytosis. The attribution of GI symptoms in patients with clonal or monoclonal mast cell activation syndromes (MMCAS) or the evolving syndrome or constellation of symptoms attributed to the idiopathic mast cell activation syndrome (MCAS) is largely inferred from the presence of well-documented GI symptoms and GI involvement in patients with systemic mastocytosis. It is important to recognize that in systemic mastocytosis, especially in mastocytosis patients with biopsy-proven disease fulfilling current World Health Organization diagnostic criteria, the mast cells are intrinsically abnormal; that is, the mast cells have the activating KIT D816V or other KIT

Disclosure Statement: The corresponding author has no relationship with a commercial company that has a direct financial interest in the subject matter or materials discussed in this article or with a company making a competing product.
Allergy and Immunology, Respiratory Institute, Cleveland Clinic, 9500 Euclid Avenue, A90, Cleveland, OH 44195, USA
E-mail address: hsiehf@ccf.org

mutations and/or a variety of other somatic cell mutations that may influence mast cell survival, proliferation, activation, and function.[1,2] It cannot be automatically assumed that patients with clonal or MMCAS (with a presumably lower level or total body load of abnormal mast cells) or with the idiopathic MCAS (where the mast cells have to date been largely identified to have a normal immunophenotype and normal cytology and c-KIT genetics) would necessarily have the same symptom complex involving any organ system, including the GI tract, as patients with systemic mastocytosis. Because GI involvement with systemic mastocytosis has been the subject of several thorough reviews,[3–6] this article briefly reviews the GI involvement with systemic mastocytosis to serve in comparison with GI involvement reported in patients with mast cell activation disorders, such as the MMCAS, and those symptoms attributed to the idiopathic MCAS.

GASTROINTESTINAL INVOLVEMENT IN SYSTEMIC MASTOCYTOSIS

The occurrence of GI symptoms in patients with systemic mastocytosis has been documented since the 1960s and the frequency of GI symptoms in patients with mastocytosis ranges from 20% to 100%, with the early mastocytosis case series documenting fewer GI-related symptoms and studies in the last 20 years or so reporting more GI symptomatology; in some studies the frequency of GI symptoms is as high as skin manifestations.[5–16] The symptoms can be severe and debilitating and are associated with a decreased quality of life.[8] A large number of GI symptoms have been attributed to systemic mastocytosis (**Table 1**). The occurrence of GI symptoms does not seem to differ based on age of onset.[8,17]

There are at least two pathophysiologic mechanisms proposed by which mastocytosis leads to GI symptoms: direct mast cell infiltration of the GI tract, and the downstream effect of mast cell mediators on the gut. Direct involvement of the GI tract by abnormal mast cells could certainly be responsible for GI symptoms and is a likely factor in some number of patients.[18,19] However, recent studies suggest that the frequency of GI symptoms apparently does not seem to correlate with the presence of the KIT D816V mutation, the absolute value of serum tryptase, or histologic findings of mast cell infiltration in the GI biopsies.[8] Indeed, there may even be an inverse correlation between the presence of the KIT D816V mutation and a high diarrhea score.[8] This suggests that perhaps a significant component of GI symptoms are related to the release of mast cell mediators, such as histamine or prostaglandins, and some studies have implicated GI peptides, such as gastrin, neurotensin, substance P, or vasoactive intestinal peptide, as also playing a role.[7,20,21] It is not clearly established whether the mediators triggering GI symptoms are derived directly from the mast cells localized to the GI tract mediators derived from mast cells at distant sites away from the GI tract.

GI involvement in mastocytosis is markedly heterogeneous with distinct variations as to the specific symptoms and severity of any given symptom with any given individual. Abdominal pain may be caused in large part by dyspepsia and peptic ulcer disease, which is associated with increased gastric acid secretion in a subset of patients and may respond to H_2 antagonists.[7] Multiple studies have suggested that patients with mastocytosis are at higher risk for gastroduodenal ulcers.[7,8,11] The pathogenesis of diarrhea in mastocytosis is also unclear, with contributions from gastric hypersecretion or prostaglandin D_2 overproduction postulated.[7,20] Malabsorption in systemic mastocytosis is rare and is not associated with pancreatic abnormalities; it may be related to small intestinal dysfunction and, again, possibly gastric hyperacidity.[6,22] Additional GI findings in systemic mastocytosis are detailed in **Table 2**.[3,5,6,8,23,24]

Table 1
Gastrointestinal symptoms reported in patients with systemic mastocytosis

Clinical Symptom (% Patients with Reported Symptom)	Demis,[9] 1963, n = 113	Mutter et al,[10] 1963, n = 29	Webb et al,[14] 1982, n = 26	Yam et al,[16] 1986, n = 13	Cherner et al,[7] 1988, n = 16	Travis et al,[12] 1988, n = 58	Horan et al,[54] 1990, n = 21	Pagano et al,[13] 2008, n = 24	Lim et al,[15] 2009, n = 342	Sokol et al,[8] 2013, n = 83	Doyle et al,[28] 2014, n = 24
Any GI symptom	—	—	—	—	—	—	—	—	65	59	—
Abdominal pain	23	48	40	46	80	35	81	17	—	27	33
Nausea and/or vomiting	23	45	28	31	—	21	57	17	—	23	25
Diarrhea	23	28	40	54	63	24	67	8	—	34	75
GI bleeding	23	24	—	8	—	7	5	—	—	19	—
Peptic ulcer disease	4	14	24	31	44	36	24	17	—	11	—
Malabsorption	—	—	—	—	25	5	24	—	—	—	—
Bloating	—	—	—	—	—	—	—	—	—	33	8
Hepatomegaly	12	83	45	77	—	41	38	46	27	—	—
Splenomegaly	11	86	50	62	—	48	19	50	37	—	—

Table 2
Gastrointestinal abnormalities reported in systemic mastocytosis

Location	Features
Esophagus	Esophagitis Esophageal stricture Esophageal varices Lower esophageal sphincter dysfunction
Stomach	Acid hypersecretion Peptic ulcer disease Gastritis Altered motility "Urticarial" lesions
Small intestine	Dilated small bowel Villous atrophy or blunting Malabsorption Mesenteric thickening Nodular mucosal densities
Large intestine	Nodular densities Polypoid lesions Intestinal telangiectasias Steatorrhea
Liver	Elevated liver function tests Hepatomegaly Portal hypertension Infiltration and liver stiffness Ascites Portal venopathy Budd-Chiari syndrome
Spleen	Splenomegaly Hypersplenism Splenic infarct
Lymph nodes	Lymphadenopathy: retroperitoneal, periportal, mesenteric

Upper and lower endoscopies are often performed with biopsies in the work-up of patients with suspected mastocytosis. Endoscopic findings may include the appearance of mucosal erythema, mucosal nodules, pigmented areas, thickened folds, and ulcerations, or may appear visually normal.[19,25,26] There remains an urgent need for additional rigorous and quantitative diagnostic criteria in the evaluation of all mast cell activation disorders, but even in the histologic evaluation of GI biopsies in systemic mastocytosis the findings are not necessarily straightforward, because mucosal mast cell quantitation in pathologic studies has reported increased, normal, or even decreased numbers of mast cells in patients with mastocytosis compared with control subjects.[8,18,27–32] Indeed, two of the more recent comprehensive pathologic studies of GI involvement in systemic mastocytosis vary significantly with regards to GI mast cell expansion in mastocytosis (**Table 3**).[8,27] The most commonly involved sites in the GI tract are the colon and ileum, with the stomach less commonly involved and the esophagus rarely involved.[28] Histologic features that can suggest a diagnosis of systemic mastocytosis in comparison with other disorders where there may a local GI mast cell tissue expansion, such as with eosinophilic GI disease, parasitic disease, and inflammatory bowel disease, include spindle-shaped mast cells in large aggregates or sheets; coexpression of CD25 on mast cells; diffuse membranous staining of KIT; and a mast cell/inflammatory cell ratio that favors mast cells (**Table 4**).[3,5,8,28]

Table 3
Recent studies quantitating mast cells in the GI tract

Anatomic Location	Hahn & Hornick,[27] 2007[a] Normal	Mastocytosis	Sokol et al,[8] 2013[b] Normal	Mastocytosis
Stomach	12 (5–21)	57 (24–90)	17.9 ± 1.8	20.5 ± 5.1
Duodenum	27 (4–51)	175 (74–339)	24.1 ± 2.7	40.3 ± 6.1
Ileum	32 (21–40)		28.4 ± 2.7	45.7 ± 3.5
Colon	21 (10–31)	209 (110–301)	14.4 ± 3.1	45.1 ± 8.8

[a] Mean/high-power field (range).
[b] Mean number of mast cells counted on five fields/high-power field.

GASTROINTESTINAL INVOLVEMENT IN THE MONOCLONAL MAST CELL ACTIVATION SYNDROME (MMCAS)

MMCAS is a term used to described patients with symptoms suggestive of mast cell activation and who do not have cutaneous findings of mastocytosis (ie, no maculopapular cutaneous mastocytosis or urticarial pigmentosa) but are found to have the KIT D816V mutation or mast cells with an aberrant immunophenotype (ie, CD2/CD25+ mast cells) in the bone marrow. These patients generally have baseline serum tryptase levels less than 20 ng/mL, have a low burden of mast cells in the marrow without immunophenotypically abnormal mast cell aggregates, and thus may have one or more World Health Organization criteria for the diagnosis of systemic mastocytosis without meeting the full diagnostic criteria for the diagnosis of systemic mastocytosis.[33] Initial reports of MMCAS included subjects who had unexplained hypotension after hymenoptera stings with negative testing for hymenoptera-specific IgE or syncopal episodes accompanied by one or more symptoms suggestive of mast cell degranulation, including the GI symptoms of abdominal pain and diarrhea.[33,34] Subsequent case reports of subjects diagnosed with MMCAS have reported multisystem reactions including hypotension plus cutaneous, respiratory, cardiovascular, and GI symptoms,[35,36] although in one report the criteria used to define MMCAS was not entirely clear.[36]

Outside of these reports there have not been extensive retrospective series describing the clinical phenotype of patients with MMCAS using uniform diagnostic criteria and no prospective reports of any significant number of patients with MMCAS with respect to natural history and disease progression. There have not been significant numbers of cases reported of MMCAS subjects who experienced multisystem

Table 4
Interpretation of GI biopsies in systemic mastocytosis

Issue	Response
Mast cell infiltrate is focal, heterogeneous, or patchy	Perform multiple biopsies, either systematic and sequential or random
Inflammatory cell infiltrates, especially eosinophils, can mask the mast cell infiltrate	Quantitate the mast cells and inflammatory cells; in mastocytosis, the mast cell/inflammatory cell infiltrate favors mast cells
CD25 coexpression is variable on mast cells	Correlate with KIT D816V status
Tryptase expression by mast cells may be weak or variable	Immunostain for CD117/c-KIT and for CD25

complaints, including GI symptoms, in the *absence* of concomitant syncope/hypotension/anaphylaxis. MMCAS subjects having the clinical presentation of venom anaphylaxis in the absence of venom-specific IgE either were not recognized as having additional mast cell–implicated clinical symptoms or were classified as having absent other mediator-related symptoms.[37,38] Based on the available clinical data it may be reasonable to find at this point in time that GI symptoms can occur in patients with MMCAS in the context of anaphylaxis with multisystem involvement (concomitant symptoms involving the cardiovascular, respiratory, skin, GI systems) but it is unclear to what extent patients with MMCAS present with GI symptoms in the absence of acute anaphylaxis.

GASTROINTESTINAL INVOLVEMENT IN THE IDIOPATHIC MAST CELL ACTIVATION SYNDROME (MCAS)

GI involvement is considered a key clinical symptom in the idiopathic MCAS. The current working criteria for diagnosing MCAS includes typical clinical symptoms; an increase in serum total tryptase by at least 20% higher than baseline + 2 ng/mL within 4 hours of a symptomatic event; and a documented clinical response of clinical symptoms to a mast cell targeting therapy, such as an H_1 or H_2 receptor blocker or cromolyn sodium. Included in the typical clinical symptoms category for diagnosis are GI symptoms, such as abdominal cramping, vomiting, and diarrhea.[39] Although not explicitly articulated in the consensus diagnostic criteria, it is assumed that the appropriate consideration or studies have been performed to exclude the possibility of a clonal disorder, such as systemic mastocytosis or MMCAS. As experience with MCAS has evolved, proposed refinements to the MCAS diagnostic criteria include an understanding of the episodic nature of the clinical symptoms consistent with mast cell activation; use of alternative tests to total serum tryptase, such as the assay of urinary histamine or prostaglandin metabolites during/after symptomatic episodes; and a requirement that there should be at least two independent measurements of elevated mast cell mediators documented with clinical symptoms.[40,41]

The evolving nature of the idiopathic MCAS diagnostic criteria is an important issue because various investigators have used different criteria to report their respective case series.[39–43] Given that one diagnostic criteria includes the presence of episodic symptoms consistent with mast cell activation, there should be some consensus as to which symptoms from the GI standpoint should be included to fulfill this criteria. Some authors have included symptoms self-reported at baseline in addition to symptoms reported with acute attacks; the appropriateness of including baseline versus acute symptoms is not resolved.[41] Some authors include GI symptoms that occur specifically during an episode of anaphylaxis, so it is not clear that GI symptoms would be reported in the absence of frank anaphylaxis. Some authors have specifically excluded an irritable bowel syndrome diagnosis or irritable bowel syndrome symptoms as a mast cell activation criterion; other authors include irritable bowel-like symptoms.[43,44] Regardless, there seems to be a rough consensus among the limited reported case series available that at least abdominal pain and cramping (from 22%–100% of cases), diarrhea (18%–67% of cases), and nausea and vomiting (25%–90%) should be included (**Table 5**).[36,43–45] Other symptoms, such as bloating (44%–100%) and reflux (44%–50%), could be considered given that patients with biopsy-proven systemic mastocytosis may also report these symptoms. Such symptoms as constipation, constipation alternating with diarrhea, dysphagia, and other findings such as abnormalities in the liver enzymes, bilirubin, or hepatomegaly and splenomegaly, likely require further investigation and replication. It is unclear that it is appropriate to

Table 5
Gastrointestinal symptoms reported in patients with the idiopathic mast cell activation syndrome

Clinical Symptom (% Patients with Reported Symptom)	Álvarez-Twose et al.[45] 2010, In-between Episodes, n = 32	Acute Episodes, n = 32	Molderings et al.[36] 2010, n = 20[a]	Hamilton et al.[44] 2011, n = 18	Ravi et al.[61] 2014, n = 25	Afrin et al.[43] 2017, n = 413[a]
Any GI symptom	16	35	—	—	—	—
Abdominal pain/cramping	—	22	100	94	52	48
Diarrhea	—	18	60	67	48	27
Nausea and vomiting	—	25	—	—	—	57
Nausea alone	—	—	90	33	—	—
Bloating	—	—	100	44	—	—
Reflux	—	—	—	44	—	50
Constipation	—	—	20	—	—	14
Diarrhea alternating with constipation	—	—	5	—	—	36
Dysphagia	—	—	—	—	—	35
Hepatic involvement						
Elevated liver enzymes	—	—	20	—	—	—
Elevated bilirubin	—	—	10	—	—	—
Organomegaly						
Hepatomegaly	—	—	5	—	—	—
Splenomegaly	—	—	10	—	—	—

[a] These studies use diagnostic criteria for mast cell activation disorders that substantively differs from the other studies listed.

assume that once the diagnosis of MCAS is made then any or all symptoms localized to the GI tract, or any other organ system for that matter, can solely be attributable to mast cell disease.

Endoscopic evaluation with mucosal biopsies is often performed in patients with GI symptoms undergoing evaluation for possible MCAS. In general, MCAS is not associated with any specific visible endoscopic abnormalities. A pathology study comparing mast cell mucosal counts from colonic biopsies of 10 subjects with idiopathic MCAS versus 100 subjects with diarrhea-predominant IBS versus 100 asymptomatic subjects found no increase in mean mast cell counts in the MCAS cohort (28 mast cells/high-power field; range, 14–48) versus the asymptomatic cohort (26 mast cells/high-power field; range, 11–55), although the degree or extent of GI symptoms in this particular MCAS group was not discussed.[28] Mast cells normally traffic to the GI tract and this normal broad variation in mast cell density in the colonic mucosa in asymptomatic individuals should be taken into consideration before claiming that GI mucosal mast cells are increased in chronic diarrhea or any other condition.[46] Regardless, the available evidence suggests that the pathogenesis of GI symptoms in MCAS is presumably caused by the effect of mast cell mediators on the GI tract because there is currently no study demonstrating immunophenotypically abnormal mast cells, abnormal mast cell positioning, or a substantial increase or infiltration of mast cells in the GI tract of patients with MCAS.

TREATMENT OF GASTROINTESTINAL SYMPTOMS IN MAST CELL ACTIVATION DISORDERS

Treatment options for GI symptoms in systemic mastocytosis include medical therapy targeting mast cell mediators to control clinical symptoms and then cytoreductive therapy for aggressive or advanced mastocytosis disease classifications, which by directly targeting mast cells and reducing mast cell load may alleviate clinical symptoms (**Table 6**).[47] H_1 and H_2 blocker antihistamines remain the mainstay of therapy and sedating and nonsedating H_1 blockers can be used and their dose titrated based on each individual patient's severity of symptoms. In addition to being an H_1 blocker, ketotifen and desloratadine may also decrease mast cell mediator release, although ketotifen has not been shown to be superior to traditional H_1 antagonists in mastocytosis.[48–50] It may be the H_2 antagonists that provide the most GI symptom relief in systemic mastocytosis; although some earlier studies have suggested that H_1 antagonists may improve GI symptoms, a more recent double-blind, placebo-controlled study of the second-generation dual H_1 receptor/platelet activating factor antagonist rupatadine in adult mastocytosis subjects found statistically significant improvement in the treatment group for a large number of clinical symptom parameters except for GI symptoms.[50–53] Abdominal cramping and diarrhea may be responsive to oral cromolyn sodium.[54] Malabsorption may respond to cromolyn sodium and low doses of oral corticosteroids.[55] Nonsteroidal anti-inflammatory drugs (NSAIDs) could be considered in the control of GI symptoms and diarrhea, but must be considered with caution because NSAIDs can also provoke anaphylactic reactions in patients with mastocytosis.[56,57] Individual case reports suggest leukotriene antagonists may improve GI symptoms in mastocytosis.[58] Several case reports describing the administration of omalizumab in patients with mastocytosis report a reduction in anaphylactic symptoms and possibly an improvement in GI symptoms.[59,60] It must be noted that most studies suggesting drug efficacy for GI symptoms in systemic mastocytosis are derived from case reports or uncontrolled and mostly retrospective case series and randomized, controlled studies are few.

Table 6
Treatment of gastrointestinal symptoms in mast cell disease–targeting mediators

Symptom	Treatment Options
General: avoidance of triggers	Possible triggers include: Physical stimuli Emotional factors Drugs/medications Venoms and toxins
Peptic ulcer disease	H_2 antagonist antihistamines Proton pump inhibitors
Nausea, vomiting, abdominal pain, cramping	H_1 and H_2 antagonist antihistamines Proton pump inhibitors Leukotriene antagonists Cromolyn sodium Low-dose corticosteroids
Diarrhea	H_2 antagonist antihistamines Cromolyn sodium Leukotriene antagonists Low-dose corticosteroids Anticholinergic therapy
Malabsorption	Cromolyn sodium Low-dose corticosteroids

Other therapies: nonsteroidal anti-inflammatory drugs may help with abdominal pain and diarrhea; consider with caution because nonsteroidal anti-inflammatory drugs may also provoke anaphylaxis. Omalizumab: case reports suggest improvement in a variety of clinical symptoms, including GI symptoms.

To date there has not been any published randomized, controlled trials for the treatment of any specific clinical aspect of idiopathic MCAS. Because a subjectively defined positive clinical response to anti–mast cell mediator therapy is a diagnostic criterion of idiopathic MCAS, there is a potential impediment to designing clinical trials of MCAS free from bias because a response to therapy is required to make the diagnosis in the first place.[41,42] Given this caveat, case series describing idiopathic MCAS report marked improvement in abdominal symptoms (82% response, 14/17 patients) with antimediator therapy with responses sustained with continuous medical therapy for up to 4 years.[44] In patients with idiopathic MCAS diagnosed based on elevated urinary prostaglandin metabolites treated with acetylsalicylic acid at doses from 81 mg to 500 mg daily, a decrease in urinary prostaglandin excretion was noted with improvement in clinical symptoms, although several subjects had GI symptoms caused by chronic NSAID therapy.[61]

SUMMARY

GI symptoms are commonly described in patients with systemic mastocytosis and idiopathic MCAS. Although GI biopsy studies have shown that some patients with systemic mastocytosis have increased mast cell numbers and abnormal immunophenotypic or structural abnormalities, the GI pathology specimens of other patients with mastocytosis contain only more subtle findings, thus suggesting that the GI symptoms may be largely caused by the effect of mast cell mediators on the GI tract. The published case series of patients with MMCAS suggest that GI symptoms in patients with MMCAS occur largely in the context of acute anaphylaxis. There remains some controversy as to what GI symptoms should be attributed to MCAS. Further studies are urgently needed in systemic mastocytosis and idiopathic MCAS to confirm and develop treatment options in mast cell patients.

REFERENCES

1. Valent P, Akin C, Hartmann K, et al. Advances in the classification and treatment of mastocytosis: current status and outlook toward the future. Cancer Res 2017; 77(6):1261–70.
2. Valent P, Akin C, Metcalfe DD. Mastocytosis: 2016 updated WHO classification and novel emerging treatment concepts. Blood 2017;129(11):1420–7.
3. Doyle LA, Hornick JL. Pathology of extramedullary mastocytosis. Immunol Allergy Clin North Am 2014;34(2):323–39.
4. Carter MC, Metcalfe DD, Komarow HD. Mastocytosis. Immunol Allergy Clin North Am 2014;34(1):181–96.
5. Sokol H, Georgin-Lavialle S, Grandpeix-Guyodo C, et al. Gastrointestinal involvement and manifestations in systemic mastocytosis. Inflamm Bowel Dis 2010; 16(7):1247–53.
6. Jensen RT. Gastrointestinal abnormalities and involvement in systemic mastocytosis. Hematol Oncol Clin North Am 2000;14(3):579–623.
7. Cherner JA, Jensen RT, Dubois A, et al. Gastrointestinal dysfunction in systemic mastocytosis: a prospective study. Gastroenterology 1988;95(3):657–67.
8. Sokol H, Georgin-Lavialle S, Canioni D, et al. Gastrointestinal manifestations in mastocytosis: a study of 83 patients. J Allergy Clin Immunol 2013;132(4): 866–73.e1-3.
9. Demis DJ. The mastocytosis syndrome: clinical and biological studies. Ann Intern Med 1963;59:194–206.
10. Mutter RD, Tannenbaum M, Ultmann JE. Systemic mast cell disease. Ann Intern Med 1963;59:887–906.
11. Horan RF, Austen KF. Systemic mastocytosis: retrospective review of a decade's clinical experience at the Brigham and Women's Hospital. J Invest Dermatol 1991;96(3 Suppl):5S–14S.
12. Travis WD, Li CY, Bergstralh EJ, et al. Systemic mast cell disease. Analysis of 58 cases and literature review. Medicine (Baltimore) 1988;67(6):345–68. Available at: http://www.ncbi.nlm.nih.gov/pubmed/3054417.
13. Pagano L, Valentini CG, Caira M, et al. Advanced mast cell disease: an Italian Hematological Multicenter experience. Int J Hematol 2008;88(5):483–8.
14. Webb TA, Li CY, Yam LT. Systemic mast cell disease: a clinical and hematopathologic study of 26 cases. Cancer 1982;49(5):927–38. Available at: http://www.ncbi.nlm.nih.gov/pubmed/6174198.
15. Lim KH, Tefferi A, Lasho TL, et al. Systemic mastocytosis in 342 consecutive adults: survival studies and prognostic factors. Blood 2009;113(23):5727–36.
16. Yam LT, Chan CH, Li CY. Hepatic involvement in systemic mast cell disease. Am J Med 1986;80(5):819–26.
17. Lanternier F, Cohen-Akenine A, Palmerini F, et al. Phenotypic and genotypic characteristics of mastocytosis according to the age of onset. PLoS One 2008;3(4): e1906.
18. Bedeir A, Jukic DM, Wang L, et al. Systemic mastocytosis mimicking inflammatory bowel disease: a case report and discussion of gastrointestinal pathology in systemic mastocytosis. Am J Surg Pathol 2006;30(11):1478–82.
19. Scolapio JS, Wolfe J 3rd, Malavet P, et al. Endoscopic findings in systemic mastocytosis. Gastrointest Endosc 1996;44(5):608–10.

20. Awad JA, Morrow JD, Roberts LJ 2nd. Detection of the major urinary metabolite of prostaglandin D2 in the circulation: demonstration of elevated levels in patients with disorders of systemic mast cell activation. J Allergy Clin Immunol 1994;93(5): 817–24.
21. Wesley JR, Vinik AI, O'Dorisio TM, et al. A new syndrome of symptomatic cutaneous mastocytoma producing vasoactive intestinal polypeptide. Gastroenterology 1982;82(5):963–7.
22. Hirschowitz BI, Groarke JF. Effect of cimetidine on gastric hypersecretion and diarrhea in systemic mastocytosis. Ann Intern Med 1979;90(5):769–71.
23. Mican JM, Di Bisceglie AM, Fong TL, et al. Hepatic involvement in mastocytosis: clinicopathologic correlations in 41 cases. Hepatology 1995;22(4 PART 1): 1163–70.
24. Adolf S, Millonig G, Seitz HK, et al. Systemic mastocytosis: a rare case of increased liver stiffness. Case Reports Hepatol 2012;2012:728172.
25. Philpott H, Gow P, Crowley P, et al. Systemic mastocytosis: a gastroenterological perspective. Frontline Gastroenterol 2012;3(1):5–9.
26. Kirsch R, Geboes K, Shepherd NA, et al. Systemic mastocytosis involving the gastrointestinal tract: clinicopathologic and molecular study of five cases. Mod Pathol 2008;21(12):1508–16.
27. Hahn HP, Hornick JL. Immunoreactivity for CD25 in gastrointestinal mucosal mast cells is specific for systemic mastocytosis. Am J Surg Pathol 2007;31(11): 1669–76.
28. Doyle LA, Sepehr GJ, Hamilton MJ, et al. A clinicopathologic study of 24 cases of systemic mastocytosis involving the gastrointestinal tract and assessment of mucosal mast cell density in irritable bowel syndrome and asymptomatic patients. Am J Surg Pathol 2014;38(6):832–43.
29. Siegert SI, Diebold J, Ludolph-Hauser D, et al. Are gastrointestinal mucosal mast cells increased in patients with systemic mastocytosis? Am J Clin Pathol 2004; 122(4):560–5.
30. Achord JL, Langford H. The effect of cimetidine and propantheline on the symptoms of a patient with systemic mastocytosis. Am J Med 1980;69(4):610–4.
31. Tebbe B, Stavropoulos PG, Krasagakis K, et al. Cutaneous mastocytosis in adults. evaluation of 14 patients with respect to systemic disease manifestations. Dermatology 1998;197(2):101–8. Available at: http://ovidsp.ovid.com/ovidweb. cgi?T=JS&PAGE=reference&D=med4&NEWS=N&AN=9732155.
32. Ferguson J, Thompson RP, Greaves MW. Intestinal mucosal mast cells: enumeration in urticaria pigmentosa and systemic mastocytosis. Br J Dermatol 1988; 119(5):573–8.
33. Akin C, Scott LM, Kocabas CN, et al. Demonstration of an aberrant mast-cell population with clonal markers in a subset of patients with "idiopathic" anaphylaxis. Blood 2007;110(7):2331–3.
34. Sonneck K, Florian S, Müllauer L, et al. Diagnostic and subdiagnostic accumulation of mast cells in the bone marrow of patients with anaphylaxis: monoclonal mast cell activation syndrome. Int Arch Allergy Immunol 2007;142(2):158–64.
35. Jagdis A, Vadas P. Omalizumab effectively prevents recurrent refractory anaphylaxis in a patient with monoclonal mast cell activation syndrome. Ann Allergy Asthma Immunol 2014;113(1):115–6.
36. Molderings GJ, Meis K, Kolck UW, et al. Comparative analysis of mutation of tyrosine kinase kit in mast cells from patients with systemic mast cell activation syndrome and healthy subjects. Immunogenetics 2010;62(11–12):721–7.

37. Zanotti R, Lombardo C, Passalacqua G, et al. Clonal mast cell disorders in patients with severe Hymenoptera venom allergy and normal serum tryptase levels. J Allergy Clin Immunol 2015;136(1):135–9.

38. Bonadonna P, Perbellini O, Passalacqua G, et al. Clonal mast cell disorders in patients with systemic reactions to Hymenoptera stings and increased serum tryptase levels. J Allergy Clin Immunol 2009;123(3):680–6.

39. Valent P, Akin C, Arock M, et al. Definitions, criteria and global classification of mast cell disorders with special reference to mast cell activation syndromes: a consensus proposal. Int Arch Allergy Immunol 2012;157(3):215–25.

40. Theoharides TC, Valent P, Akin C. Mast cells, mastocytosis, and related disorders. N Engl J Med 2015;373(2):163–72.

41. Akin C. Mast cell activation syndromes. J Allergy Clin Immunol 2017;140(2): 349–55.

42. Akin C, Valent P, Metcalfe DD. Mast cell activation syndrome: proposed diagnostic criteria. J Allergy Clin Immunol 2010;126(6):1099–104.e4.

43. Afrin LB, Self S, Menk J, et al. Characterization of mast cell activation syndrome. Am J Med Sci 2017;353(3):207–15.

44. Hamilton MJ, Hornick JL, Akin C, et al. Mast cell activation syndrome: a newly recognized disorder with systemic clinical manifestations. J Allergy Clin Immunol 2011;128(1):147–52.

45. Álvarez-Twose I, González de Olano D, Sánchez-Muñoz L, et al. Clinical, biological, and molecular characteristics of clonal mast cell disorders presenting with systemic mast cell activation symptoms. J Allergy Clin Immunol 2010;125(6): 1269–78.e2.

46. Jakate S, Demeo M, John R, et al. Mastocytic enterocolitis: increased mucosal mast cells in chronic intractable diarrhea. Arch Pathol Lab Med 2006;130(3): 362–7.

47. Escribano L, Akin C, Castells M, et al. Mastocytosis: current concepts in diagnosis and treatment. Ann Hematol 2002;81(12):677–90.

48. Klooker TK, Braak B, Koopman KE, et al. The mast cell stabiliser ketotifen decreases visceral hypersensitivity and improves intestinal symptoms in patients with irritable bowel syndrome. Gut 2010;59(9):1213–21.

49. Weller K, Maurer M. Desloratadine inhibits human skin mast cell activation and histamine release. J Invest Dermatol 2009;129(11):2723–6.

50. Kettelhut BV, Berkebile C, Bradley D, et al. A double-blind, placebo-controlled, crossover trial of ketotifen versus hydroxyzine in the treatment of pediatric mastocytosis. J Allergy Clin Immunol 1989;83(5):866–70.

51. Siebenhaar F, Fortsch A, Krause K, et al. Rupatadine improves quality of life in mastocytosis: a randomized, double-blind, placebo-controlled trial. Allergy 2013;68(7):949–52.

52. Nurmatov UB, Rhatigan E, Simons FER, et al. H $_1$-antihistamines for primary mast cell activation syndromes: a systematic review. Allergy 2015;70(9):1052–61.

53. Friedman BS, Santiago ML, Berkebile C, et al. Comparison of azelastine and chlorpheniramine in the treatment of mastocytosis. J Allergy Clin Immunol 1993;92(4):507–12.

54. Horan RF, Sheffer AL, Austen KF. Cromolyn sodium in the management of systemic mastocytosis. J Allergy Clin Immunol 1990;85(5):852–5.

55. Friedman BS, Metcalfe DD. Effects of tixocortol pivalate on gastrointestinal disease in systemic mastocytosis: a preliminary study. Clin Exp Allergy 1991; 21(2):183–8.

56. Butterfield JH. Survey of aspirin administration in systemic mastocytosis. Prostaglandins Other Lipid Mediat 2009;88(3–4):122–4.
57. Moreno-Borque R, Matito A, Álvarez-Twose I, et al. Response to celecoxib in a patient with indolent systemic mastocytosis presenting with intractable diarrhea. Ann Allergy Asthma Immunol 2015;115(5):456–7.
58. Turner PJ, Kemp AS, Rogers M, et al. Refractory symptoms successfully treated with leukotriene inhibition in a child with systemic mastocytosis. Pediatr Dermatol 2012;29(2):222–3.
59. Carter MC, Robyn JA, Bressler PB, et al. Omalizumab for the treatment of unprovoked anaphylaxis in patients with systemic mastocytosis. J Allergy Clin Immunol 2007;119(6):1550–1.
60. Lieberoth S, Thomsen SF. Cutaneous and gastrointestinal symptoms in two patients with systemic mastocytosis successfully treated with omalizumab. Case Rep Med 2015;2015:903541.
61. Ravi A, Butterfield J, Weiler CR. Mast cell activation syndrome: improved identification by combined determinations of serum tryptase and 24-hour urine 11β-prostaglandin2α. J Allergy Clin Immunol Pract 2014;2(6):775–8.

Bone Disease in Mastocytosis

Giovanni Orsolini, MD[a],*, Ombretta Viapiana, MD, PhD[a], Maurizio Rossini, MD, PhD[a], Massimiliano Bonifacio, MD[b], Roberta Zanotti, MD[b]

KEYWORDS

- Mastocytosis • Osteoporosis • Osteosclerosis • Fracture • Bone mineral density
- Bone turnover markers

KEY POINTS

- Systemic mastocytosis often involves bone, mainly as osteoporosis and fragility fractures.
- In patients with otherwise unexplained osteoporosis or fragility fractures, systemic mastocytosis should be ruled out.
- Risk for vertebral fractures is high, especially in men.
- Bone turnover markers and bone mineral density must be evaluated in each patient, and radiographs of the axial skeleton should be performed to screen for vertebral fracture.
- Traditional risk factors for osteoporosis should be corrected.
- Currently bisphosphonates are the first-line pharmacologic treatment of osteoporosis.

EPIDEMIOLOGY

Bone involvement is one of most common expressions of systemic mastocytosis (SM) in adults. The range of clinical pictures is wide: from osteoporosis with fragility fractures and poorly localized bone pain to asymptomatic osteolytic and/or focal sclerotic lesions and diffuse osteosclerosis. Despite the importance of these aspects, it has only been in the last few years that large epidemiologic studies have been published,[1–7] also supported by ever increasing extensive use of the dual-energy X-ray absorptiometry (DXA) technique, the gold standard for assessing bone mineral density (BMD).[8]

The prevalence of osteoporosis as defined by the World Health Organization (T score, standard deviation [SD] below the mean of young healthy adults less than -2.5)[8] in SM varies from 8% to 41% (**Fig. 1**). It must be emphasized that most of these studies included elderly patients, and this could be a possible confounder

[a] Rheumatology Unit, University of Verona, Verona, Italy; [b] Hematology Unit, University of Verona, Verona, Italy
* Corresponding author. Rheumatology Unit, Policlinico G.B. Rossi, Piazzale L. Scuro 10, Verona 37134, Italy.
E-mail address: giovanniorsolini@gmail.com

Immunol Allergy Clin N Am 38 (2018) 443–454
https://doi.org/10.1016/j.iac.2018.04.013   immunology.theclinics.com
0889-8561/18/© 2018 Elsevier Inc. All rights reserved.

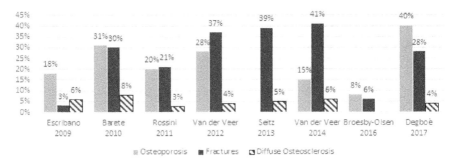

Fig. 1. Prevalence of main bone manifestation in the largest related available studies.

of the real prevalence esteem. Other possible biases could come from data obtained by the health care system, where only clinical evident fractures and osteoporosis were reported,[7] or from cohorts including a significant proportion of advanced SM (advSM).[6]

The Z score (SD less than the age- and gender-matched mean reference value) is the most appropriate parameter of bone involvement in secondary osteoporosis, as stated by the International Society for Clinical Bone Densitometry.[9] An inappropriate low bone mass in this case is defined as a Z score lower than −2.

In the authors' 2011 study on indolent SM (ISM), the prevalence of T scores defined as osteoporosis was 20%, whereas using Z score less than −2 was 9% in women and 28% in men.[3] This gender difference has been reported by others,[1,5] and, interestingly, a study involving men with idiopathic osteoporosis who underwent bone biopsy found a 9% prevalence of SM.[10]

The use of Z score helps to correct the above-mentioned confounder, and it changes the proportions, showing a much higher prevalence of inappropriately low BMD in men (**Fig. 2** relative to an updated authors' cohort). Data on BMD, a surrogate of bone fragility, confirm data on vertebral fractures that are significantly more prevalent in men than women (20% vs 14%, see **Fig. 2**), as also reported in other populations.[1,3,5]

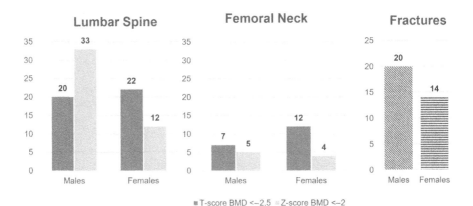

Fig. 2. Prevalence of mastocytosis-related low bone mass, osteoporosis, and fractures according to different criteria in authors' cohort. (*Adapted from* Rossini M, Zanotti R, Viapiana O, et al. Bone involvement and osteoporosis in mastocytosis. Immunol Allergy Clin N Am 2014;34(2):385; with permission.)

The prevalence, which included all types of bone involvement, in the authors' series of ISM was 36%; this is lower than that reported by Barete and colleagues[4] or Degboe and colleagues,[6] which also included advSM, which has a more extensive systemic burden and poorer prognosis. Interestingly, in the authors' experience, patients without a history of anaphylaxis showed a lower total hip Z score than patients with a history of anaphylaxis, possibly reflecting a higher diagnosis delay due to the lack of revealing symptoms.[11]

A study reporting data of a Danish cohort[2] composed of 157 patients with ISM also described a high incidence of vertebral fractures. Variables associated with fractures and thus inserted in a risk calculator were higher age, male gender, high serum C-terminal telopeptide of collagen I (CTX), lower hip T score, absence of urticaria pigmentosa (UP), and alcohol consumption.[1,3,5]

These data on UP could find its explanation in an earlier diagnosis of patients with UP and thus a lesser bone burden of disease. However, other investigators did not report the same association.[6]

A rarer bone manifestation of SM is osteosclerosis, which could be local or diffuse, with a total prevalence of the diffuse form ranging from 2.5% to 8%,[1–5,12] and with a strong predominance among women.[13] Its prevalence is probably underestimated because of the absence of symptoms and the need for whole skeleton radiographs for detection.

So far there have been no reports of fragility fractures in patients with the sclerotic ISM-related form. However, a coexistence of focal lytic and sclerotic lesions is possible.[2,4] In a study including 75 adult patients with SM, a mixed pattern was seen in 4%.[14]

A limitation in the evaluation of the bone burden of the disease lies also with the fact that almost all the available studies have a cross-sectional design. Longitudinal studies need to be carried out in order to understand the evolution of bone involvement in SM.

Another point that needs to be investigated is bone health in patients with nonclonal mast cell (MC) disorder (mast cell activation syndrome). Data on osteoporosis and fractures prevalence in this subset of MC disease are almost nonexistent, but it is possible that this population also has an increased risk of bone loss and fractures because of the effect of mediators on bone. The only data available are from Alvarez-Twose and colleagues[15] with a 10% prevalence (2 out of 20 patients) of osteoporosis compared with 24% in ISM without skin lesions and 16% of ISM with skin lesions (P = NS), but the numbers are too small to draw any conclusions.

PATHOPHYSIOLOGY

Bone loss seems to affect trabecular bone more than cortical bone, as demonstrated by a higher prevalence of osteoporosis identified at the lumbar spine than at hip (see **Fig. 2**) and by a much higher rate of vertebral rather than nonvertebral fractures. The reason of predilection for trabecular bone probably resides in direct colonization of bone marrow by MC with local effects, or the mediators may influence the type of bone more with greater metabolic activity. However, cortical bone can also be affected,[6] with data reporting a high incidence of nonvertebral fractures as well.[1]

The hypothesized mechanisms of bone loss in SM vary and could be related either to total number or to higher activity of MC.[16]

Among the mediators released by MC are histamine, heparin, tryptase, and cytokines, such as tumor necrosis factor-α, interleukin-1 (IL-1), IL-17, and IL-6, with effects on both osteoblasts and osteoclasts.[14,17–20] Increased serum levels of IL-6 have been reported to correlate with disease progression,[21] which is also associated with a higher bone burden.

Histamine is one of the distinguishing products of MC, and it is not only involved in the pathophysiology of many SM extraskeletal manifestations but also affects osteoclasts and their precursors, by autocrine and paracrine signaling.[19,20] Mice knocked-out for an enzyme key for histamine production were protected from postovariectomy bone loss and showed a reduced number of osteoclasts.[22] A positive correlation has also been reported between histamine metabolites and risk of osteoporotic manifestations.[1,5]

Male gender has been reported as a risk factor for osteoporosis and fractures in ISM,[1,3] suggesting that the mediators could act differently depending on the gender hormonal environment.

Bone histomorphometric data are scarce; however, the little evidence available reports an increased[12,23] or normal[24] number of osteoclasts. A quantitative histomorphometric evaluation applied to a large population of patients with ISM[12] found a decrease in bone trabeculae and an increase in osteoid and bone cellularity (osteoclasts and osteoblasts) that was similar in patients with or without skin involvement.

SM-induced osteoporosis shares some histomorphometric features with the much more common glucocorticoid-induced osteoporosis (GIOP). In fact, in both there is a reduction in the number and the thickness of trabeculae. However, in GIOP, osteoblasts are reduced, whereas in ISM-related osteoporosis, they are not, and bone turnover is significantly increased instead. Of great interest is that osteoclast and osteoblast numbers increase not only with the number of MC but also with the tendency of MC to create granuloma-like groups rather than to be scattered.[12]

Recently, studies on the bone marrow niche suggest a defect of bone marrow stromal cells due to either c-kit mutation of stromal cells as well, or an impaired differentiation toward the osteogenic lineage but not toward the adipogenic one.[25,26]

Even if histomorphometric analysis is the gold standard for bone metabolism evaluation, in clinical practice, serum bone turnover markers (BTM) are widely used as surrogates. Systemic bone remodeling activity is evaluated through bone formation markers, such bone alkaline phosphatase (bAP), osteocalcin and N-terminal of procollagen type I, and bone resorption markers such as CTX.

In postmenopausal osteoporosis, these markers have been shown to have a good correlation with BMD and fracture.[27] In a previous study on patients with ISM-related osteoporosis,[3] those markers were within the normal range in most of the cases, and there was no correlation with BMD Z score (**Fig. 3**). The investigators but also other researchers[12] failed to find a predictive value for vertebral fracture of these markers.

Conversely, another study with 45 subjects also involving advSM[11] reported increased values of CTX, deoxypyridinoline, bAP, and osteoprotegerin (OPG), although with a wide range of values probably due to the presence of both indolent and aggressive types. In fact, CTX and OPG were higher in patients with advSM rather than ISM and also correlated with serum tryptase.[11] Furthermore, a study by van der Veer and colleagues[5] identified elevated serum CTX levels as a predictive risk factor for fragility fracture and included it in their fracture risk score.

Effectively, in a recent longitudinal study in patients with ISM, the authors found that serum CTX at baseline could predict BMD change, being negatively correlated to BMD change at lumbar spine over the following 30 months (see **Fig. 3**).[28]

The correlation between tryptase, BTM, and aggressiveness of SM is in line with the hypothesis of a number-dependent effect of MC on bone metabolism. Of interest is the strong independent correlation in the population of Degboe and colleagues,[6] between bone marrow tryptase level and fragility fractures; this bone marrow level rather

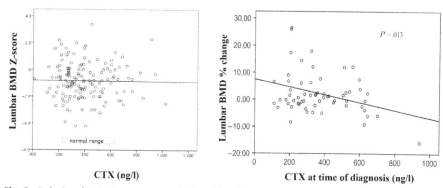

Fig. 3. Relationship between serum CTX and lumbar BMD among patients with ISM, and between baseline CTX and lumbar BMD change over 30 months after diagnosis in nonosteoporotic patients with ISM. (*Adapted from* Rossini M, Zanotti R, Viapiana O, et al. Bone involvement and osteoporosis in mastocytosis. Immunol Allergy Clin N Am 2014;34(2):385; and Artuso A, Caimmi C, Tripi G, et al. Longitudinal evaluation of bone mineral density and bone metabolism markers in patients with indolent systemic mastocytosis without osteoporosis. Calcif Tissue Int 2017;100(1):40–6; with permission.)

than the serum level could help to identify patients at higher risk of fracture and recently has also been proposed as a more reliable diagnostic tool.[29]

On the other hand, there are reports of elevated tryptase levels being associated with greater bone density in patients with SM.[30] The authors also observed in their patients with ISM that a positive correlation existed between tryptase levels, Z score BMD, and bAP, thus showing a correlation with bone formation.[31] In accordance with these data, the authors noticed that patients with diffuse osteosclerosis were characterized by very high tryptase levels and high BTM levels, reflecting the image at bone scintigraphy of a diffuse hyper-uptake (superscan).[3] It is known that MC can also stimulate osteoblasts, maybe through tryptase, and osteoblasts can thus increase production of OPG, limiting the activity of osteoclasts.[32]

The data reported above give an idea of the complexity of the pathophysiology of bone involvement in SM, with implication of both bone formation and resorption. However, the factors that determine the direction toward the osteoporotic or the osteosclerotic form still remains obscure. It is reasonable to think that the different bone phenotypes are expressions of the relative predominance of one pathway over the others or the presence or absence of permitting or inhibiting cofactors or could also be related to the total number of MC or their activation status, due to aggressiveness of the disease.

There are reports of increased OPG and RANKL in MS. There are reports of MC production of OPG and RANKL production, suggesting a strong role of this pathway in SM bone involvement[11,33]; as mentioned above, in one of these experiences,[11] OPG, BTM, and tryptase were positively correlated.

The canonical Wnt acts, together with bone morphogenetic proteins, predominantly on osteoblasts, to enhance their differentiation and activity, but also it exerts an inhibitory effect on osteoclasts.[34]

The Wnt system is constitutively activated, and thus, it is regulated by inhibitory modulators; the most known and studied are Dickkopf-1 (Dkk1) and Sclerostin (SOST).[34]

A German study showed an increase of SOST but not of Dkk1.[33] This datum is coherent with a negative effect on bone formation (with bone turnover imbalance toward bone loss), even if it is known that SOST increases with age and the SM population was older than controls in that study. In the authors' patients with ISM, the authors failed to find any difference of SOST with matched population, but did find higher Dkk1 serum levels, which correlated with parathyroid hormone, CTX, and bAP.[35] However, histomorphometric studies report a higher osteoid presence, higher cellularity, and thus higher Dkk1 seems related more to bone turnover alterations and increased number of osteoblast. Therefore, in the authors' opinion, the pathogenetic role of Wnt pathway is negligible or marginal in SM.[35,36]

CLINICAL FEATURES

Most of the patients obtain a diagnosis of SM with a delay of years from onset even if most of the time the presenting symptoms leading to diagnosis are the most evident ones, such as skin lesions (eg, maculopapular cutaneous mastocytosis) or anaphylactic reactions.[37] The principal clinical bone manifestations are fragility fractures or poorly localized bone pain that is often misdiagnosed because of the rarity of SM. This rarity is probably the reason why among male patients at time of diagnosis, 20% already have multiple vertebral deformities, typically fish-shaped in nature, as seen in GIOP or osteomalacia (**Fig. 4**). Also to be noted is that the cervical spine can be involved by vertebral fractures, a fact that is quite uncommon in primary osteoporosis.

It is important to highlight that in the Verona ISM cohort, 36% of patients presenting with a history of fractures suffered from nonvertebral ones,[3] meaning that cortical bone is also involved, and clinicians should also consider SM in unexplained nonvertebral fractures.

Bone pain is a complaint in 54% of the patients, 18% of which describe it as severe or intolerable.[38]

Concomitant osteolytic and osteosclerotic lesions are frequent and suggestive of mastocytosis bone involvement.

The clinical meaning of focal bone lesions, especially sclerotic ones, is still uncertain because of the lack of studies on their evolution over time. Similarly, the diffuse osteosclerotic type is usually asymptomatic, and its clinical implication is also still uncertain; in the authors' opinion, it might predispose a more accelerated osteoarthritis.

DIAGNOSIS

Diagnosis in the absence of anaphylactic reaction or skin lesions can be really challenging. Osteoporosis and fragility fractures are common in SM, particularly in men and patients without skin involvement.[3,5] Osteoporotic fractures are rarely not the only presenting manifestation; thus, it is crucial to investigate this possibility in otherwise unexplained fractures or osteoporosis, especially in men. In patients without typical skin lesions, the flow chart diagnostic algorithm proposed by the authors could be of help (**Fig. 5**).

In patients diagnosed with SM, it is recommended that a careful screen for bone manifestation be performed.

First, a BMD measurement at lumbar spine and femur (neck and total) by DXA should be obtained and T score and Z score should be considered according to the sex of the patient. However, there is wide variability, and half of the patients have a fragility fracture without a pathologic BMD value.[3,5] This variability limits the use of DXA as a predictor of fracture, but BMD still remains a key determinant in evaluation.[5,6] The authors usually perform a DXA scan once a year until stability is achieved and less frequently (between 12 and 24 months) thereafter in osteoporotic patients depending on the case.[39] In particular, the authors' data show that patients without

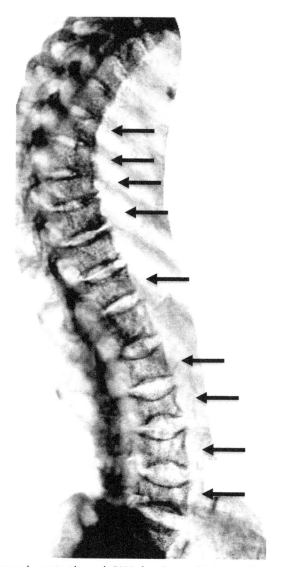

Fig. 4. Vertebral morphometry through DXA showing multiple vertebral fractures (*arrows*).

osteoporosis and with normal serum CTX do not require DXA before an interval of 2 years.[28] Thus, in osteopenic patients without particular risk factors and with normal CTX, a DXA evaluation every 24 to 36 months is deemed sufficient.

Because BMD is partially reliable for assessing bone health in SM, a total spine radiography is strongly recommended for early detection of vertebral asymptomatic fractures. A whole skeleton radiograph might be suggested to exclude other focal lytic or sclerotic lesions.

Vertebral fractures should be classified accordingly to the Genant criteria,[40] because a loss in height greater than 20% with a grade score of 3, based on the entity of height reduction: grade I from 20% to 24%, grade II from 25% to 40%, grade III greater than 40%.

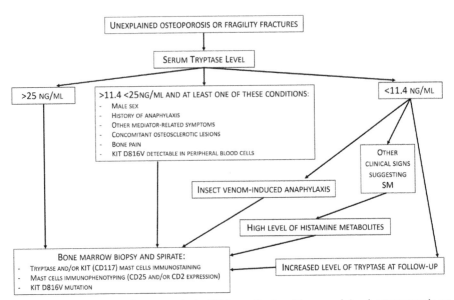

Fig. 5. Diagnostic algorithm to exclude SM in patients with unexplained osteoporosis or fragility fracture but without typical skin lesions. (*Adapted from* Rossini M, Zanotti R, Orsolini G, et al. Prevalence, pathogenesis, and treatment options for mastocytosis-related osteoporosis. Osteoporos Int 2016;27(8):2411–21; with permission.)

DXA technology has recently become very useful in outpatient clinical practice because it combines the possibility of having a BMD measure and a vertebral fractures assessment as well through vertebral morphometry (see **Fig. 4**), using low radiographs exposition.

In the diagnostic process of unexplained osteoporosis or fractures in the absence of typical skin lesions of mastocytosis, the measurement of serum tryptase seems to be a good screening tool (see **Fig. 5**), considering that about 95% of patients with SM have above normal serum tryptase levels. It must be said that false positives exist (eg, chronic urticaria, renal insufficiency, other hematologic diseases, Onchocerciasis, ischemic myocardial disease, presence of heterophilic antibodies), and thus, consequently, bone marrow biopsy is mandatory, because it represents the gold standard for diagnosis and the core of diagnostic criteria. Bone marrow biopsy should be considered also in patients with normal tryptase if there are other clinical signs suggesting SM.

Currently, the role of BTM in clinical practice is not clear. Not infrequently the patient with SM with vertebral fractures will have normal BTM, whereas very high BTM serum levels are typically present in diffuse osteosclerosis. In patients with high BTM, a bone scintigraphy could be helpful to detect focal asymptomatic bone lesions and target radiographs examination.[41]

The very rare occurrence of large osteolytic lesions leads to the diagnosis of an aggressive SM variant, but if this finding does not correlate with other clinical and laboratory parameters, a histologic evaluation is recommended in order to exclude an associated hematological neoplasm or a solid cancer.[42]

MANAGEMENT

In patients with ISM, a high prevalence of vitamin D deficiency has been reported[28]: therefore, the first level of therapy is vitamin D supplementation. The other important traditional risk factors for osteoporosis and fractures should be taken into consideration and effectively corrected (alcohol consumption, corticosteroids, smoking, calcium intake, and so forth).

Considering the potential pathogenetic role of histamine and other MC mediators, antimediator therapy has been proposed as a therapeutic approach for bone involvement as well[43]; however, conclusive evidence is still lacking.

The most studied approach for the treatment of mastocytosis-related osteoporosis is the use of antiresorptive drugs, bisphosphonates, with the rationale of preventing bone loss determined by an absolute or relative predominance of osteoclast activity. In particular, different aminobisphosphonates have been used, both oral and parenteral (oral alendronate 70 mg/wk, oral risedronate 35 mg/wk, intra or endovenous pamidronate 90 mg/mo), with a positive effect on lumbar spine BMD but much less on the femoral one.[4,44–46] Tolerance and adherence to therapy are relevant issues in the general population, and this is even more important in patients with SM that often have gastrointestinal disturbances because of the disease itself. Parenteral administration should then be favored, and the least frequent administration possible would guarantee the best adherence and tolerance. In the authors' experience with ISM, one infusion of zoledronate 5 mg obtained a mean increase in BMD (at both lumbar and femoral sites) double that observed with oral alendronate or pamidronate, along with a reduction of BTM lasting for at least 1 year.[47] The gain in BMD and suppression of BTM are surrogate markers of anti–fracture efficacy, and therefore, yearly infusions of zoledronate in patients with ISM with nonsevere osteoporosis might be sufficient. However, in patients with previous vertebral fractures, more frequent administration of zoledronate should be recommended.

The authors recently administered denosumab in a few patients refractory or intolerant to bisphosphonates, with the regimen for postmenopausal osteoporosis treatment. The choice was made based on pathophysiologic data on the RANKL/RANK role. In these patients, denosumab was well tolerated and showed positive results on BMD along with a reduction of serum levels of BTM and tryptase.[48]

A rational approach, especially in the presence of low bone formation markers, might be osteoblasts stimulation with teriparatide, the 1 to 34 active fragment of parathyroid hormone. However, no experiences with the use of this anabolic treatment have been reported until now, and the description of an increase in MC in parathyroid bone disease[49] suggests some safety concerns in SM. In the authors' opinion and based on current knowledge, the use of teriparatide should not be proposed as an alternative approach in the management of mastocytosis-related osteoporosis because this treatment might further enhance the growth and proliferation of abnormal MC and induce more aggressive forms of SM.

In refractory or intolerant patients, the use of cytoreductive drugs has also been suggested as a rescue treatment.[50] There are studies reporting the use of a combined therapy with interferon-α (IFN-α) and bisphosphonates for cases refractory to bisphosphonates alone.[39,51–55] This combination appears effective in increasing BMD but is poorly tolerated by the side effects of IFN. Cladribine can be used in patients with SM who are refractory to IFN-α.[56] Tyrosine kinase inhibitors, such as Midostaurin, are a group of drugs indicated in aggressive forms of SM because they target KIT[57]; currently, there are no data on their effects on BTM, BMD, and fracture risk. There is a case report of one patient with advSM and diffuse osteosclerosis who did not respond to stem cell transplantation but did respond clinically to cytarabine and midostaurin, with resolution of osteosclerosis after midostaurin.[58]

However, in the authors' opinion, more longitudinal data are needed for a better understanding of bone involvement evolution and the impact of treatments in SM.

ACKNOWLEDGMENTS

The authors acknowledge Prof Mark Newman, native English speaker and medical writer.

REFERENCES

1. van der Veer E, van der Goot W, de Monchy JG, et al. High prevalence of fractures and osteoporosis in patients with indolent systemic mastocytosis. Allergy 2012;67(3):431–8.
2. Escribano L, Alvarez-Twose I, Sanchez-Munoz L, et al. Prognosis in adult indolent systemic mastocytosis: a long-term study of the Spanish Network on Mastocytosis in a series of 145 patients. J Allergy Clin Immunol 2009;124(3):514–21.
3. Rossini M, Zanotti R, Bonadonna P, et al. Bone mineral density, bone turnover markers and fractures in patients with indolent systemic mastocytosis. Bone 2011;49(4):880–5.
4. Barete S, Assous N, de Gennes C, et al. Systemic mastocytosis and bone involvement in a cohort of 75 patients. Ann Rheum Dis 2010;69(10):1838–41.
5. van der Veer E, Arends S, van der Hoek S, et al. Predictors of new fragility fractures after diagnosis of indolent systemic mastocytosis. J Allergy Clin Immunol 2014;134(6):1413–21.
6. Degboe Y, Eischen M, Nigon D, et al. Prevalence and risk factors for fragility fracture in systemic mastocytosis. Bone 2017;105:219–25.
7. Broesby-Olsen S, Farkas DK, Vestergaard H, et al. Risk of solid cancer, cardiovascular disease, anaphylaxis, osteoporosis and fractures in patients with systemic mastocytosis: a nationwide population-based study. Am J Hematol 2016;91(11):1069–75.
8. Kanis JA. Assessment of fracture risk and its application to screening for postmenopausal osteoporosis: synopsis of a WHO report. WHO Study Group. Osteoporos Int 1994;4(6):368–81.
9. Baim S, Binkley N, Bilezikian JP, et al. Official positions of the International Society for Clinical Densitometry and executive summary of the 2007 ISCD position development conference. J Clin Densitom 2008;11(1):75–91.
10. Brumsen C, Papapoulos SE, Lentjes EG, et al. A potential role for the mast cell in the pathogenesis of idiopathic osteoporosis in men. Bone 2002;31(5):556–61.
11. Guillaume N, Desoutter J, Chandesris O, et al. Bone complications of mastocytosis: a link between clinical and biological characteristics. Am J Med 2013;126(1):75.e1-7.
12. Seitz S, Barvencik F, Koehne T, et al. Increased osteoblast and osteoclast indices in individuals with systemic mastocytosis. Osteoporos Int 2013;24(8):2325–34.
13. Travis WD, Li CY, Bergstralh EJ, et al. Systemic mast cell disease. Analysis of 58 cases and literature review. Medicine (Baltimore) 1988;67(6):345–68.
14. Kanzaki S, Takahashi T, Kanno T, et al. Heparin inhibits BMP-2 osteogenic bioactivity by binding to both BMP-2 and BMP receptor. J Cell Physiol 2008;216(3):844–50.
15. Alvarez-Twose I, Gonzalez de Olano D, Sanchez-Munoz L, et al. Clinical, biological, and molecular characteristics of clonal mast cell disorders presenting with systemic mast cell activation symptoms. J Allergy Clin Immunol 2010;125(6):1269–78.e2.
16. Gulen T, Moller Westerberg C, Lyberg K, et al. Assessment of in vivo mast cell reactivity in patients with systemic mastocytosis. Clin Exp Allergy 2017;47(7):909–17.
17. Metcalfe DD. Mast cells and mastocytosis. Blood 2008;112(4):946–56.
18. Theoharides TC, Boucher W, Spear K. Serum interleukin-6 reflects disease severity and osteoporosis in mastocytosis patients. Int Arch Allergy Immunol 2002;128(4):344–50.

19. Dobigny C, Saffar JL. H1 and H2 histamine receptors modulate osteoclastic resorption by different pathways: evidence obtained by using receptor antagonists in a rat synchronized resorption model. J Cell Physiol 1997;173(1):10–8.

20. Biosse-Duplan M, Baroukh B, Dy M, et al. Histamine promotes osteoclastogenesis through the differential expression of histamine receptors on osteoclasts and osteoblasts. Am J Pathol 2009;174(4):1426–34.

21. Mayado A, Teodosio C, Garcia-Montero AC, et al. Increased IL6 plasma levels in indolent systemic mastocytosis patients are associated with high risk of disease progression. Leukemia 2016;30(1):124–30.

22. Fitzpatrick LA, Buzas E, Gagne TJ, et al. Targeted deletion of histidine decarboxylase gene in mice increases bone formation and protects against ovariectomy-induced bone loss. Proc Natl Acad Sci U S A 2003;100(10):6027–32.

23. de Gennes C, Kuntz D, de Vernejoul MC. Bone mastocytosis. A report of nine cases with a bone histomorphometric study. Clin Orthop Relat Res 1992;(279):281–91.

24. Delling G, Ritzel H, Werner M. Histological characteristics and prevalence of secondary osteoporosis in systemic mastocytosis. A retrospective analysis of 158 cases. Pathologe 2001;22(2):132–40 [in German].

25. Garcia-Montero AC, Jara-Acevedo M, Alvarez-Twose I, et al. KIT D816V-mutated bone marrow mesenchymal stem cells in indolent systemic mastocytosis are associated with disease progression. Blood 2016;127(6):761–8.

26. Nemeth K, Wilson TM, Ren JJ, et al. Impaired function of bone marrow stromal cells in systemic mastocytosis. Stem Cell Res 2015;15(1):42–53.

27. Garnero P. The utility of biomarkers in osteoporosis management. Mol Diagn Ther 2017;21(4):401–18.

28. Artuso A, Caimmi C, Tripi G, et al. Longitudinal evaluation of bone mineral density and bone metabolism markers in patients with indolent systemic mastocytosis without osteoporosis. Calcif Tissue Int 2017;100(1):40–6.

29. Bulai Livideanu C, Apoil PA, Lepage B, et al. Bone marrow tryptase as a possible diagnostic criterion for adult systemic mastocytosis. Clin Exp Allergy 2016;46(1):133–41.

30. Kushnir-Sukhov NM, Brittain E, Reynolds JC, et al. Elevated tryptase levels are associated with greater bone density in a cohort of patients with mastocytosis. Int Arch Allergy Immunol 2006;139(3):265–70.

31. Rossini M, Zanotti R, Viapiana O, et al. Bone involvement and osteoporosis in mastocytosis. Immunol Allergy Clin North Am 2014;34(2):383–96.

32. Chiappetta N, Gruber B. The role of mast cells in osteoporosis. Semin Arthritis Rheum 2006;36(1):32–6.

33. Rabenhorst A, Christopeit B, Leja S, et al. Serum levels of bone cytokines are increased in indolent systemic mastocytosis associated with osteopenia or osteoporosis. J Allergy Clin Immunol 2013;132(5):1234–7.e7.

34. Spencer GJ, Utting JC, Etheridge SL, et al. Wnt signalling in osteoblasts regulates expression of the receptor activator of NFkappaB ligand and inhibits osteoclastogenesis in vitro. J Cell Sci 2006;119(Pt 7):1283–96.

35. Rossini M, Viapiana O, Zanotti R, et al. Dickkopf-1 and sclerostin serum levels in patients with systemic mastocytosis. Calcif Tissue Int 2015;96(5):410–6.

36. Rossini M, Adami S, Zanotti R, et al. Serum levels of bone cytokines in indolent systemic mastocytosis associated with osteopenia or osteoporosis. J Allergy Clin Immunol 2014;133(3):933–5.

37. Pieri L, Bonadonna P, Elena C, et al. Clinical presentation and management practice of systemic mastocytosis. A survey on 460 Italian patients. Am J Hematol 2016;91(7):692–9.

38. Hermine O, Lortholary O, Leventhal PS, et al. Case-control cohort study of patients' perceptions of disability in mastocytosis. PLoS One 2008;3(5):e2266.
39. Pardanani A. How I treat patients with indolent and smoldering mastocytosis (rare conditions but difficult to manage). Blood 2013;121(16):3085–94.
40. Genant HK, Wu CY, van Kuijk C, et al. Vertebral fracture assessment using a semiquantitative technique. J Bone Miner Res 1993;8(9):1137–48.
41. Chen CC, Andrich MP, Mican JM, et al. A retrospective analysis of bone scan abnormalities in mastocytosis: correlation with disease category and prognosis. J Nucl Med 1994;35(9):1471–5.
42. Bonifacio M, Zanotti R, Guardalben E, et al. Multiple large osteolytic lesions in a patient with systemic mastocytosis: a challenging diagnosis. Clin Case Rep 2017;5(12):1988–91.
43. Graves L, Stechschulte DJ, Morris DC, et al. Inhibition of mediator release in systemic mastocytosis is associated with reversal of bone changes. J Bone Miner Res 1990;5(11):1113–9.
44. Cundy T, Beneton MN, Darby AJ, et al. Osteopenia in systemic mastocytosis: natural history and responses to treatment with inhibitors of bone resorption. Bone 1987;8(3):149–55.
45. Brumsen C, Hamdy NA, Papapoulos SE. Osteoporosis and bone marrow mastocytosis: dissociation of skeletal responses and mast cell activity during long-term bisphosphonate therapy. J Bone Miner Res 2002;17(4):567–9.
46. Marshall A, Kavanagh RT, Crisp AJ. The effect of pamidronate on lumbar spine bone density and pain in osteoporosis secondary to systemic mastocytosis. Br J Rheumatol 1997;36(3):393–6.
47. Rossini M, Zanotti R, Viapiana O, et al. Zoledronic acid in osteoporosis secondary to mastocytosis. Am J Med 2014;127(11):1127.e1-4.
48. Orsolini G, Gavioli I, Tripi G, et al. Denosumab for the treatment of mastocytosis-related osteoporosis: a case series. Calcif Tissue Int 2017;100(6):595–8.
49. Turner RT, Iwaniec UT, Marley K, et al. The role of mast cells in parathyroid bone disease. J Bone Miner Res 2010;25(7):1637–49.
50. Pardanani A. Systemic mastocytosis in adults: 2017 update on diagnosis, risk stratification and management. Am J Hematol 2016;91(11):1146–59.
51. Weide R, Ehlenz K, Lorenz W, et al. Successful treatment of osteoporosis in systemic mastocytosis with interferon alpha-2b. Ann Hematol 1996;72(1):41–3.
52. Lehmann T, Lammle B. IFNalpha treatment in systemic mastocytosis. Ann Hematol 1999;78(10):483–4.
53. Butterfield JH. Interferon treatment for hypereosinophilic syndromes and systemic mastocytosis. Acta Haematol 2005;114(1):26–40.
54. Laroche M, Bret J, Brouchet A, et al. Clinical and densitometric efficacy of the association of interferon alpha and pamidronate in the treatment of osteoporosis in patients with systemic mastocytosis. Clin Rheumatol 2007;26(2):242–3.
55. Laroche M, Livideanu C, Paul C, et al. Interferon alpha and pamidronate in osteoporosis with fracture secondary to mastocytosis. Am J Med 2011;124(8):776–8.
56. Tefferi A, Li CY, Butterfield JH, et al. Treatment of systemic mast-cell disease with cladribine. N Engl J Med 2001;344(4):307–9.
57. Verstovsek S. Advanced systemic mastocytosis: the impact of KIT mutations in diagnosis, treatment, and progression. Eur J Haematol 2013;90(2):89–98.
58. Ustun C, Courville EL. Resolution of osteosclerosis after alloHCT in systemic mastocytosis. Blood 2016;127(14):1836.

Hymenoptera Anaphylaxis as a Clonal Mast Cell Disorder

Patrizia Bonadonna, MD[a,b,*], Luigi Scaffidi, MD[b,c]

KEYWORDS

- Systemic mastocytosis ● Monoclonal mast cell activation syndrome
- Hymenoptera venom allergy ● Anaphylaxis ● Tryptase ● Clonal mast cell disease

KEY POINTS

- Up to 7% of adult patients with Hymenoptera venom allergy may simultaneously suffer from a clonal mast cell disease.
- Patients with clonal mast cell disease and Hymenoptera venom anaphylaxis are commonly males, without skin lesions, and anaphylaxis is characterized by hypotension and syncope in the absence of urticaria and angioedema.
- A normal value of tryptase (≤11.4 ng/mL) in these patients does not exclude a mastocytosis.
- The diagnosis of a mast cell disease leads to several therapeutic consequences concerning the treatment of Hymenoptera venom allergy.
- These patients have to undergo long-life venom immunotherapy to prevent further, potentially fatal severe reactions.

INTRODUCTION

Mastocytosis is a clonal mast cell disorder (CMD) that encompasses a heterogeneous group of clonal disorders characterized by the proliferation and accumulation of mast cells (MC) in different tissues, with a preferential localization in the bone marrow (BM) and skin.[1] Subjects with mastocytosis can experience symptoms owing to a massive MC activation and release of mediators.

Systemic symptoms may include hypotension and anaphylactic shock, flushing, headache, itching, abdominal pain, dyspepsia, diarrhea, and bone and soft tissue pain.[2]

CMD includes cases not fulfilling sufficient criteria for systemic mastocytosis (SM) but showing MC clonality markers by expression CD25/CD2 on immunophenotyping

Disclosure: The authors have no conflict of interest to declare.
[a] Allergy Unit, Azienda Ospedaliera Universitaria Integrata di Verona, Piazzale Stefani 1, Verona 37126, Italy; [b] Multidisciplinary Outpatients Clinic for Mastocytosis (GISM), Azienda Ospedaliera Universitaria Integrata di Verona, Piazzale Stefani 1, Verona 37126, Italy; [c] Department of Medicine, Section of Hematology, Azienda Ospedaliera Universitaria Integrata di Verona, Piazzale L. A. Scuro 10, Verona 37134, Italy
* Corresponding author. Allergy Unit, Azienda Ospedaliera Universitaria Integrata di Verona, Piazzale Stefani 1, Verona 37126, Italy.
E-mail address: patrizia.bonadonna@aovr.veneto.it

Immunol Allergy Clin N Am 38 (2018) 455–468
https://doi.org/10.1016/j.iac.2018.04.010
0889-8561/18/© 2018 Elsevier Inc. All rights reserved.

immunology.theclinics.com

and/or a KIT mutation at codon 816 on molecular analysis. These latter patients may have a limited, prediagnostic form of SM, also indicated as monoclonal MC activation syndrome (MMAS), but their risk of developing severe life-threatening anaphylaxis is similar to patients with SM.[2–4]

The prevalence of anaphylaxis in patients with mastocytosis is much higher than the 0.05% to 2.00% estimated frequency of anaphylaxis in the general population[5,6] and has been reported to be between 22% and 49% in adults[7–9] and between 6% and 9% in children[7,8]; discrepancies between different studies might be a result of the heterogeneity of patient cohorts, the definition of anaphylaxis, and the sensitivity of diagnostic techniques.

A wide variety of stimuli (venom, drug, or food) can trigger anaphylaxis in patients with mastocytosis, but for certain patients no eliciting factors can be identified despite a comprehensive allergy workup and, therefore, we use the term idiopathic anaphylaxis. All epidemiologic studies have shown that Hymenoptera stings represent the most common trigger of anaphylaxis in subjects with mastocytosis.[7–10]

Hymenoptera Venom Allergy

Hymenoptera venom allergy (HVA) is a typical immunoglobulin (Ig)E-mediated disease, whose clinical manifestations are the result of the MC degranulation, which is triggered by the binding of the venom allergens to specific IgE (sIgE). Severity can vary from large local reactions to systemic anaphylaxis. The reactions are classified according to Mueller's scale with 4° of increasing severity.[11] Diagnostic procedures include skin prick and intradermal tests and serum-sIgE essays.

The insects responsible for allergic reactions are Hymenoptera belonging to the suborder Aculeate, which includes the Apidae, Vespidae, and Formicidae families (**Fig. 1**). The Apidae family includes *Apis mellifera* and *bombus*. The Vespidae family takes in the Vespinae subfamilies (*Vespula* species and *Vespa crabro*) and Polistinae subfamilies (*Polistes* species), among which *Polistes dominulus* is widespread especially in the Mediterranean area.[12] There is no preventive pharmacologic treatment

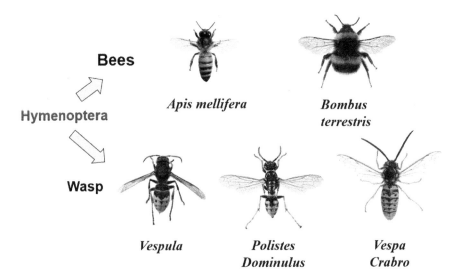

Bees

Hymenoptera

Apis mellifera

Bombus terrestris

Wasp

Vespula

Polistes Dominulus

Vespa Crabro

Fig. 1. Hymenoptera venom allergy and clonal mast cell disorders (CMD). (*Courtesy of* Anallergo, Scarperia e San Piero FI, Italy.)

available for HVA. These patients should carry a self-administration emergency kit that includes oral antihistamines and corticosteroids as well as self-injectable epinephrine. Venom immunotherapy (VIT) represents a safe and effective treatment that decreases the risk of subsequent systemic reactions and reduces morbidity and mortality.[13] VIT is prescribed to all subjects with a clear history of systemic reaction and positive skin test or venom sIgE in serum.

Hymenoptera Venom Allergy and Clonal Mast Cell Disease

During the last few years it has increasingly been realized that there is a preferential association between HVA and mastocytosis. First, the most common trigger of anaphylaxis in patients with mastocytosis is Hymenoptera venom. In 3 large case series that evaluated the causes of anaphylaxis in patients with mastocytosis, HVA was reported to range from 22% to 53% of the subjects[7–9]; in contrast, in children with mastocytosis, Hymenoptera stings played no role in eliciting anaphylaxis.[7,8]

Second, the association is also confirmed because the prevalence of CMD in patients with HVA is greater than in general population. As a matter of fact, according to the literature, between 1.0% and 7.9% of patients with HVA have a CMD (**Table 1**). The lower prevalence rate reported in some study could be explained by the low sensitivity of the screening test used,[14] by the lack of a BM evaluation,[15] or the evaluation of CD25/CD2 MC coexpression by flow cytometry and/or Kit mutation.[16–18]

Formerly, systemic or anaphylactic reactions after Hymenoptera stings were described in case reports or in a small series of patients with cutaneous mastocytosis or SM (**Table 2**).[19–22]

The first report of a routine BM evaluation of patients with HVA and raised tryptase showed 7.9% of CMD among all the patients with systemic reactions to Hymenoptera venom, regardless of serum basal tryptase (SBT) level.[23] In this series, 88% of the patients who underwent BM evaluation (for SBT >11.4 ng/mL; n = 34) were diagnosed with a CMD: indolent SM (ISM) in 21 subjects (62.%), where 14 patients fulfilled both major and minor criteria, and 7 satisfied 3 minor criteria and MMAS in 9 subjects (26%). Therefore, 16 ISM/MMAS cases (47%) would not have been diagnosed without flow cytometry KIT mutation analysis, or both. Increased SBT seems to be a useful criterion for selecting patients eligible for BM evaluation when SM is suspected[23,24];

Table 1
Prevalence of CMD in patients with. Systemic reactions to Hymenoptera venom, screened on the basis of elevated tryptase[a]

	Patients	Raised Tryptase (%)	CMD	%
Haeberli et al,[15] 2003[b]	259	19 (7.3)	3 CM	1
Dubois,[14] 2004[c]	2375	32 (1.3)	22 SM	1
Rueff et al,[16] 2006[e]	1102	106 (9.6)	21 CM + 8 SM	2.6
Bonadonna et al,[23] 2009	379	44 (11.6)	21 ISM + 9 MMAS	7.9
Potier et al,[17] 2009[e]	138	22 (15.9)	1 CM + 5 SM	4.4
Guenova et al,[18] 2010[d,e]	274	30 (10.9)	1 CM + 3 ISM	1.5

Abbreviations: BM, bone marrow; CM, cutaneous mastocytosis; CMD, clonal mast cell disease; ISM, indolent systemic mastocytosis; MMAS, monoclonal mast cell activation syndrome; SBT, serum basal tryptase level; SM, systemic mastocytosis.

[a] SBT > 11.4 ng/mL.
[b] BM evaluation not performed.
[c] Screening with urinary Histamine metabolite.
[d] BM performed if SBT > 15 ng/mL.
[e] Evaluation of CD25/CD2 MC coexpression and Kit mutation not performed or reported.

Table 2
Characteristics of the majority of reported MCD presenting systemic reactions to Hymenoptera sting

	Patients (n)	Diagnosis	Male/Female	Median Age, y (Range)	Tryptase <20 ng/mL, n (%)	Without Skin Involvement, n (%)
Müller et al,[20] 1983	3	2 CM[a] + 1 SM	1/2	34 (32–50)	Not reported	0
Kors et al,[66] 1993	5	2 ISM (−) 3 ISM (+)	0/5	49 (20–71)	Not reported	2 (40)
Fricker et al,[33] 1997	10	7 CM[a] 3 SM	4/6	39 (29–51)	5 (50)	0
Oude Elberink et al,[22] 1997	2	2 ISM	0/2	44–43	Not reported	0
Dubois,[14] 2004	17	17 SM	—	—	—	8 (47)
González de Olano et al,[7] 2007	21	21 SM	17/4	50 (29–74)	2 (9)	16 (76)
Potier et al,[17] 2009[b]	1 CM + 4 ISMs(+) 2 ISMs(−)	6/1	45 (29–59)	1 (14)	2 (28)	—
Bonadonna et al,[23] 2009	30	21 SM 9 MMAS	13/8 9/0	48 (19–76) 51 (32–69)	6 (29) 6 (67)	26 (87)
Alvarez-Twose et al,[34] 2014	150	143 ISMs(−) 7 ISMs(+)	111/32	44 (16–76)	54 (38)	143 (95)
Bonadonna et al,[10] 2016	219	171 ISMs(−) 48 ISMs(+)	—	—	—	171 (78)
Rietveld et al,[57] 2016	9	4 ISMs(−) 5 ISMs(+)	05/04/18	52 (36–72)	—	4 (44)
Michel et al,[47] 2016	27	5 CM 4 MIS 8 ISMs(+) 9 ISMs(−) 1 MMAS	1/4 3/1 4/4 3/6 1/0	44 (31–56) 39 (26–49) 61 (41–76) 55 (46–59) —	4 (80) 0 1 (12) 4 (44) 0	8 (30)
Total	500	15 CM 4 MIS 140 ISMs(+) 331 ISMs(−) 10 MMAS	184/87 (ratio 2.11)	—	90/238 (38)	380 (76)

Abbreviations: BM bone marrow; CM, cutaneous mastocytosis; CMD, clonal mast cell disease; ISM, indolent systemic mastocytosis; ISMs(−), indolent systemic mastocytosis skin negative; ISMs(+), indolent systemic mastocytosis skin positive; MMAS, monoclonal mast cell activation syndrome; SM, systemic mastocytosis.

[a] BM evaluation not performed or in a portion of cases.

[b] BM histology without evaluation of CD25/CD2 MC expression.

nevertheless, a CMD cannot be excluded in subjects with systemic severe HVA but with normal SBT.[25]

In a retrospective analysis of 142 subjects without skin lesions who were investigated for suspected CMD, none of the 44 patients with a SBT of less than 10 ng/mL confirmed a diagnosis of CMD.[26]

However, a failure to identify a CMD in patients with normal SBT could be possibly related to the technical approach used. In fact, BM MC immunophenotyping with only 300,000 events, as well as the KIT-D816 V mutation detection by techniques less sensitive than reverse transcriptase qualitative polymerase chain reaction cannot be sufficient to identify atypical MC in patients with very low MC burden. In a recent study, 22 patients with at least 1 episode of anaphylaxis with ascertained hypotension after Hymenoptera sting, normal SBT and the absence of urticaria pigmentosa underwent BM evaluation. The diagnosis of ISM was established in 16 patients and MMAS in 1 patient. Notably, in all cases the diagnosis of ISM was based only on minor criteria because BM biopsy specimens did not show compact MC aggregates.[27]

Several years ago, a Spanish group identified 4 clinical elements (male sex, presyncopal and/or syncopal episodes, absence of urticarial/angioedema, and serum tryptase >25 ng/mL) as independent predictive factors of CMD in patients suffering from insect bite anaphylaxis without mastocytosis in the skin.[4] The evaluation of these parameters—the so-called REMA score—provides a good tool for screening patients with suspected mastocytosis for severe mediator symptoms but without typical skin lesions.[28] An early diagnosis of CMD in patients with normal tryptase and severe HVA would represent a substantial advantage for several reasons. One-quarter of these patients had evidence of osteoporosis[27] and early therapy can prevent vertebral fractures.[29] Some fatal sting reactions have been described in patients with SM with HVA after stopping VIT[22,30]; thus, an accurate diagnosis is essential in recommending life-long treatment. Another category of patients with HVA has been shown very recently in which there is cause to suspect a CMD: those who experienced severe reactions at re-sting after VIT discontinuation[31]; as a matter of fact, the authors confirmed that 95% of these patients, when investigated thoroughly by the most sensitive available techniques, resulted to be affected by a CMD.

Clinical Characteristics of Patients with Hymenoptera Venom Allergy and Clonal Mast Cell Disease

For years, the diagnostic workup for SM in patients with HVA has been usually limited to those with urticaria pigmentosa, because cutaneous mastocytosis or SM with skin involvement was believed to represent the majority of these patients.[16,20,22,32,33] Instead, in later years, it has been shown that HVA is more frequent in patients with mastocytosis without skin involvement[7,10,23,34] (see **Table 1**).

Surprisingly, progression to aggressive mastocytosis or an associated hematologic malignancy has not been yet reported in patients with SM with HVA[35] and, as a consequence, HVA seems to be absent in patients with the aggressive subtypes of SM, who harbor the highest MC load.[36,37]

It has been reported that patients with mastocytosis who experience anaphylaxis with 1 trigger do not react to others.[9] This issue has been confirmed more recently, where 90% of ISM skin negative patients diagnosed after HVA do not refer anaphylaxis with other triggers.[10]

Another important characteristic of patients with HVA and ISM skin negative disease is the male predominance, a significantly lower MC burden, lower levels of serum tryptase, and a lower frequency of dense compact MC aggregates in BM sections than in ISM skin positive patients. They also frequently show coexisting populations of phenotypically normal and aberrant MC in BM and a lower frequency of multilineage KIT mutation.[4,28]

The majority of patients do not report MC activation symptoms between acute episodes; therefore, most of these patients may have HVA severe reactions as the sole clinical manifestation of mastocytosis.

The anaphylactic reactions of patients with CMD and HVA are characterized in most cases by the absence of angioedema and erythema, and the predominance of cardiovascular symptoms, such as hypotension, leading to loss of consciousness.[27,34]

Management of Patients with Hymenoptera Venom Allergy and Clonal Mast Cell Disease

Diagnosis

The diagnosis of HVA is based on the combination of a history of reactions to stings and positive IgE antibodies, which can be revealed by intradermal testing with venom or by measurement of sIgE in serum.[38]

Current guidelines indicate that the diagnostic tests should be performed only on patients who have suffered from anaphylactic reaction.[13,38] In fact, asymptomatic sensitization to bee and wasp venom occurs frequently with in vitro tests, and 27.1% to 40.7% of the general population is reported to have detectable sIgE to Hymenoptera venom.[39,40] One of the main causes of asymptomatic sensitization is the presence of sIgE to cross-reactive carbohydrate determinants in the serum[41,42]; these carbohydrate structures are present in plants and invertebrates and IgE antibodies against cross-reactive carbohydrate determinants are found in patients allergic to pollen or insect venom. Nevertheless, a large portion of subjects sensitized to nonglycosylated venom allergens tolerate Hymenoptera stings well.

A recent study of a group of subjects who tolerated Hymenoptera sting and with detectable sIgE showed that only 5.3% of sensitized patients had severe systemic reactions (SSRs) after the sting challenge. These subjects presented a 9.5-fold higher risk than the general population for large local reactions but not for SSRs. Therefore, the frequency of reactors seems to be comparable with the risk of the general population and far less than the risk for a re-sting reaction in allergic patients, which was reported to be between 25% and 52% after deliberate sting challenges.[43]

History

For an accurate diagnosis, it is important first to identify the culprit insect, even though there are numerous allergy-eliciting Hymenoptera species with overlapping phenotypes and, as a consequence, sometimes it is hard to discriminate between them; in fact, although it is easy to recognize the honey bee because it usually loses its stinger after sting or the *Vespa crabro* because it is very big and the nests are very typical, the same is not true in the case of wasps (yellow jacket and polistes), because they are very similar in shape and in behavior.

Tests

Skin tests, such as in vitro tests, should be done 4 weeks after the reaction; if negative, the test can be easily repeated because, in some cases, it becomes positive a few weeks later.[44] In contrast, if the time period between the sting and the test is longer, the result may be falsely negative.

In vivo tests

Skin prick tests are performed with a standard concentration of insect venom ranging from 1 to 100 μg/mL. If skin prick tests are negative, intradermal tests are then performed with concentrations of 0.001 to 1.000 μg/mL. Higher concentrations may lead to false-positive results.[45] The extracts usually used for the all diagnostic procedures (in vivo and in vitro tests)[38] are *Apis mellifera, Vespa crabro, Polistes dominulus*, and *Vespula vulgaris.* In fact, is very important for a correct diagnosis and the subsequent prescription of immunotherapy, to include *Polistes dominulus*, which is largely diffused in Europe,[12] especially in the Mediterranean areas (Italy, Greece, Spain, France, and North Africa).

The safety of skin tests was confirmed in many studies, which did not report any reaction in patients with mastocytosis and HVA.[7,23,45–47]

In vitro test

The first level test is the detection of sIgE against major natural allergens of venom (CAP assay). Thanks to modern molecular biology technology and the increasing knowledge about venom composition on a molecular level, in the last decade it has become possible to develop an advanced molecular or component-resolved diagnostics approach to HVA, which has largely contributed to solving many diagnostic challenges.[48] The detection of these recombinants allowed a more precise diagnosis with the identification of the causative venom in patients with apparent double sensitization to yellow jacket and wasp (*Polistes*) venom or to honeybee and yellow jacket venom.[49] The Hymenoptera venom allergens currently available on various diagnostic platforms are for honey bees (*Apis*; Api m 1, Api m 2, APi m 3, Api m 4, Api m 5, and Api m 10), for yellow jacket (*Vespula vulgaris*; Ves v1, Ves V 5), and for European paper asp (*Polistes domunulus*; Pol d 1 and Pol d 5).

More recently, some authors used Ves v 1 and Ves v 5 (Immulite system) to diagnose 27 patients with yellow jacket venom allergy and 53 patients with yellow jacket venom allergy and mastocytosis and/or elevated baseline serum tryptase.[47] This study confirmed that the analyses of sIgE reactivity on a component-resolved level revealed no obvious differences in the reactivity profiles of Hymenoptera venom-allergic patients of 2 groups; in contrast, it showed that a diagnostic sensitivity of 100% was reached in the mastocytosis group using the recombinant allergens an the cutoff of 0.10 kUA/L, instead of the cutoff of 0.35 kUA/L. Other authors more recently confirmed in a study that, with the lower cutoff, the diagnostic sensitivity improved but specificity did not; therefore, they showed that the optimal combined diagnostic sensitivity and specificity of sIgE was found at a cutoff level of 0.21 kUA/L (82.1% and 87.5%, respectively). However, because missing the diagnosis of yellow jacket venom allergy could have serious consequences, a lower cutoff level of 0.17 kUA/L is preferable, which gives a sensitivity and specificity of 83.6% and 85.0%, respectively.[50]

Basophil activation test

The basophil activation test (BAT) has been proposed as a useful adjunct in the diagnosis of allergic disease, especially in patients with negative or contradictory conventional tests.[51] In the BAT, basophils are used as an in vitro model for MCs because both contain granules of preformed molecules that can cause an anaphylactic reaction after degranulation. Using the BAT, both IgE-mediated and IgE-independent type 1 hypersensitivity can be measured in vitro.[52] In patients with HVA, the BAT was proposed as a third-level test for selected cases, and it can be useful in polysensitization patients.[53–55] Regarding patients with mastocytosis, the role and usefulness of the BAT remains a topic of discussion in the current literature, with earlier studies reporting conflicting evidence. The first study, which evaluated the value of BAT in patients with mastocytosis,[56] confirmed that in 11 patients with SM who had specific sIgE against Hymenoptera venom and an evaluable BAT, BAT was found to be positive in 9 patients. Additionally, a positive BAT was detected in 3 of 7 patients who had no sIgE. A further study that evaluated 7 patients with SM with reactions to Hymenoptera stings and negative tests confirmed that 6 of these patients with SM were also negative with the BAT; therefore, the authors confirmed that this test did not add valuable information, because it was invariably negative when the standard diagnostic tests were negative.[45] More recently, some authors evaluated 29 patients with SM, 9 of whom had a history of HVA, and sIgE was detected in 6 patients with HVA. The BAT was positive in only 1 patient, for whom the skin test and sIgE were also positive[57]; therefore, the authors confirmed the data from previous study[45]: the BAT is not a reliable tool for randomly screening patients with SM for HVA.

Based on these data from the literature, we therefore postulate that the BAT does not add useful information to the conventional diagnostic tests for HVA.

Immunotherapy

The only curative treatment that is effective in reducing the risk of subsequent systemic reactions and improving the patients' quality of life is VIT. VIT in the general population is reported to be effective in 77% to 84% of patients treated with honeybee venom and in 91% to 96% of patients receiving vespid venom.[58]

After some debate, mainly owing to safety concerns,[22] it is now generally accepted that VIT is clinically justified in those patients with severe HVA and documented mastocytosis. In fact, it is now generally accepted that VIT should be given always. Based on the data from the literature available to date, the effectiveness of treatment in patients with mastocytosis with standard doses is slightly lower than in the general population (**Table 3**). Recently however, more robust recommendations have been

Table 3
Immunotherapy in patients with mastocytosis

| Author | Diagnosis | Patients with Mastocytosis, n (%) | | | Cumulative Reactions to Re-sting, n/N (%) |
| | | Total | Side Effects | | |
			System		
Engler,[61] 1994	4 UP, 1 ISM	2 (33)	2 (33)		0/1
Fricker,[33] 1997	3 ISM + UP, 3 ISM − UP +, 4 UP no BM diagnosis	2 (20)	1 (10)		1/6 (16)
Haeberli,[15] 2003	10 patients with tryptase >13.5 μg/L and sting challenge performed	1 (10)	1 (10)		4/10 (40)
Dubois,[14] 2004	7 SM	6 (85)	6 (85)		6/7 (85)
Rueff,[16] 2006	48 patients with mastocytosis	9 (18.8) built up phase of VIT	9 (18.8) built up phase of VIT		7/33 (21.6)
González De Olano,[7] 2007	21 ISM (5 UP+, 16 UP-)	6 (29) 3 built up, 3 maintenance phase of VIT	5 (24)		3/12 (25)
Bonadonna,[23] 2009	16 ISM (2 UP+, 14 UP-)	2 (12.5)	0		2/13 (15)
Bonadonna,[46] 2013	77 ISM (12UP+, 65 UP-) MMAS 7	10 (8.4)	4 (built up) (4.8)		7/50 (14)
Total	201	38 (18.9)	28 (13.9)		30/132 (22.7)

Abbreviations: BM bone marrow; ISM, indolent systemic mastocytosis; MMAS, monoclonal mast cell activation syndrome; SM, systemic mastocytosis; UP, urticaria pigmentosa; VIT, venom immunotherapy.

provided for the use of VIT in patients with SM and HVA. By joining together 2 homogeneous populations of patients from Italy and Spain, the authors had a relatively large number of patients with HVA and SM.[46] In this study, VIT was well-tolerated, although a slightly higher number of adverse events were seen with the rush-modified induction regimen. Thus, although a statistical significance was not seen, it would be reasonable to suggest a less aggressive induction in patients with SM. Despite previous reports,[59] none of the patients discontinued the treatment owing to VIT-related side effects, and no reaction was observed during the maintenance period. In addition, in patients with HVA and SM not fully protected at field re-stings, an increase of the maintenance dose to 200 μg of venom could be recommended.[46] The study also confirmed that VIT conferred a full protection in the majority (86%) of re-stung patients, although this percentage is slightly smaller than that reported in patients without SM.[60]

Furthermore, in patients with mastocytosis, a pretreatment with an H1 antihistamine can be used to decrease the number and severity of large local reactions and mild SRs to VIT, such as urticaria and angioedema.[13,61] More recently, several case reports showed that pretreatment with anti-IgE monoclonal antibodies may permit more rapid and higher doses of allergen immunotherapy: patients with ISM who experienced SRs to VIT were able to tolerate immunotherapy after pretreatment with omalizumab.[35,62–65]

In the normal HVA population, the literature confirmed that a minimum of a 5-year treatment is better for long-term effectiveness[58] and life-long therapy should be considered in patients with severe initial SSRs, systemic adverse events during VIT, and patients allergic to honeybee venom allergic with a high risk of future honeybee stings. In the literature, there are some case reports showing that patients with mastocytosis and HVA, who were protected during VIT, can have very severe reactions after VIT discontinuation.[22,66]

Very recently, some authors performed a retrospective multicenter study evaluating patients with HVA who underwent a 4- to 11-year course of VIT for previous severe reactions. For the analysis, they considered patients who experienced severe reactions at re-sting after VIT discontinuation. None of them had a previous ascertained diagnosis of mastocytosis, and in fact, in all but 1 tryptase evaluation was not performed before VIT because in that time (before 2007) tryptase dosage was not routinely evaluated.

Importantly, 95% of these patients were thoroughly investigated by the most sensitive available techniques and found to be affected by a CMD. The results obtained in these selected patients clearly documented that the probability of having mastocytosis (in any form) is quite high when VIT protection is lost after treatment. This finding would suggest that patients with HVA-induced anaphylaxis who lose protection after a proper course of VIT should be investigated for mastocytosis. These data also confirmed that, when a diagnosis of mastocytosis is established, these patients should continue life-long VIT31, therefore, from a practical point of view, regardless of the tryptase value, we would suggest an accurate hematologic workup be performed before stopping immunotherapy in those patients with very severe reactions with hypotension and without urticaria and angioedema to exclude CMD. In these patients, it is very important to use a highly sensitive multiparameter flow cytometry approach to stain BM cells, using a combination of 5 monoclonal antibodies—CD45, CD117, CD34, CD25, and CD2—and with at least 1 to 3 million events acquired to detect atypical MC in these patients who have a very low MC burden.[27]

In general, to improve the compliance of patients in the HVA population who have to continue life-long injections, a 3- to 4-month extended interval can be proposed, and this schedule, adopted after 5 years of immunotherapy, seems to be safe and effective.[67] We can hypothesize that patients with mastocytosis can also adopt this schedule even if up to now there have been no studies about the efficacy and protection in case of re-sting.

All patients with mastocytosis who undergo VIT, even in the maintenance phase, should carry epinephrine self-injectors because of the persistent risk of SSR and the possibility that SSR may also occur after a sting of an insect whose venom was not used for VIT.[30]

Emergency treatment
Patients with CMD a should carry with them an emergency kit irrespective of tests result. Moreover, patients with mastocytosis who have experienced SSRs should carry 2 or more epinephrine self-injectors. In a recent position paper from the European Academy, this precaution is also advised for all patients with mastocytosis treated with VIT, even if they had reached the maintenance dose.[68]

KEY MESSAGES

- HVA represents the most common trigger of anaphylaxis in subjects with mastocytosis.
- The majority of patients with HVA and SM are diagnosed as SM lacking skin lesions and this is called BM mastocytosis.
- There is a strong association between Hymenoptera anaphylaxis with a negative allergy study and the presence of an underlying SM.
- Anaphylaxis manifestations in HVA and CMD are characterized by an absence of angioedema and erythema, and the predominance of cardiovascular symptoms.
- The characteristics of severe HVA episodes, with hypotension in the absence of urticaria and or angioedema, may represent the most relevant factor in identifying those patients with HVA and CMD, regardless of baseline tryptase levels.
- In cases of systemic reaction after Hymenoptera sting in patients with CMD, it is mandatory to perform in vivo and in vitro tests to identify the culprit insect venom and then start correct immunotherapy, which must to be continued for life.
- The only therapy effective in patients with HVA and CMD is immunotherapy, which is generally well-tolerated. VIT must be continued for life.
- The probability of having SM (in any form) is quite high when VIT protection is lost after treatment. It can be hypothesized that patients with no skin involvement, normal SBT levels, and anaphylaxis with certain hypotension and loss of consciousness caused by Hymenoptera stings should undergo a BM examination to detect a possible CMD before stopping immunotherapy.

REFERENCES

1. Horny HP, Metcalfe DD, Bennett JM, et al, editors. WHO classification of tumors of hematopoietic and lymphoid tissues. 4th edition. Lyon (France): IARC Press; 2008. p. 54–63.
2. Valent P, Akin C, Escribano L, et al. Standards and standardization in mastocytosis: consensus statements on diagnostics, treatment recommendations and response criteria. Eur J Clin Invest 2007;37:435–53.
3. Akin C, Valent P, Metcalfe DD. Mast cell activation syndrome: proposed diagnostic criteria. J Allergy Clin Immunol 2010;126:1099–104.
4. Alvarez-Twose I, Gonzalez de Olano D, Sanchez-Munoz L, et al. Clinical, biological and molecular characteristics of systemic mast cell disorders presenting with severe mediator-related symptoms. J Allergy Clin Immunol 2010;125:1269–78.

5. Lieberman P, Camargo CA Jr, Bohlke K, et al. Epidemiology of anaphylaxis: findings of the American College of Allergy, Asthma and Immunology Epidemiology of Anaphylaxis Working Group. Ann Allergy Asthma Immunol 2006;97:596–602.

6. Muraro A, Werfel T, Hoffmann-Sommergruber K, et al, EAACI Food Allergy and Anaphylaxis Guidelines Group. Anaphylaxis: guidelines from the European Academy of Allergy and Clinical Immunology. Allergy 2014;69:1026–45.

7. González de Olano D, de la Hoz Caballer B, Núñez López R, et al. Prevalence of allergy and anaphylactic symptoms in 210 adult and pediatric patients with mastocytosis in Spain: a study of the Spanish Network on Mastocytosis (REMA). Clin Exp Allergy 2007;37(10):1547–55.

8. Brockow K, Jofer C, Behrendt H, et al. Anaphylaxis in patients with mastocytosis: a study on history, clinical features and risk factors in 120 patients. Allergy 2008; 63:226–32.

9. Gulen T, Hagglund H, Dahlen B, et al. High prevalence of anaphylaxis in patients with systemic mastocytosis: a single-centre experience. Clin Exp Allergy 2014; 44:121–9.

10. Bonadonna P, Bonifacio M, Lombardo C, et al. Hymenoptera allergy and mast cell activation syndromes. Curr Allergy Asthma Rep 2016;16(1):5.

11. Mueller H. Diagnosis and treatment of insect sensitivity. J Asthma Res 1966;3: 331.

12. Severino MG, Campi P, Macchia D, et al. European polistes venom allergy. Allergy 2006;61(7):860–3.

13. Bonifazi F, Jutel M, Biló BM, et al, EAACI Interest Group on insect venom hypersensitivity. Prevention and treatment of Hymenoptera venom allergy: guidelines for clinical practice. Allergy 2005;60:1459–70.

14. Dubois AE. Mastocytosis and Hymenoptera allergy. Curr Opin Allergy Clin Immunol 2004;4(4):291–5.

15. Haeberli G, Bronnimann M, Hunziker T, et al. Elevated basal serum tryptase and Hymenoptera venom allergy: relation to severity of sting reactions and to safety and efficacy of venom immunotherapy. Clin Exp Allergy 2003;33:1216–20.

16. Rueff F, Placzek M, Przybilla B. Mastocytosis and Hymenoptera venom allergy. Curr Opin Allergy Clin Immunol 2006;6:284–8.

17. Potier A, Lavigne C, Chappard D, et al. Cutaneous manifestations in Hymenoptera and Diptera anaphylaxis: relationship with basal serum tryptase. Clin Exp Allergy 2009;39:717–25.

18. Guenova E, Volz T, Eichner M, et al. Basal serum tryptase as risk assessment for severe Hymenoptera sting reactions in elderly. Allergy 2010;65(7):919–23.

19. Biedermann T, Rueff F, Sander CA, et al. Mastocytosis associated with severe wasp sting anaphylaxis detected by elevated serum mast cell tryptase levels. Br J Dermatol 1999;141:1110–2.

20. Müller UR, Horat W, Wuthrich B, et al. Anaphylaxis after Hymenoptera stings in three patients with urticaria pigmentosa. J Allergy Clin Immunol 1983;72(6):685–9.

21. Florian S, Krauth MT, Simonitsch-Klupp I, et al. Indolent systemic mastocytosis with elevated serum tryptase, absence of skin lesions, and recurrent severe anaphylactoid episodes. Int Arch Allergy Immunol 2005;136(3):273–8.

22. Oude Elberink JN, de Monchy JG, Kors JW, et al. Fatal anaphylaxis after a yellow jacket sting, despite venom immunotherapy, in two patients with mastocytosis. J Allergy Clin Immunol 1997;99:153–4.

23. Bonadonna P, Perbellini O, Passalacqua G, et al. Clonal mast cell disorders in patients with systemic reactions to Hymenoptera stings and increased serum tryptase levels. J Allergy Clin Immunol 2009;123:680–6.

24. Schwartz LB. Diagnostic value of tryptase in anaphylaxis and mastocytosis. Immunol Allergy Clin North Am 2006;26:451–63.
25. Metcalfe DD, Schwart LB. Assessing anaphylactic risk? Consider mast cell clonality. J Allergy Clin Immunol 2009;123:687–8.
26. Van Doormaal JJ, van der Veer E, van Voorst Vader PC, et al. Tryptase and histamine metabolites as diagnostic indicators of indolent systemic mastocytosis without skin lesions. Allergy 2012;67:683–90.
27. Zanotti R, Lombardo C, Passalacqua G, et al. Clonal mast cell disorders in patients with severe Hymenoptera venom allergy and normal serum tryptase levels. J Allergy Clin Immunol 2015;136(1):135–9.
28. Alvarez-Twose I, Bonadonna P, Matito A, et al. Systemic mastocytosis as a risk factor for severe Hymenoptera sting-induced anaphylaxis. J Allergy Clin Immunol 2013;13:614–5.
29. Rossini M, Zanotti R, Viapiana O, et al. Bone involvement and osteoporosis in mastocytosis. Immunol Allergy Clin North Am 2014;34(2):383–96.
30. Reimers A, Muller U. Fatal outcome of a Vespula sting in a patient with mastocytosis after specific immunotherapy with honey bee venom. Swiss Med Wkly 2005; 135(suppl 144):S14.
31. Bonadonna P, Zanotti R, Pagani M, et al. Anaphylactic reactions after discontinuation of Hymenoptera venom immunotherapy: a clonal mast cell disorder should be suspected. J Allergy Clin Immunol Pract 2017 [pii:S2213-2198(17) 30913-3].
32. Ludolph-Hauser D, Ruëff F, Fries C, et al. Constitutively raised serum concentrations of mast-cell tryptase and severe anaphylactic reactions to Hymenoptera stings. Lancet 2001;357(9253):361–2.
33. Fricker M, Helbling A, Schwartz L, et al. Hymenoptera sting anaphylaxis and urticaria pigmentosa: clinical findings and results of venom immunotherapy in ten patients. J Allergy Clin Immunol 1997;100:11–5.
34. Alvarez-Twose I, Zanotti R, González-de-Olano D, et al. Non aggressive systemic mastocytosis (SM) without skin lesions associated with insect-induced anaphylaxis shows unique features versus other indolent SM. J Allergy Clin Immunol 2014;133:520–8.
35. Castells MC, Hornick JL, Akin C. Anaphylaxis after Hymenoptera sting: is it venom allergy, a clonal disorder, or both? J Allergy Clin Immunol Pract 2015;3(3):350–5.
36. Van Anrooij B, van der Veer E, de Monchy JG, et al. Higher mast cell load decreases the risk of Hymenoptera venom-induced anaphylaxis in patients with mastocytosis. J Allergy Clin Immunol 2013;132:125–30.
37. Wimazal F, Geissler P, Shnawa P, et al. Severe life-threatening or disabling anaphylaxis in patients with systemic mastocytosis: a single-center experience. Int Arch Allergy Immunol 2011;25(157):399–405.
38. Bilò BM, Rueff F, Mosbech H, et al. Diagnosis of Hymenoptera venom allergy. Allergy 2005;60:1339–49.
39. Schafer T, Przybilla B. IgE antibodies to Hymenoptera venoms in the serum are common in the general population and are related to indications of atopy. Allergy 1996;51:372–7.
40. Sturm GJ, Schuster C, Kranzelbinder B, et al. Asymptomatic sensitization to Hymenoptera venom is related to total immunoglobulin E levels. Int Arch Allergy Immunol 2008;148:261–4.
41. Sturm GJ, Jin C, Kranzelbinder B, et al. Inconsistent results of diagnostic tools hamper the differentiation between bee and vespid venom allergy. PLoS One 2011;6:e20842.

42. Hemmer W, Focke M, Kolarich D, et al. Antibody binding to venom carbohydrates is a frequent cause for double positivity to honeybee and yellow jacket venom in patients with stinging-insect allergy. J Allergy Clin Immunol 2001;108:1045–52.

43. Sturm GJ, Kranzelbinder B, Christian S, et al. Sensitization to Hymenoptera venoms is common, but systemic sting reactions are rare. J Allergy Clin Immunol 2014;133:1635–43.

44. Przybilla B, Rueff F. Insect stings: clinical features and management. Dtsch Arztebl Int 2012;109:238–48.

45. Bonadonna P, Zanotti R, Melioli G, et al. The role of basophil activation test in special populations with mastocytosis and reactions to Hymenoptera sting. Allergy 2012;67:962–5.

46. Bonadonna P, Gonzalez-de-Olano D, Zanotti R, et al. Venom Immunotherapy in patients with clonal mast cell disorders: efficacy, safety, and practical considerations. J Allergy Clin Immunol Pract 2013;1:474–8.

47. Michel J, Brockow K, Darsow U, et al. Added sensitivity of component-resolved diagnosis in Hymenoptera venom-allergic patients with elevated serum tryptase and/or mastocytosis. Allergy 2016;71(5):651–60.

48. Blank S, Bilò MB, Ollert M. Component-resolved diagnostics to direct in venom immunotherapy: important steps towards precision medicine. Clin Exp Allergy 2018;48(4):354–64.

49. Caruso B, Bonadonna P, Bovo C, et al. Wasp venom allergy screening with recombinant allergen testing. Diagnostic performance of rPol d 5 and rVes v 5 for differentiating sensitization to Vespula and Polistes subspecies. Clin Chim Acta 2016;453:170–3.

50. Vos BJPR, van Anrooij B, van Doormaal JJ, et al. Fatal anaphylaxis to yellow jacket stings in mastocytosis: options for identification and treatment of at-risk patients. J Allergy Clin Immunol Pract 2017;5(5):1264–71.

51. Hoffmann HJ, Santos AF, Mayorga C, et al. The clinical utility of basophil activation testing in diagnosis and monitoring of allergic disease. Allergy 2015;70: 1393–405.

52. De Weck AL, Sanz ML. Flow cytometric cellular allergen stimulation test (FAST/ Flow- CAST): technical and clinical evaluation of a new diagnostic test in allergy and pseudo-allergy. ACI Int 2002;14:204–15.

53. Sturm GJ, Böhm E, Trummer M, et al. The CD63 basophil activation test in Hymenoptera venom allergy: a prospective study. Allergy 2004;59:1110–7.

54. Eberlein-Konig B, Rakoski J, Behrendt H, et al. Use of CD63 expression as marker of in vitro basophil activation in identifying the culprit in insect venom allergy. J Investig Allergol Clin Immunol 2004;14:10–6.

55. Dubois AE, van der Heide S. Basophil-activation tests in Hymenoptera allergy. Curr Opin Allergy Clin Immunol 2007;7:346–9.

56. Gonzalez-de-Olano D, Alvarez-Twose I, Morgado JM, et al. Evaluation of basophil activation in mastocytosis with Hymenoptera venom anaphylaxis. Cytometry B Clin Cytom 2011;80:167–75.

57. Rietveld MJ, Schreurs MW, Gerth van Wijk R, et al. The basophil activation test is not a useful screening tool for Hymenoptera venom-related anaphylaxis in patients with systemic mastocytosis. Int Arch Allergy Immunol 2016;169(2):125–9.

58. Sturm GJ, Varga EM, Roberts G, et al. EAACI guidelines on allergen immunotherapy: Hymenoptera venom allergy. Allergy 2018;73(4):744–64.

59. Niedoszykto M, DeMonchy J, vanDoormal JJ, et al. Mastocytosis and insect venom allergy: diagnosis, safety and efficacy of venom immunotherapy. Allergy 2009;64:1237–45.

60. Incorvaia C, Frati F, Dell'Albani I, et al. Safety of Hymenoptera venom immuno-therapy: a systematic review. Expert Opin Pharmacother 2011;12:2527–32.
61. Engler RJ, Davis WS. Rush Hymenoptera venom immunotherapy: successful treatment in a patient with systemic mast cell disease. J Allergy Clin Immunol 1994;94:556–9.
62. Galera C, Soohun N, Zankar N, et al. Severe anaphylaxis to bee venom immuno-therapy: efficacy of pretreatment and concurrent treatment with omalizumab. J Investig Allergol Clin Immunol 2009;19:225–9.
63. Kontou-Fili K, Filis CI. Prolonged high-dose omalizumab is required to control re-actions to venom immunotherapy in mastocytosis. Allergy 2009;64(9):1384–5.
64. da Silva EN, Randall KL. Omalizumab mitigates anaphylaxis during ultrarush hon-ey bee venom immunotherapy in monoclonal mast cell activation syndrome. J Allergy Clin Immunol Pract 2013;1(6):687–8.
65. Sokol KC, Ghazi A, Kelly BC, et al. Omalizumab as a desensitizing agent and treatment in mastocytosis: a review of the literature and case report. J Allergy Clin Immunol Pract 2014;2(3):266–70.
66. Kors JW, van Doormaal JJ, de Monchy JG. Anaphylactoid shock following Hyme-noptera sting as a presenting symptom of systemic mastocytosis. J Intern Med 1993;233(3):255–8.
67. Simioni L, Vianello A, Bonadonna P, et al. Efficacy of venom immunotherapy given every 3 or 4 months: a prospective comparison with the conventional regimen. Ann Allergy Asthma Immunol 2013;110:51–4.
68. Bilò MB, Cichocka-Jarosz E, Pumphrey R, et al. Self-medication of anaphylactic reactions due to Hymenoptera stings-an EAACI task force consensus statement. Allergy 2016;71(7):931–43.

Nonclonal Mast Cell Activation Syndrome

A Growing Body of Evidence

Matthew J. Hamilton, MD

KEYWORDS

- Mast cell activation syndrome • Tryptase • Histamine • Prostaglandin
- Mastocytosis • Mast cell • Flushing

KEY POINTS

- Patients who present with typical features of mast cell activation with laboratory confirmation and without evidence of a clonal mast cell disorder or other medical condition should be initiated on medical treatment to block mast cells and their mediators.
- If a major response is achieved, a diagnosis of nonclonal mast cell activation syndrome (NC-MCAS) is likely and treatment should be optimized, including management of any associated conditions.
- In this review, the latest evidence with regard to the diagnosis and treatment of NC-MCAS is presented.

INTRODUCTION

Over the last decade, recognition of a unique syndrome has emerged in clinical practices and in the literature. These patients present with a unique constellation of signs and symptoms suggesting primary mast cell activation, such as systemic mastocytosis (SM), but without fulfilling the established criteria (**Fig. 1**). Furthermore, these patients do not have primary allergic disorders to better explain their presentation, such as immunoglobulin E (IgE)–mediated allergy, chronic idiopathic urticaria, or idiopathic anaphylaxis (examples of secondary mast cell activation). Other medical inflammatory conditions, autoimmune diseases, malignant processes, and infections have been ruled out. Although objective markers for this disorder are lacking at this time, patients are diagnosed with idiopathic mast cell activation syndrome (MCAS) and have greatly benefitted from specific treatments that work to block the mast cell mediators. In this review, the diagnosis and treatment of nonclonal idiopathic MCAS (NC-MCAS) are discussed.

Disclosure Statement: The author has no relevant disclosures to declare.
Division of Gastroenterology, Hepatology, and Endoscopy, Harvard Medical School, Brigham and Women's Hospital, 75 Francis Street, Boston, MA 02115, USA
E-mail address: mjhamilton@bwh.harvard.edu

Immunol Allergy Clin N Am 38 (2018) 469–481
https://doi.org/10.1016/j.iac.2018.04.002

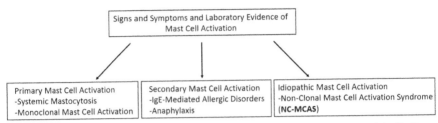

Fig. 1. Classification schemes of mast cell activation disorders. IgE, immunoglobulin E.

BACKGROUND AND PROPOSED MECHANISMS

The mast cell is a complex immune cell that in its mature form resides in the tissues that interact with the external environment, such as the air passageway, skin, and gastrointestinal tract. Although best known for its central role in allergy, anaphylaxis, and asthma, mast cells primarily function in host defense to bacteria, parasites, and viruses (reviewed in[1]). Although a full explanation for the mechanisms that drive activation of mast cells is beyond the scope of this review, it is important to highlight the diversity of receptors and mediators that mast cells may release that characterize the diverse aspects of mast cell activation. Although mast cells exhibit plasticity in development and in response to various stimuli, they generally express the high affinity IgE receptor and low affinity IgG receptor, receptors for complement, proteinase-activating receptors, and pathogen-specific receptors, such as toll-like receptors. On activation, mast cells release a variety of preformed mediators housed in the cytosol granules, including proteases (tryptase, chymase), histamine, newly generated lipid mediators including prostaglandins and leukotrienes, and more than 30 cytokines and chemokines that may be synthesized and released (reviewed in[2]). These mediators that are released either in total (eg, anaphylaxis) or piecemeal[3] carry out a wide array of pathophysiologic functions, including dilation of blood vessels, stimulatory and inhibitory interactions with nerves, physiologic shifts in electrolytes and fluids, and serving as a chemoattractant for other immune cells (eg, neutrophils).

The pathologic hallmark of NC-MCAS is inappropriate activation of mast cells to stimuli that otherwise would be tolerated if not in the activated or reactive state. This inappropriate activation may occur because of altered threshold for activation, aberrant expression of receptors and mediators shifted toward an allergic immune response, or changes in the tissue environment that affect the expression and function of the mediators.[4] There may also exist defects or changes in downstream signaling pathways for mast cell activation (reviewed in[5]). The genetic basis for NC-MCAS is not well understood, but a team of investigators has identified many mutations in the KIT receptor (responsible for proliferation and retention of mast cells in the tissues) and alternative splicing variants in the CD117+ peripheral blood cells of patients with NC-MCAS.[6]

CLINICAL FEATURES

It has become apparent that there is a typical constellation of signs and symptoms of mast cell activation that suggest NC-MCAS and then a smattering of other features that may be more unique to an individual. Many of these classic symptoms have been long appreciated in patients with SM. These symptoms are necessary for the diagnosis (**Box 1**) and include signs and symptoms involving the skin (flushing, pruritis, urticaria, sweating, localized swelling), the air passageway and lungs (rhinitis, throat

---

Box 1

Typical presenting features of nonclonal mast cell activation syndrome

Typical Mast Cell Activation Symptoms

Skin-flushing, pruritis, sweating, urticaria

Air passageway: rhinitis, throat itching and swelling, dyspnea, wheeze

Gastrointestinal: abdominal pain, diarrhea, nausea, bloating

Cardiac: palpitations, tachycardia, presyncope

Neurologic: headache, paresthesias, memory and concentration difficulties

Typical Mast Cell Activation Signs

Skin: dermatographism, flushing (face and chest)

Gastrointestinal: bloat, abdominal tenderness

Cardiac: tachycardia

Typical Mast Cell Activation Triggers

Heat and temperatures changes

Stress

Alcohol

Certain drugs: morphine, NSAIDs, antibiotics

Strong odors: perfumes, smoke, cleaning agents

Typical Demographics

Female

Age: fifth and sixth decade

Caucasian

Typical Associated Conditions

POTS: adrenergic type

Ehlers-Danlos syndrome: hypermobility type

Abbreviations: NSAIDs, nonsteroidal antiinflammatory drugs; POTS, postural orthostatic tachycardia syndrome.

---

tightness, wheezing, dyspnea), the gastrointestinal tract (intermittent abdominal pain and cramping, loose stools and diarrhea, abdominal bloating, nausea, reflux), the neurologic system (headaches, difficulty with concentration and memory [brain fog], tingling in the extremities), and the cardiovascular system (palpitations, fast heart rate, presyncope, hypotension, and syncope). More atypical signs and symptoms may exist in any other organ systems, such as various aches and pains; however, patients and providers should hesitate to attribute all of their symptoms to mast cell activation, especially when they are not relieved with medications that block the mast cell mediators or that occur in isolation of the other symptoms.

Although triggers for mast cell activation in an individual with NC-MCAS may be numerous, particularly when in an activated state, there are a set of triggers commonly experienced in these patients. In a cross-sectional survey filled out by patients with mast cell disorders, including those with SM, cutaneous mastocytosis, and NC-MCAS, heat was the most common trigger reported in 82%, followed by stress (81%), exercise (63%), alcohol (54%), medications (53%), and odors (48%).[7]

Several recent studies have attempted to identify clinical characteristics of patients with presumed NC-MCAS. In a population of 83 patients who presented to an allergy clinic for further evaluation of "severe and systemic" mast cell activation symptoms, 39% did not have evidence for a clonal mast cell population on bone marrow biopsy and were labeled NC-MCAS.[8] The investigators in this study aimed to compare the clinical, biological, and molecular characteristics of this identified population with NC-MCAS compared with the patients diagnosed with a primary clonal form of mast cell disorder. When compared with the clonal mast cell disorder groups, the patients with NC-MCAS had significantly more urticaria and angioedema, were more often female, and were triggered more by drugs. In addition, the patients with NC-MCAS were triggered less by insect stings and had less presyncope and syncope. In keeping with the diagnostic criteria, patients with NC-MCAS also had lower tryptase levels and no evidence of clonal mast cells as assessed by serum KIT mutations and presence of CD25 on bone marrow examination.

The clinical manifestations of a cohort of patients referred to a center with expertise in mast cell disorders and diagnosed with NC-MCAS (classic symptoms and signs of mast cell activation, an elevated mast cell mediator on laboratory testing, positive response to anti–mast cell mediator therapy, and without other medical conditions to explain the symptoms) were evaluated. In this select group of 18 patients, gastrointestinal symptoms were prominent, with abdominal pain and diarrhea present in 17 (94%) and 12 (67%) of patients, respectively. The skin manifestations of flushing and dermatographism were each present in 16 (89%) of patients, whereas headache and poor concentration and memory were observed in 15 (83%) and 12 (67%).

The reported signs and symptoms of mast cell activation in NC-MCAS are remarkably similar to published cohorts of patients with SM ([9–12] and reviewed in[13]).

In the published cohort studies of NC-MCAS, there is a female predominance with a peak age of diagnosis in the fifth and sixth decades, although many of the patients had experienced signs and symptoms for many years before diagnosis.[14] Most patients diagnosed with NC-MCAS are Caucasian, but there is little published about the incidence in non–North American and European populations. The overall prevalence of NC-MCAS is unknown but is thought to be perhaps 10-fold higher than SM by many experts studying this disorder.

DIAGNOSTIC GUIDELINES

Although no consensus diagnostic criteria exist for NC-MCAS, proposed diagnostic criteria have been published[15,16] and then discussed at a working conference of experts in 2012.[17] Important to the panel set of guidelines[17] is the "accepted, objective, easily measurable, and commonly applicable parameters and criteria." By these guidelines and in order to satisfy the criteria, typical symptoms (as described earlier) must be present and intermittent or persistent and involving 2 or more organ systems. The objective piece for the diagnosis is a documented increase in easily and reproducibly measurable mediators over baseline during a period of increased symptoms attributable to mast cell activation. The preferred mediator is the mast cell–specific serum tryptase, and other acceptable mediators include 24-hour urine tests for metabolites to histamine and prostaglandin D2 (see diagnostic testing discussed later). The third criterion is a major response (>50% reduction) in mast cell activation symptoms with medications that block the production or activity of mast cell mediators. It is noted that the medications used to treat mast cell activation may have actions on other cell types and factors so that the medication response is only considered supportive to the diagnosis.

Important to the criteria port forth by Akin and colleagues[15] is the fourth criterion, which is to rule out other causes of mast cell activation and those medical conditions that may present with overlapping signs and symptoms. There are 2 primary causes of mast cell activation that must be considered and ruled out before diagnosing patients with NC-MCAS. One is SM, a proliferative mast cell disorder characterized by specific clonal mutations most often in the KIT gene (eg, D816 V) and defined by a set of criteria including one major and 4 minor criteria.[18] The other is monoclonal MCAS whereby there are clonal populations of mast cells but without abnormal proliferation or clustering of mast cells, overall satisfying 1 or 2 minor and no major criteria for SM.[19] Medical conditions that may be associated with evidence of secondary mast cell activation include atopic disease and allergy mediated by IgE, autoimmune disorders and autoimmune urticaria, neoplasms, drug allergies, chronic infections, and chronic inflammatory conditions, such as rheumatoid arthritis and inflammatory bowel disease.

Although no subclassifications of NC-MCAS currently exist, one possible subgroup of patients has been recently described who have elevated serum levels of alpha tryptase due to duplications and triplications in the specific tryptase gene.[20] They exhibit many clinical features of NC-MCAS, and this specific disorder is inherited with variable penetrance.

DIAGNOSTIC TESTING

As mentioned, laboratory testing can help confirm the diagnosis of NC-MCAS. Detection of serum tryptase is an important screening tool in the evaluation of patients with a suspected mast cell disorder and is a highly reliable and reproducible test. Mast cells in the tissue produce and constitutively release the alpha form of tryptase, which can be detected by a commercial fluoro-immune enzyme assay. A specialized assay can detect the beta form of tryptase that is released from the granules on anaphylaxis or certain types of mast cell activation.[21] The median baseline alpha tryptase level for heathy human individuals is approximately 5 ng/mL, and most laboratories consider a level less than 11.4 ng/mL to be normal.[22] A level greater than 20 ng/mL is a minor criterion for the diagnosis of SM,[18] and a baseline level greater than 11.4 and less than 20.0 ng/mL is suggestive of a diagnosis of NC-MCAS. Elevation of serum tryptase is detected during or within 4 hours of a reaction (reviewed in[23]), and the expert panel on the diagnostic criteria of NC-MCAS agreed that a 20%+ 2 ng/mL increase from the baseline level constitutes mast cell activation.[17] It is important to note that false-positive elevations in serum tryptase may exist, including chronic end-stage kidney disease and certain hematologic malignancies (reviewed in[24]).

Histamine metabolites in a 24-hour urine specimen (N-methyl histamine) are also a reliable marker of mast cell activation in certain patients albeit less specific than mast cell tryptase given that basophils also produce and release histamine. The third suggested laboratory test to confirm mast cell activation is prostaglandin D2 or its metabolite 11-beta prostaglandin F2-alpha in a 24-hour urine specimen.

In a study that showed the utility of the measurement of metabolites for histamine and prostaglandin to detect mast cell activation using urine assays, the investigators found differences between a group of patients with chronic urticaria with hypersensitivity to aspirin and food additives who were challenged compared with a group that was not sensitive to aspirin and food additives who were challenged.[25]

Other laboratory assessments that have been used in MCAS include chromogranin A, a member of the granin family of neuroendocrine secretory proteins. This test is not specific to mast cells and may be affected by cardiac and renal failure and medications, namely, proton pump inhibitors. Plasma heparin may be a strong marker of mast cell activation and was positive more often than the traditional markers mentioned earlier in a study of 257 patients with MCAS and SM,[26] but current clinical assays are not sensitive enough to detect the low levels that may be released. A urine test for the detection of leukotriene E4 is being developed, which could also serve as a helpful diagnostic tool to detect mast cell activation.[27]

The assessment of tissue biopsies is an important part of the diagnostic workup of patients with NC-MCAS, mainly to rule out other primary causes of mast cell activation and medical conditions, such as inflammatory disorders and malignancies. Criteria have been established for the indications to perform a bone marrow biopsy on patients suspected of having a clonal mast cell disorder; these include individually or a combination of the following: presence of urticaria pigmentosa skin lesions, tryptase greater than 15 ng/mL, unexplained anaphylaxis, REMA (Spanish Network on Mastocytosis) score greater than 2,[28] and presence of typical mast cell symptoms. In the absence of any of these factors, the diagnostic yield of biopsies for clonal mast cells in the bone marrow or other organs is thought to be low. In the intestine, patients with NC-MCAS have normal findings at endoscopy and the mast cells on histology are single and dispersed and found in similar numbers compared with a healthy control population.[14] In a study that compared 100 patients with irritable bowel syndrome (IBS) with 100 healthy controls and 10 patients with MCAS, there was no clinically meaningful difference in the numbers of mast cells in the intestinal mucosa between any of the groups. Future studies may help to determine whether there are subtypes of NC-MCAS that may indeed have significantly elevated mast cells, as 30% of the patients with NC-MCAS had "increased mast cells " (>25 per high power field) compared with 16% of controls.[29]

A highly sensitive and specific, noninvasive screening test for primary clonal mast cell disorders is a peripheral blood test to detect the KIT D816 V mutation.[30] A positive result for this test when a clonal mast cell disorder is strongly suspected is a minor diagnostic criterion for SM.[18]

ASSOCIATED CONDITIONS

Although not well reported in the literature, it is becoming apparent that there are certain conditions that present in association with NC-MCAS. What is not known is how or why these associations occur and how mast cell activation may or may not specifically play a role. One such condition is the postural orthostatic tachycardia syndrome (POTS). In a small study, patients with POTS and mast cell activation, defined as elevated histamine levels and presence of flushing, had more adrenergic features of POTS compared with subjects with POTS without mast cell activation and healthy controls.[31] These features included orthostatic tachycardia and elevated blood pressure in the upright position. Another condition that is frequently present in association with NC-MCAS is the connective tissue disorder Ehlers-Danlos syndrome, particularly the hypermobility subtype. In the cohort of patients with symptoms attributable to mast cell activation and inherited duplications of the tryptase gene leading to alpha hypertryptasemia, there was an associated prevalence of POTS and joint hypermobility.[20]

In the current proposed guidelines for NC-MCAS, patients with anaphylaxis are best characterized as idiopathic anaphylaxis, although there may be a spectrum of the disorders whereby some patients have prominent MCAS manifestations in between anaphylactic episodes and may be better characterized as NC-MCAS with anaphylaxis (reviewed in[32]).

Not surprisingly, allergic disorders and specific IgE-mediated allergies to environmental factors and foods are prominent in patients with NC-MAS and should be weighed in the context of the presenting manifestations to decide whether secondary mast cell activation due to allergy is the more appropriate diagnosis. Furthermore, the presence of NC-MCAS may increase the severity of allergic reactions as was shown in a cohort of patients with NC-MCAS and allergy to amoxicillin.[33]

Patients with NC-MCAS have numerous non–IgE-mediated intolerances to foods and drugs that provoke various symptoms. A possible mechanism for the idiosyncratic, non–IgE-mediated reactions to drugs was recently identified. Investigators showed that many basic secretagogues, such as inflammatory peptides, and drugs can activate the mast cell surface receptor Mrgprb2 that is the orthologue of the G-coupled receptor MRGPRX2.[34]

TREATMENT OPTIONS

The successful treatment of patients with NC-MCAS requires a multimodal approach to address the multitude of triggers, reactions, and intermittent and chronic symptoms (**Box 2**). It is possible that patients with NC-MCAS experience heightened reactivity states that increase with each individual reaction, a state that may be highest around the time of diagnosis. Therefore, a key arm of treatment is an understanding of the triggers for each individual followed by strict avoidance. Unfortunately, there is no clinically validated test for the non–IgE-mediated reactions that patients with NC-MCAS may experience. Although there is a host of classic triggers (outlined earlier), an individual may experience unique triggers that are only identified after an exposure and subsequent reaction.

The next step in treatment management is the initiation and titration of medications that target mast cells and their mediators in order to break the cycle of reactivity. In general, a combination of medications are used in a stepwise approach and adjusted to maximal efficacy, tolerance, and safety for each individual. Because of the reactivity

---

Box 2
The phases of diagnosis and treatment of patients with nonclonal mast cell activation syndrome

Phase 1

Establishing diagnosis-typical symptoms, laboratory tests, ruling out other conditions (provider)

Trial of medications to block mast cells and mediators (provider and patient)

Learning individual triggers for mast cell activation (patient)

Phase 2

Adding mast cell blocking medications in a stepwise manner (provider)

Discerning which symptoms are due to mast cell activation and which are not (patient)

Managing how to avoid triggers: environmental, diet (patient)

Phase 3

Adjusting dosing of mast cell blocking medications (provider)

Adding in complementary therapies: stress reduction, exercise (provider and patient)

Reassessing any new symptoms or signs not typical of mast cell activation (provider)

---

of patients with NC-MCAS, it is advised to start with low doses of each new medication and titrate to the recommended daily maintenance doses. It is also important to note that in the United States there are no medications that are approved by the Food and Drug Administration for the treatment of NC-MCAS, so the recommendations discussed later are considered off-label use.

The first-line medication is often the combination of nonsedating H1 antihistamines (eg, cetirizine, loratadine, and fexofenadine) and H2 antihistamines (eg, ranitidine and famotidine). The antivasodilatory effects of type 1 and 2 antihistamines may work best when used in combination. Their dosages are adjusted to the minimum effective amount so as to prevent tachyphylaxis and side effects, such as sedation and dry mouth. It is important for patients with NC-MCAS to have on-demand treatment of significant reactions and could include short-acting H1 blockers, such as a sublingual form of loratadine or traditional diphenhydramine.

Although the H1 type of antihistamines are considered first-line agents in most published guidelines, there is little published evidence of efficacy; most trials were conducted several decades ago with small numbers of patients with SM (reviewed in[35]). In a more recent trial, investigators enrolled 33 patients with systemic and cutaneous mastocytosis to receive the second-generation H1 antihistamine rupatadine versus placebo. They found significant improvements in itching, flushing, skin reactivity, headache, and tachycardia. Quality of life was also improved.[36]

A key maintenance medication most often used in combination with antihistamines is cromolyn sodium. Although the exact mechanisms of action of this drug are not fully known, one study showed that cromolyn acts as an agonist for the G-protein-coupled 35 receptor expressed in human mast cells and alters calcium flux, a process thought to be necessary for the release of the cytosolic granule mediators once the mast cell is activated.[37] This medication has been used with good effect to treat the gastrointestinal manifestations of SM, including abdominal pain and cramping, loose stools and diarrhea, abdominal bloating, and nausea.[38] A more recent study was designed to evaluate the ability of cromolyn to treat patients with diarrhea-predominant IBS, a functional disorder of the gut with a similar intestinal symptom profile as mastocytosis and whereby mast cell activation is known to play a role.[39–41] The investigators determined that cromolyn reduced gastrointestinal symptoms and markers of mast cell activation, such as luminal tryptase and ultrastructure changes showing degranulation of mast cells. Although cromolyn is thought to have poor intestinal absorption, patients may report improvement in symptoms outside of the gastrointestinal tract; it may be considered to be a first-line therapy. A case report details the added symptom benefit of inhaled cromolyn for symptoms attributed to mast cell activation.[42]

Another medication that has been used for the treatment of anaphylaxis and extended to the treatment of NC-MCAS is ketotifen, which is thought to have both antihistamine and mast cell–stabilizing properties. In a study to assess the effect of treatment with ketotifen on patients with IBS characterized by increased visceral hypersensitivity in the rectum, patients with IBS had improvement in the hypersensitivity as well as other symptoms of IBS and quality of life. The investigators in this study, however, did not detect changes in the release of histamine or tryptase in the rectal biopsies, so the exact mechanism of action of ketotifen was not determined.[43] In one small, blinded, placebo-controlled study comparing treatment with ketotifen with hydroxyzine over 12 weeks in patients with pediatric mastocytosis and mediator-related symptoms, 7 of 8 patients had a greater reduction in symptoms with hydroxyzine.[44]

If symptoms persist, other medications may be added in a stepwise approach. The cysteinyl leukotriene receptor blockers (eg, montelukast) and 5-lipoxygenase inhibitors (eg, zileuton) may be especially effective for pulmonary and airway symptoms in keeping with their primary indication in asthma.

Aspirin has been proposed as a treatment of patients with NC-MCAS with elevated urine prostaglandin metabolites. In a small case series, baseline levels of prostaglandin were restored to normal and symptoms were prevented.[45] To achieve therapeutic targets, high doses of aspirin were needed (325 mg to 650 mg daily but as high as 1950 mg in one patient), which may limit their use because of the bleeding risk and gastrointestinal toxicity. In another study of patients with MC-MCAS at the Mayo Clinic, 9 patients with elevated prostaglandin levels were treated with aspirin therapy, 8 had normalization of urine prostaglandin levels, and 6 out of 9 experienced symptom improvement (flushing and pruritis were the most common symptoms in this subset).[46]

Corticosteroids are given for refractory cases but ideally in short effective courses so as to limit steroid side effects. They may be used in the acute setting for severe reactions and before diagnostic studies or procedures when severe reactions are anticipated. All patients with NC-MCAS should be asked about episodes of anaphylaxis and prescribed injectable epinephrine if there is any suspicion. This treatment is potentially lifesaving.

Flavonoids including quercetin are compounds with antioxidant and antiinflammatory properties that have been shown to inhibit the release of cytokines and proteases from cultured human mast cells.[47] In a publication comparing the use of the flavonoid quercetin with cromolyn, quercetin more effectively blocked inflammatory cytokine release and reduced symptoms of contact dermatitis and photosensitivity in a small, pilot, nonblinded clinical trial.[48]

Lastly, omalizumab, a monoclonal antibody to IgE that may increase the threshold for mast cell mediator release, has had efficacy in refractory cases of patients presenting with mast cell activation. In a small, nonblinded, observational study of patients with SM, treatment with omalizumab resulted in a complete or major reduction in the physician global assessment of symptoms in more than half of the patients. Treatment efficacy was best with skin manifestations and episodes of anaphylaxis at the various time points with a median duration of follow-up of 17 months.[49] Although the experience with omalizumab for the treatment of NC-MCAS is less studied and published, there are reports of treatment success for this patient population.[50]

There are very limited published data on the response to medical therapies for NC-MCAS. In a nonblinded and non–placebo-controlled trial using standardized treatment response criteria established for SM,[14] 12 of 18 patients with NC-MCAS had a complete or major (>50%) regression in symptoms after 12 months of standard anti–mast cell medical therapy. There were no patients who had no regression in symptoms.

OTHER TREATMENTS

Specific dietary interventions for the treatment of symptoms have not been studied in patients with mast cell disorders. In practice, the single most important dietary recommendation is to avoid known triggers. Other recommendations may include avoiding foods known to be high in histamine content and poorly tolerated, processed and preserved foods; inflammatory foods, such as sugars and foods high in omega-6 fatty acid content and alcohol. Several dietary factors that have been shown to suppress mast cell activation include vitamin C (reviewed in[51]) and curcumin.[52] Gluten has been shown to stimulate mast cell activation,[53] and many patients with NC-MCAS report improvement in symptoms with gluten avoidance.

Numerous studies have examined the relationship between depression, anxiety, and psychological stress with mast cell activation and mast cell disorders (reviewed in[54,55]). To round out the treatment of patients with NC-MCAS, medical and behavioral therapy should be directed at the coexisting psychiatric symptoms. Patients are encouraged to pursue activities for stress reduction, such as yoga, meditation, and exercise.

SUMMARY AND FUTURE PERSPECTIVES

In this review, the characteristic clinical presentation of patients with NC-MCAS is highlighted and that includes atypical features that may characterize an individual's symptom profile. The greatest challenge for the treating provider is to correctly attribute signs and symptoms to the disorder and to appropriately workup any other features that may not fit or may overlap with other diseases. As emphasized in this review, objective markers for the disorder are lacking and every effort must be made to obtain confirmatory laboratory evidence and to rule out other conditions with appropriate testing. If the diagnosis is suspected and other more likely conditions have been ruled out, directed medical therapies targeting mast cell mediators can not only help to confirm the diagnosis but can also provide relief to the significant burden of illness.

The development of objective markers of disease may lead to a diagnostic test or tests and established guidelines for treatment that may easily be followed by the wide array of providers seeing these patients. Once established, clinical studies and clinical trials will be possible to build on the foundation of our current understanding of the disorder and its treatment. Drug discovery may also be advanced to include curative therapies that reset the hyperactive and inappropriate immune response. Although there is a lot of work to be done, these future developments are obtainable and begin with increased awareness among the medical and scientific research communities of the many complex features of NC-MCAS.

REFERENCES

1. Theoharides TC, Valent P, Akin C. Mast cells, mastocytosis, and related disorders. N Engl J Med 2015;373:1885–6.
2. Douaiher J, Succar J, Lancerotto L, et al. Development of mast cells and importance of their tryptase and chymase serine proteases in inflammation and wound healing. Adv Immunol 2014;122:211–52.
3. Dvorak AM, McLeod RS, Onderdonk A, et al. Ultrastructural evidence for piecemeal and anaphylactic degranulation of human gut mucosal mast cells in vivo. Int Arch Allergy Immunol 1992;99:74–83.
4. Maintz L, Novak N. Histamine and histamine intolerance. Am J Clin Nutr 2007;85: 1185–96.
5. Gilfillan AM, Tkaczyk C. Integrated signalling pathways for mast-cell activation. Nat Rev Immunol 2006;6:218–30.
6. Molderings GJ, Meis K, Kolck UW, et al. Comparative analysis of mutation of tyrosine kinase kit in mast cells from patients with systemic mast cell activation syndrome and healthy subjects. Immunogenetics 2010;62:721–7.
7. Jennings S, Russell N, Jennings B, et al. The Mastocytosis Society survey on mast cell disorders: patient experiences and perceptions. J Allergy Clin Immunol Pract 2014;2:70–6.
8. Alvarez-Twose I, Gonzalez de Olano D, Sanchez-Munoz L, et al. Clinical, biological, and molecular characteristics of clonal mast cell disorders presenting with systemic mast cell activation symptoms. J Allergy Clin Immunol 2010;125: 1269–78.e2.

9. Castells M, Austen KF. Mastocytosis: mediator-related signs and symptoms. Int Arch Allergy Immunol 2002;127:147–52.

10. Cherner JA, Jensen RT, Dubois A, et al. Gastrointestinal dysfunction in systemic mastocytosis. A prospective study. Gastroenterology 1988;95:657–67.

11. Sokol H, Georgin-Lavialle S, Canioni D, et al. Gastrointestinal manifestations in mastocytosis: a study of 83 patients. J Allergy Clin Immunol 2013;132:866–73.e1-3.

12. Pieri L, Bonadonna P, Elena C, et al. Clinical presentation and management practice of systemic mastocytosis. A survey on 460 Italian patients. Am J Hematol 2016;91:692–9.

13. Butterfield JH. Systemic mastocytosis: clinical manifestations and differential diagnosis. Immunol Allergy Clin North Am 2006;26:487–513.

14. Hamilton MJ, Hornick JL, Akin C, et al. Mast cell activation syndrome: a newly recognized disorder with systemic clinical manifestations. J Allergy Clin Immunol 2011;128:147–52.e2.

15. Akin C, Valent P, Metcalfe DD. Mast cell activation syndrome: proposed diagnostic criteria. J Allergy Clin Immunol 2010;126:1099–104.e4.

16. Molderings GJ, Homann J, Raithel M, et al, Interdisciplinary Multicenter Research Group on Systemic Mast Cell Activation Disease, Germany. Toward a global classification of mast cell activation diseases. J Allergy Clin Immunol 2011;127:1311 [author reply: 1311–2].

17. Valent P, Akin C, Arock M, et al. Definitions, criteria and global classification of mast cell disorders with special reference to mast cell activation syndromes: a consensus proposal. Int Arch Allergy Immunol 2012;157:215–25.

18. Valent P, Akin C, Escribano L, et al. Standards and standardization in mastocytosis: consensus statements on diagnostics, treatment recommendations and response criteria. Eur J Clin Invest 2007;37:435–53.

19. Akin C, Scott LM, Kocabas CN, et al. Demonstration of an aberrant mast-cell population with clonal markers in a subset of patients with "idiopathic" anaphylaxis. Blood 2007;110:2331–3.

20. Lyons JJ, Yu X, Hughes JD, et al. Elevated basal serum tryptase identifies a multisystem disorder associated with increased TPSAB1 copy number. Nat Genet 2016;48:1564–9.

21. Schwartz LB. Tryptase: a clinical indicator of mast cell-dependent events. Allergy Proc 1994;15:119–23.

22. Sperr WR, El-Samahi A, Kundi M, et al. Elevated tryptase levels selectively cluster in myeloid neoplasms: a novel diagnostic approach and screen marker in clinical haematology. Eur J Clin Invest 2009;39:914–23.

23. Schwartz LB. Diagnostic value of tryptase in anaphylaxis and mastocytosis. Immunol Allergy Clin North Am 2006;26:451–63.

24. Valent P, Sperr WR, Sotlar K, et al. The serum tryptase test: an emerging robust biomarker in clinical hematology. Expert Rev Hematol 2014;7:683–90.

25. Di Lorenzo G, Pacor ML, Vignola AM, et al. Urinary metabolites of histamine and leukotrienes before and after placebo-controlled challenge with ASA and food additives in chronic urticaria patients. Allergy 2002;57:1180–6.

26. Vysniauskaite M, Hertfelder HJ, Oldenburg J, et al. Determination of plasma heparin level improves identification of systemic mast cell activation disease. PLoS One 2015;10:e0124912.

27. Lueke AJ, Meeusen JW, Donato LJ, et al. Analytical and clinical validation of an LC-MS/MS method for urine leukotriene E4: a marker of systemic mastocytosis. Clin Biochem 2016;49:979–82.

28. Alvarez-Twose I, Gonzalez-de-Olano D, Sanchez-Munoz L, et al. Validation of the REMA score for predicting mast cell clonality and systemic mastocytosis in patients with systemic mast cell activation symptoms. Int Arch Allergy Immunol 2012;157:275–80.
29. Doyle LA, Sepehr GJ, Hamilton MJ, et al. A clinicopathologic study of 24 cases of systemic mastocytosis involving the gastrointestinal tract and assessment of mucosal mast cell density in irritable bowel syndrome and asymptomatic patients. Am J Surg Pathol 2014;38:832–43.
30. Kristensen T, Vestergaard H, Bindslev-Jensen C, et al. Sensitive KIT D816V mutation analysis of blood as a diagnostic test in mastocytosis. Am J Hematol 2014; 89:493–8.
31. Shibao C, Arzubiaga C, Roberts LJ 2nd, et al. Hyperadrenergic postural tachycardia syndrome in mast cell activation disorders. Hypertension 2005;45:385–90.
32. Akin C. Mast cell activation syndromes presenting as anaphylaxis. Immunol Allergy Clin North Am 2015;35:277–85.
33. Pastorello EA, Stafylaraki C, Mirone C, et al. Anti-amoxicillin immunoglobulin E, histamine-2 receptor antagonist therapy and mast cell activation syndrome are risk factors for amoxicillin anaphylaxis. Int Arch Allergy Immunol 2015;166:280–6.
34. McNeil BD, Pundir P, Meeker S, et al. Identification of a mast-cell-specific receptor crucial for pseudo-allergic drug reactions. Nature 2015;519:237–41.
35. Nurmatov UB, Rhatigan E, Simons FE, et al. H1-antihistamines for primary mast cell activation syndromes: a systematic review. Allergy 2015;70:1052–61.
36. Siebenhaar F, Fortsch A, Krause K, et al. Rupatadine improves quality of life in mastocytosis: a randomized, double-blind, placebo-controlled trial. Allergy 2013;68:949–52.
37. Yang Y, Lu JY, Wu X, et al. G-protein-coupled receptor 35 is a target of the asthma drugs cromolyn disodium and nedocromil sodium. Pharmacology 2010;86:1–5.
38. Horan RF, Sheffer AL, Austen KF. Cromolyn sodium in the management of systemic mastocytosis. J Allergy Clin Immunol 1990;85:852–5.
39. Guilarte M, Santos J, de Torres I, et al. Diarrhoea-predominant IBS patients show mast cell activation and hyperplasia in the jejunum. Gut 2007;56:203–9.
40. Barbara G, Stanghellini V, De Giorgio R, et al. Activated mast cells in proximity to colonic nerves correlate with abdominal pain in irritable bowel syndrome. Gastroenterology 2004;126:693–702.
41. Barbara G, Wang B, Stanghellini V, et al. Mast cell-dependent excitation of visceral-nociceptive sensory neurons in irritable bowel syndrome. Gastroenterology 2007;132:26–37.
42. Edwards AM, Hagberg H. Oral and inhaled sodium cromoglicate in the management of systemic mastocytosis: a case report. J Med Case Rep 2010;4:193.
43. Klooker TK, Braak B, Koopman KE, et al. The mast cell stabiliser ketotifen decreases visceral hypersensitivity and improves intestinal symptoms in patients with irritable bowel syndrome. Gut 2010;59:1213–21.
44. Kettelhut BV, Berkebile C, Bradley D, et al. A double-blind, placebo-controlled, crossover trial of ketotifen versus hydroxyzine in the treatment of pediatric mastocytosis. J Allergy Clin Immunol 1989;83:866–70.
45. Butterfield JH, Weiler CR. Prevention of mast cell activation disorder-associated clinical sequelae of excessive prostaglandin D(2) production. Int Arch Allergy Immunol 2008;147:338–43.
46. Ravi A, Butterfield J, Weiler CR. Mast cell activation syndrome: improved identification by combined determinations of serum tryptase and 24-hour urine 11beta-prostaglandin2alpha. J Allergy Clin Immunol Pract 2014;2:775–8.

47. Weng Z, Patel AB, Panagiotidou S, et al. The novel flavone tetramethoxyluteolin is a potent inhibitor of human mast cells. J Allergy Clin Immunol 2015;135: 1044–52.e5.
48. Weng Z, Zhang B, Asadi S, et al. Quercetin is more effective than cromolyn in blocking human mast cell cytokine release and inhibits contact dermatitis and photosensitivity in humans. PLoS One 2012;7:e33805.
49. Broesby-Olsen S, Vestergaard H, Mortz CG, et al. Omalizumab prevents anaphylaxis and improves symptoms in systemic mastocytosis: efficacy and safety observations. Allergy 2018;73:230–8.
50. Molderings GJ, Raithel M, Kratz F, et al. Omalizumab treatment of systemic mast cell activation disease: experiences from four cases. Intern Med 2011;50:611–5.
51. Johnston CS. The antihistamine action of ascorbic acid. Subcell Biochem 1996; 25:189–213.
52. Kinney SR, Carlson L, Ser-Dolansky J, et al. Curcumin ingestion inhibits mastocytosis and suppresses intestinal anaphylaxis in a murine model of food allergy. PLoS One 2015;10:e0132467.
53. Lavo B, Knutson L, Loof L, et al. Challenge with gliadin induces eosinophil and mast cell activation in the jejunum of patients with celiac disease. Am J Med 1989;87:655–60.
54. Skaper SD, Facci L, Giusti P. Mast cells, glia and neuroinflammation: partners in crime? Immunology 2014;141:314–27.
55. Theoharides TC. Neuroendocrinology of mast cells: challenges and controversies. Exp Dermatol 2017;26:751–9.

Hereditary Alpha Tryptasemia

Genotyping and Associated Clinical Features

Jonathan J. Lyons, MD

KEYWORDS

- Mast cell activation • Hypertryptasemia • Autosomal dominant • Genotyping

KEY POINTS

- Hereditary alpha tryptasemia is a genetic trait that leads to elevated basal serum tryptase.
- Some individuals with hereditary alpha tryptasemia present with a syndrome comprised of multisystem complaints.
- Increased *TPSAB1* copy number encoding alpha-tryptase on a single allele is the cause of hereditary alpha tryptasemia.
- A gene-dosage effect exists between number of additional *TPSAB1* copies, basal serum tryptase levels, and severity of clinical symptoms in affected individuals.
- Complex structural variation at the tryptase locus prevents identification of increased *TPSAB1* copy number by conventional exome or genome sequencing.

INTRODUCTION

Tryptase is a protein expressed by mast cells and basophils.[1,2] Mature, enzymatically active tryptases are tetrameric serine proteases that are stored in mast cell secretory granules and contribute to allergic inflammation.[3] Experiments inhibiting mature tryptases have demonstrated their role in promoting inflammatory cell recruitment, vascular permeability, and airway hypersensitivity and remodeling, in animal models. However, the specific contribution of mature tryptases to allergic reactions in humans is less clear.[4] Pro-tryptases, which have not undergone enzymatic conversion into mature tetrameric tryptases, are constitutively secreted into serum in their monomeric form, and provide the vast majority of measured basal serum tryptase (BST) in healthy individuals[5,6] (**Fig. 1**). Pro-tryptases are also the predominant forms of tryptase

Disclosure Statement: The author declares no competing or conflicting interests.
Funding: This research was supported by the Division of Intramural Research of the National Institute of Allergy and Infectious Diseases, NIH.
Laboratory of Allergic Diseases, National Institute of Allergy and Infectious Diseases, National Institutes of Health, Building 10, Room 11N240 MSC 1889, 10 Center Drive, Bethesda, MD 20892, USA
E-mail address: jonathan.lyons@nih.gov

Immunol Allergy Clin N Am 38 (2018) 483–495
https://doi.org/10.1016/j.iac.2018.04.003
0889-8561/18/Published by Elsevier Inc.

immunology.theclinics.com

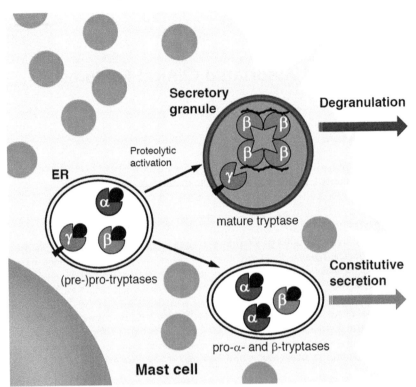

Fig. 1. Schematic of tryptase secretion from human mast cells. Pro-tryptases generated in mast cells undergo sequential proteolytic cleavage to become mature tetrameric tryptase, stabilized by heparin, and stored in secretory granules (*top*) awaiting appropriate stimuli to induce degranulation. Alternatively, pro-tryptases can be secreted constitutively into serum as enzymatically inactive pro-peptides (*bottom*). ER, endoplasmic reticulum. (*Adapted from* Caughey GH. Tryptase genetics and anaphylaxis. J Allergy Clin Immunol 2006;117(6):1412; with permission.)

present in the serum from patients with systemic mastocytosis.[7,8] During mast cell degranulation, as occurs during immunoglobulin (Ig)E-mediated immediate hypersensitivity reactions, mature tryptases are released with other mast cell mediators and contribute to symptoms of type I allergic reactions. Thus, serum tryptase in this setting is a useful biomarker for the clinical diagnosis of anaphylaxis.[9]

However, elevated BST, currently defined clinically as >11.4 ng/mL, appears to be quite common, being reported in 4% to 6% of the general population.[10,11] Although in some individuals reported increases may be due to end-stage renal disease or clonal expansion of myeloid or mast cells, including mastocytosis,[12–14] it has recently been discovered that a number of individuals with elevated BST inherit this trait.[15–18] Further, in the small cohorts studied thus far, the data suggest that this trait may also be relatively common, and frequently the cause for elevated BST in the general population.[16,18] The focus of this review is to discuss the details of this genetic trait and the complexities surrounding genotyping patients, as well as the associated clinical features and management approaches for patients with the multisystem complaints associated with hereditary alpha tryptasemia.

TRYPTASE LOCUS AND ISOTYPE DIFFERENCES

The tryptase locus contains 4 tryptase-encoding genes (*TPSG1*, *TPSB2*, *TPSAB1*, and *TPSD1*) and is present on the distal portion of the short arm of chromosome 16 at position p13.3 (**Fig. 2**). One additional human tryptase (epsilon) encoded by *PRSS22* also exists on 16p just outside of this cluster. Although all of these genes encode tryptases, only *TPSB2* and *TPSAB1* encode the secreted isoforms of tryptase that are measured and reported as serum tryptase by clinical laboratories.[19]

Although *TPSB2* is believed to encode only beta-tryptase isoforms (β), the *TPSAB1* locus encodes either alpha (α) or beta (β) isoforms[20] (see **Fig. 2**). Each of these isoforms is remarkably similar, being at least 97% identical, making detection of distinct tryptase isoforms extremely difficult. Recent publications have clarified a number of misconceptions about the biology of alpha-tryptase isoforms encoded at *TPSAB1*. We now know that alpha pro-tryptase can be processed into mature tryptase.[21] Further, the monoclonal tryptase antibody (G5 clone), which has been reported to distinguish alpha-tryptases from beta-tryptases, is now know to recognize any tryptase, including alpha-tryptase, which has been processed to maturity. This includes destabilized monomers that had previously been tetrameric enzyme.[6] There is still no antibody that can differentiate alpha-tryptase or beta-tryptase protein. Despite our limitations in detecting protein differences in vivo, a number of important functional distinctions have been identified between alpha-tryptase and beta-tryptase isoforms in vitro. Importantly, alpha-tryptase sequences contain 2 isoform-defining variants: one that may promote constitutive secretion, and a second at the enzymatic active site that appears to eliminate functional activity of homo-tetrameric alpha-tryptases.[22–24]

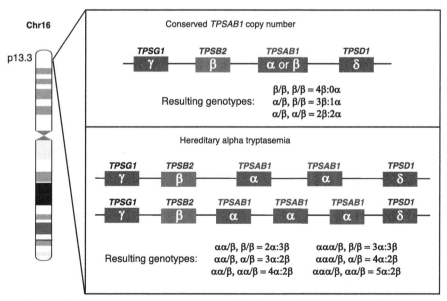

Fig. 2. Identified tryptase genotypes encoded at *TPSAB1* and *TPSB2*. Canonical alpha-tryptase and beta-tryptase genotypes based on conserved copy number (*top*) and those identified resulting from increased *TPSAB1* copy number encoding 1 or 2 additional alpha-tryptase copies on single alleles (*bottom*). Additional genotypes are likely to be identified, and other variant beta isoforms that have already been identified[19] are excluded for simplicity.

Until recently, it was believed that individuals have 1 copy each of *TPSB2* and *TPSAB1*. Based on the tryptase isoform expression at these 2 genetic loci, there have been 3 canonical genotypes described in the literature with a total tryptase gene number of 4: 0α:4β, 1α:3β, and 2α:2β (see **Fig. 2**). Importantly, among individuals with a 2α:2β genotype, the 2 alpha-tryptase copies are on opposite alleles (1 being inherited from each parent), and do not represent increased *TPSAB1* copy number. However, we now know that increased *TPSAB1* copy number encoding alpha-tryptase can occur on a single allele, and when present leads to elevated BST; duplications and triplications have thus far been identified[16] (see **Fig. 2**). Altered *TPSB2* or *TPSAB1* copy number encoding beta-tryptase has not been reported, but may also occur, and any associated biochemical findings or clinical phenotypes have yet to be described.

Several individuals have been reported with inherited *TPSAB1* duplications on both alleles (ie, both parents carried duplications and passed them to these individuals) suggesting that hereditary alpha tryptasemia may be relatively common. Complete segregation of elevated BST with increased *TPSAB1* copy number in the 2 unselected populations that have been studied[16] and the relatively high prevalence of elevated BST in multiple populations[10,11] also suggest this trait may be a common cause for elevated BST. Additional population-based studies are required to establish the prevalence of increased *TPSAB1* copy as the cause for elevated BST in the general population.

How increased mono-allelic *TPSAB1* copy number leads to increased BST and the clinical features associated with hereditary alpha tryptasemia remains unknown. However, it appears that mast cells and basophils overexpress and secrete pro-tryptase(s) in excess when increased alpha-encoding *TPSAB1* copies are present. A greater number of extra copies leads to higher BST and more reported symptoms, or an observed gene-dosage effect. However, total tryptase within basophils and mast cells does not appear to be increased, although this has not been studied in detail. Although alpha-tryptase tetramers do not exhibit the trypsin-like protease activity of their beta-tryptase counterparts,[22] the potential effects of alpha-tryptase overexpression on mature tryptases has not previously been studied and is an area of active investigation. There is limited evidence to support non-enzymatic activity of tryptases through unknown mechanisms; enzymatically inactivated human tryptases can exhibit mitogenic activity on human lung fibroblasts.[25] Ongoing investigations into the effects of altered tryptase gene expression and increased BST levels may provide new insights into the mechanisms underlying the clinical symptoms associated with hereditary alpha tryptasemia.

GENOTYPING STRATEGIES

Complex structural variation at the tryptase locus has thus far precluded its direct sequencing. The few published human genome assemblies, derived from single-molecule real-time sequencing, a technology that allows very large contiguous reads, have demonstrated remarkable structural diversity at this locus, even among ostensibly healthy individuals.[26] Because of the high degree of structural variation present and conservation of sequence between tryptase isoforms, clinically available exome or genome sequencing data do not identify increased *TPSAB1* copy number. Further limiting conventional mapping and interpretation of genetic sequence is copy number variation of wild-type *TPSAB1*, in which unaffected individuals may have 0, 1, or even 2 copies of alpha-encoding sequence on opposing alleles. There are several published approaches that have been applied to overcome these obstacles and establish alpha-encoding *TPSAB1* copy number in silico or in vitro.[16,20,27]

Relative Tryptase Gene Quantitation by Sanger Sequencing and Modified Southern Blotting

Two of the original methods described for tryptase genotyping (**Fig. 3**) provide relative quantification of alpha-tryptase and beta-tryptase encoding copies at *TPSAB1* and *TPSB2* (**Fig. 3**A–C). Both approaches rely on the calculated ratio between alpha-tryptase and beta-tryptase genomic sequences. The first method uses Sanger gene sequencing of the tryptase locus (**Fig. 3**B). To accomplish this, corresponding regions of *TPSAB1* and *TPSB2* are amplified in a single reaction, and sequenced using the chain termination (Sanger) method. Peak heights observed in the resulting chromatograms at nucleic acid residues that are only present in either alpha-tryptase or beta-tryptase sequences are directly measured, and the ratios of the 2 different nucleic acid signals are determined to provide relative quantitation of alpha-tryptases and beta-tryptases.[20]

The second method uses a similar strategy in which homologous genomic DNA from both *TPSAB1* and *TPSB2* is amplified. However, to determine the relative prevalence of sequences, the investigators took advantage of a conserved alpha-specific variant that results in the introduction of a new restriction site. Treating the amplified DNA from *TPSAB1* and *TPSB2* with the restriction enzyme EcoRV results in cleavage of only alpha-tryptase amplicons. Gel electrophoresis and Southern blotting is then performed on the digested DNA (or undigested DNA in the case of beta-sequences) (**Fig. 3**C). Alpha-sequences result in a smaller-sized band, whereas beta-sequences

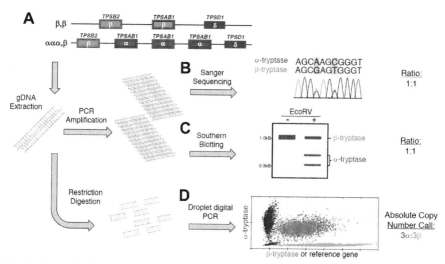

Fig. 3. Strategies for tryptase genotyping. (*A*) Two alleles in an individual with hereditary alpha tryptasemia: 1 allele with 2 beta-tryptase sequences at *TPSAB1* and *TPSB2* (*top*), and the second trait-associated allele with 3 alpha-tryptase encoding *TPSAB1* copies and a single beta-tryptase encoding *TPSB2* copy (*bottom*). Genomic DNA (gDNA) extracted from cells from this individual, containing these 6 different alpha-tryptase or beta-tryptase sequences are either amplified or restriction digested. The amplified gDNA can then either be (*B*) Sanger sequenced, or (*C*) treated with the restriction enzyme EcoRV and Southern blotted to perform relative quantitation of alpha- and beta-tryptases. In both cases, the ratio of alpha-tryptase to beta-tryptase calculated would be 1:1. (*D*) Unamplified digested gDNA is assayed by ddPCR, which allows for absolute copy number detection of alpha-tryptase and beta-tryptase sequences, yielding the genotype determination 3α:3β.

remain as an uncut larger band. Band signal intensities are then quantified to determine a relative quantity of alpha-tryptase and beta-tryptases.[27]

A major drawback of both of these methods is that they rely on conservation of both *TPSAB1* and *TPSB2* copy number to determine genotype. Therefore, with these methods, an individual with a *TPSAB1* triplication and an $\alpha\alpha\alpha/\beta{:}\beta/\beta$ genotype would not be distinguished from an individual without increased *TPSAB1* copy number and alpha-sequences on both alleles (or the $\alpha/\beta{:}\alpha/\beta$ genotype); both individuals would have equal quantities of alpha-tryptase and beta-tryptase sequences (see **Fig. 3**). Moreover, both methods rely on amplification of genomic DNA, and subtle differences in efficiency resulting from unique alpha-tryptase and beta-tryptase sequences potentially limit the precision required to distinguish individuals with *TPSAB1* duplications and an $\alpha\alpha/\beta{:}\beta/\beta$ genotype from those with an $\alpha/\beta{:}\alpha/\beta$ genotype.

Bioinformatic Realignment and Copy Number Determination

Conventional exome or genome sequencing relies on sequencing of small fragments of DNA in massive parallel (sizes typically range from 50 to 500 bp in length). Because the sequences at *TPSAB1* and *TPSB2* have a very high degree of homology, and *TPSD1* sequences also have areas of significant homology with these genes, small fragments from all 6 loci, or more in the case of hereditary alpha tryptasemia, are frequently misaligned to any of these 3 reference genes. There are several publicly available algorithms designed to resolve highly complex loci that can be adapted to circumvent this issue.[28] The strategy we developed used de novo assembly of unselected sequences (from genome sequencing data) that mapped to the tryptase locus. We defined an approximately 500-bp tryptase "consensus" sequence with a number of unique identifiers that could distinguish alpha-tryptase, beta-tryptase, and delta-tryptase from one another; gamma-tryptase was not homologous enough to require deconvolution.

To perform genotyping, all reads from exome and genome sequencing that map to *TPSAB1*, *TPSB2*, or *TPSD1* are realigned to this "consensus" sequence using an algorithm, and the number of reads assigned to each isoform (coverage) is used to estimate relative copy number.[16] There are several major limitations to this and similar approaches. First, this process is highly dependent on the quality and quantity (or depth of coverage) at the locus. Poor capture is particularly problematic with older exon capture kits, in which probes designed to extract the exome (coding DNA sequence) do not fully cover the tryptase locus, leaving gaps in the genes. Genome sequencing avoids this issue, but the locus is also highly repetitive and GC-rich, which can cause dimerization and stem-loop formation of DNA, both of which can hinder DNA amplification and/or extension still leading to poor coverage. Second, this method is still only a relative quantitation of copy. While coverage can be normalized to the average genomic coverage in the areas around the locus, the precision observed with these methods remains moderate. Because of this, the problem remains that an individual with an $\alpha\alpha/\beta{:}\beta/\beta$ genotype can be difficult to distinguish from an individual with an $\alpha/\beta{:}\alpha/\beta$ using this method.

TPSAB1 and TPSB2 Allele-Specific Genotyping by Droplet Digital Polymerase Chain Reaction

To overcome the issues of *TPSAB1* copy number variation and reliance on relative quantitation, we developed a droplet digital polymerase chain reaction (ddPCR)-based assay.[16] This platform allows for more precise and absolute quantification of alpha-tryptase–specific and beta-tryptase–specific sequences. Within the identified tryptase "consensus" sequence, we identified a region in exon 3 of tryptase-encoding genes, which allowed us to distinguish alpha-tryptase, beta-tryptase, and delta-tryptase from one another, and designed probes for each.

To accomplish genotyping, unamplified genomic DNA is restriction digested to separate each copy of tryptase sequence and then partitioned into droplets with 2 multiplexed primer/probe sets: one specific for alpha-tryptase and the other for beta-tryptase or a copy number reference gene. The samples are then placed on a thermal cycler in a process very similar to real-time PCR. However, rather than determining cycle time, all reactions are taken to completion (maximal fluorescence) and then run through a flow-based detector system much like a flow cytometer. Based on the number of positive and negative droplets, a Poisson distribution–based calculation is used to absolutely quantify copy number, yielding highly reproducible and accurate quantification of tryptase genotype (**Fig. 3**D).

Manipulation of DNA digestion strategies can further resolve monoallelic copy number changes. Two copies of alpha-tryptase or beta-tryptase sequence on the same allele are in close proximity, and without DNA shearing or digestion, do not randomly segregate into droplets. Therefore, the resulting copy number call for alpha-tryptase or beta-tryptase is suppressed when the allelic copy number is increased; this is normalized with digestion. By comparing the results of the assay using digested DNA with those results obtained without restriction digestion, allows for confirmation that alpha-tryptase or beta-tryptase sequences exist on the same allele (allele specificity). Although there are some limitations to this assay, including the inability to resolve certain allelic genotypes displaying increased copy number without sequencing of additional family members (eg, individuals with $4\alpha{:}2\beta$ genotypes cannot be further resolved as $\alpha\alpha\alpha/\beta,\alpha/\beta$ or $\alpha\alpha/\beta,\alpha\alpha/\beta$), it accurately determines absolute *TPSAB1* and *TPSB2* alpha-tryptase and beta-tryptase encoding copy number, including theoretic copy number loss, and accurately determines most allelic genotypes. Efforts are under way to make this assay available clinically.

ASSOCIATED CLINICAL FEATURES

All individuals identified to date with increased alpha-encoding *TPSAB1* copy number have basal serum tryptases above 8 ng/mL (average BST caused by a duplication is 15 ± 5 ng/mL, and a triplication is 24 ± 6 ng/mL); on this basis, hereditary alpha tryptasemia is currently believed to be a fully penetrant genetic trait. The expressivity of associated clinical phenotypes reported has been more variable, with some individuals reporting few if any symptoms. However, a number of symptoms are frequently reported by individuals with hereditary alpha tryptasemia (**Table 1**). Many of these phenotypes have also been reported in association with elevated BST in unselected cohorts, strengthening the clinical association between clinical features and increased *TPSAB1* copy number.[10,16,17,29–31]

Among the most commonly reported clinical symptoms among individuals with hereditary alpha tryptasemia are functional gastrointestinal complaints. A number of these, such as dyspepsia and odynophagia without observable pathology can be hard to characterize or quantify. However, irritable bowel syndrome (IBS), which has a number of validated measures, has been reported in approximately half of affected individuals within highly symptomatic families, and in a third of unselected individuals, using the Rome III criteria. This prevalence is approximately 2 to 5 times the estimated population prevalence in North America.[32]

Half of individuals in selected and unselected populations with *TPSAB1* duplications were reported with recurrent cutaneous symptoms that include flushing and pruritus; induration, angioedema, and urticaria were less commonly present. In some

Table 1
Clinical features reported in association with hereditary alpha tryptasemia

Manifestation	Reported Prevalence,[a] %	Association Supported in an Unselected Cohort[b]
Basal serum tryptase >8 ng/mL	100	Yes
Chronic gastroesophageal reflux symptoms	56–77	No
Arthralgia	44–45	No
Body pain/headache	33–47	No
Flushing/pruritus	32–55	Yes
Irritable bowel syndrome (Rome III)	28–49	Yes
Sleep disruption	22–39	No
Systemic immediate hypersensitivity reaction	21–28	No
Retained primary dentition	20–33	Yes
Systemic venom reaction	14–22	Yes
Congenital skeletal abnormality	11–26	No
Joint hypermobility	0–28	No
Positive Tilt-table test	0–11	No

[a] In order of reported prevalence, ranges are derived from available data in 3 reports.[14,15,17]
[b] Finding was identified as significantly associated with increased *TPSAB1* copy number in an unselected volunteer adult population.

individuals, these symptoms were spontaneous; however, vibration or minor trauma, such as hand clapping, were frequently reported triggers. Although these symptoms are suggestive of mast cell mediator release, few of these patients had identifiable evidence of chronic mast cell mediator release, and symptomatic events were not sufficiently studied to confirm these symptomatic episodes were mast cell–related.

Systemic reactions consistent with IgE-mediated immediate hypersensitivity to stinging insects (eg, Hymenoptera or honey bee) have been reported in approximately 20% of patients with hereditary alpha tryptasemia. This prevalence is threefold to fourfold that of what has been reported in the general population.[33] Although the established association between elevated BST and severe anaphylaxis to stinging insects has been largely attributed to clonal mast cell disease,[34] these independent findings of an association between elevated BST caused by hereditary alpha tryptasemia and stinging insect allergy suggest some of this signal may come from increased *TPSAB1* copy number, and requires further study.

Several additional clinical manifestations have been reported in association with hereditary alpha tryptasemia, including connective tissue abnormalities, such as joint hypermobility; retained primary dentition, and congenital abnormalities; symptoms suggestive of autonomic dysfunction, such as orthostatic hypotension, palpitations, tachycardia, presyncope, and syncope; and constitutional symptoms, such as chronic pain and fatigue. Many of these symptoms are difficult to characterize or quantify and require additional validation. Finally, eosinophilic gastrointestinal disease, multiple food intolerances, failure to thrive, and IgE-mediated allergy have been observed in a small number of highly symptomatic families with increased *TPSAB1* copy number. Whether these findings are generalizable to all individuals with hereditary alpha tryptasemia also remains to be determined.

Despite the fact that tryptase genotype has not been evaluated extensively, several independent studies have examined the relationship between elevated BST, ostensibly in the absence of clonal mast cell disease or mastocytosis, and many of the clinical phenotypes observed in association with hereditary alpha tryptasemia. In addition to the well-documented association of elevated BST and severe anaphylaxis to stinging insects,[10,30,34–36] a recent publication demonstrated an association between elevated BST and anaphylaxis in children with food allergy.[31] In this study, a BST greater than 14.5 ng/mL had a 90% positive predictive value for severe anaphylaxis.

In a separate, case-control study of patients in a clinical practice in Austria, 100 individuals with elevated BST and 100 individuals with BST less than 11.4 ng/mL (mean BST 3.7 ng/mL) were administered a questionnaire that evaluated a number of the symptoms later reported in individuals with hereditary alpha tryptasemia. Significant associations were observed between elevated BST and cutaneous symptoms (flushing, angioedema), gastrointestinal symptoms (abdominal pain, nausea, meteorism, diarrhea), symptoms suggestive of autonomic dysfunction (tachycardia, palpitations, vertigo) and collapse of unclear eitiology; fatigue, pain symptoms, and mood alterations were also reported to be associated with increased BST.[10]

In a third study examining patients with chronic idiopathic urticaria (CIU) who experience systemic symptoms during disease flares (n = 155), BST greater than 8.2 ng/mL was not observed in patients without systemic complaints. The complaints reported included gastrointestinal symptoms, flushing, joint pain or swelling, cardiovascular manifestations, respiratory symptoms, and other constitutional complaints. Overall, significantly higher BSTs were observed in patients with systemic symptoms, and were associated with significantly more severe urticaria (determined by several validated measures). Further, examining patients with BST $\geq$10 ng/mL in this cohort, the mean itch score was nearly twice what was reported in the remainder of individuals.[29]

In a final report, a 3-generation Belgian family was described with dominantly inherited BST elevations associated with severe episodic gastrointestinal cramping and diarrhea. Serum tryptase levels were observed to rise in association with symptomatic events. In one affected individual, evidence of clonal mast cell disease was also reported (hepatosplenomegaly and the missense *KIT* p.[D816V] in bone marrow) consistent with the diagnosis of monoclonal mast cell activation syndrome.[17]

MANAGEMENT APPROACHES

Clinical treatment approaches for patients with hereditary alpha tryptasemia are currently personalized based on symptoms. Like other patients with the kinds of multisystem complaints reported by individuals with hereditary alpha tryptasemia, responses to therapy are often mixed and variable from person-to-person. As there are few data to support a particular strategy, and no prospective studies on which to rely, the following management approaches are based solely on the limited clinical experience at the National Institutes of Health Clinical Center, and focus on the commonest symptoms.

For cutaneous and gastrointestinal symptoms, we recommend trials of maximal antihistamine therapy targeting both H1 and H2 receptors twice daily, as used in CIU or indolent forms of mastocytosis.[37,38] We also prescribe oral cromolyn sodium if gastrointestinal symptoms are severe. Although our center does not have access to oral ketotifen, a number of patients have also reported some improvement with this medication. However, the overall clinical responses to these mast cell–directed therapies have been disappointing. Although 1 patient reported complete resolution of diarrhea, abdominal pain, dysphagia, and migraine headaches with addition of oral ketotifen to maximal twice daily antihistamines, most others have reported only modest benefit of mast cell stabilizers, and even responses to antihistamines have been mixed. Anecdotally, a few patients who have received omalizumab for allergic asthma or CIU have reported improvement in some additional symptoms.

For individuals with recurrent severe systemic symptoms and/or anaphylaxis, triggers should be identified and avoided, and epi-pens should be provided, as is the standard of care. However, many systemic events in these patients are difficult to characterize, and in some cases may not represent immediate hypersensitivity reactions. Regardless of etiology, particularly when anxiety plays a large contributing role, biofeedback, as frequently used in management of patients with mastocytosis, has proven beneficial in many patients.

Several other medications that have been anecdotally observed as beneficial for symptoms in some patients include tricyclic antidepressants, clemastine fumarate, and gabapentin. More effective medications are greatly needed for the symptoms associated with hereditary alpha tryptasemia, and prospective clinical trials are critically lacking to evaluate the efficacy of current treatment approaches in these difficult-to-treat patients.

SUMMARY

In summary, hereditary alpha tryptasemia is a relatively common genetic trait caused by increased copies of TPSAB1 encoding alpha-tryptase on a single allele, and is inherited in an autosomal dominant manner. Affected individuals have elevated BST and may present with multisystem complaints, both of which positively correlate with the number of additional TPSAB1 copies, in a gene-dose manner. A number of questions remain around the clinical phenotypes associated with hereditary alpha tryptasemia and whether this trait may play a causative or modifying role in the findings that have been reported. A common haplotype reported to be coinherited with increased TPSAB1 copy number in approximately two-thirds of individuals was recently characterized.[18] Additional variants in TPSG1 encoding gamma-tryptase and partial gain-of-function variants in CACNA1H encoding a T-type voltage gated calcium channel were identified. Although no effect on clinical phenotype could be observed, the CACNA1H variants are quite intriguing, as this channel has been implicated in nociception and IBS in animal models.[39,40]

Given that hereditary alpha tryptasemia appears to be a common cause for elevated BST, TPSAB1 copy number should be considered in the clinical evaluation of patients with BST greater than 8 ng/mL. Once clinically available, tryptase genotyping of patients will likely be a useful tool for evaluation of patients with suspected clonal mast cell disease and other myeloid abnormalities that can also be associated with elevated BST. The normal reference range for BST also bears reevaluation in this context. Currently the upper limit of normal is assigned as 11.4 ng/mL, somewhat arbitrarily. Now that a genetic basis has been established that appears to explain a large number of individuals with BST greater than 10 ng/mL, a rationally identified upper limit of normal at 8 to 10 ng/mL should be considered, and has been suggested in the literature.[30]

As more individuals and larger cohorts are genotyped, and the association between elevated BST and increased TPSAB1 copy number at the population level is clarified, the strength of association between hereditary alpha tryptasemia and the multiple clinical phenotypes that have been reported will no doubt evolve. Further, as the functional effects of elevated BST and/or altered tryptase gene expression are elucidated, potential mechanisms for causation and/or modification of clinical disease are likely to be elucidated. Once identified, these findings will provide a rationale for future therapeutic intervention in these patients, and potentially others with similar clinical presentations.

ACKNOWLEDGMENTS

The author is grateful to Kelly Stone, MD, PhD, for his thoughtful comments on the article.

REFERENCES

1. Theoharides TC, Valent P, Akin C. Mast cells, mastocytosis, and related disorders. N Engl J Med 2015;373(2):163–72.
2. Foster B, Schwartz LB, Devouassoux G, et al. Characterization of mast-cell tryptase-expressing peripheral blood cells as basophils. J Allergy Clin Immunol 2002; 109(2):287–93.
3. Schwartz LB, Lewis RA, Seldin D, et al. Acid hydrolases and tryptase from secretory granules of dispersed human lung mast cells. J Immunol 1981;126(4): 1290–4.
4. Caughey GH. Mast cell tryptases and chymases in inflammation and host defense. Immunol Rev 2007;217:141–54.
5. Schwartz LB, Sakai K, Bradford TR, et al. The alpha form of human tryptase is the predominant type present in blood at baseline in normal subjects and is elevated in those with systemic mastocytosis. J Clin Invest 1995;96(6):2702–10.
6. Schwartz LB, Min HK, Ren S, et al. Tryptase precursors are preferentially and spontaneously released, whereas mature tryptase is retained by HMC-1 cells, Mono-Mac-6 cells, and human skin-derived mast cells. J Immunol 2003; 170(11):5667–73.
7. Kanthawatana S, Carias K, Arnaout R, et al. The potential clinical utility of serum alpha-protryptase levels. J Allergy Clin Immunol 1999;103(6):1092–9.
8. Akin C, Soto D, Brittain E, et al. Tryptase haplotype in mastocytosis: relationship to disease variant and diagnostic utility of total tryptase levels. Clin Immunol 2007;123(3):268–71.
9. Schwartz LB. Diagnostic value of tryptase in anaphylaxis and mastocytosis. Immunol Allergy Clin North Am 2006;26(3):451–63.
10. Fellinger C, Hemmer W, Wohrl S, et al. Clinical characteristics and risk profile of patients with elevated baseline serum tryptase. Allergol Immunopathol (Madr) 2014;42(6):544–52.
11. Gonzalez-Quintela A, Vizcaino L, Gude F, et al. Factors influencing serum total tryptase concentrations in a general adult population. Clin Chem Lab Med 2010;48(5):701–6.
12. Sirvent AE, Gonzalez C, Enriquez R, et al. Serum tryptase levels and markers of renal dysfunction in a population with chronic kidney disease. J Nephrol 2010; 23(3):282–90.
13. Valent P, Akin C, Metcalfe DD. Mastocytosis: 2016 updated WHO classification and novel emerging treatment concepts. Blood 2017;129(11):1420–7.
14. Valent P, Sperr WR, Sotlar K, et al. The serum tryptase test: an emerging robust biomarker in clinical hematology. Expert Rev Hematol 2014;7(5):683–90.
15. Lyons JJ, Sun G, Stone KD, et al. Mendelian inheritance of elevated serum tryptase associated with atopy and connective tissue abnormalities. J Allergy Clin Immunol 2014;133(5):1471–4.

16. Lyons JJ, Yu X, Hughes JD, et al. Elevated basal serum tryptase identifies a multisystem disorder associated with increased TPSAB1 copy number. Nat Genet 2016;48(12):1564–9.

17. Sabato V, Van De Vijver E, Hagendorens M, et al. Familial hypertryptasemia with associated mast cell activation syndrome. J Allergy Clin Immunol 2014;134(6): 1448–50.e3.

18. Lyons JJ, Stotz SC, Chovanec J, et al. A common haplotype containing functional CACNA1H variants is frequently coinherited with increased TPSAB1 copy number. Genet Med 2018;20(5):503–12.

19. Caughey GH. Tryptase genetics and anaphylaxis. J Allergy Clin Immunol 2006; 117(6):1411–4.

20. Trivedi NN, Tamraz B, Chu C, et al. Human subjects are protected from mast cell tryptase deficiency despite frequent inheritance of loss-of-function mutations. J Allergy Clin Immunol 2009;124(5):1099–105.e1-4.

21. Le QT, Min HK, Xia HZ, et al. Promiscuous processing of human alphabetaprotryptases by cathepsins L, B, and C. J Immunol 2011;186(12):7136–43.

22. Huang C, Li L, Krilis SA, et al. Human tryptases alpha and beta/II are functionally distinct due, in part, to a single amino acid difference in one of the surface loops that forms the substrate-binding cleft. J Biol Chem 1999;274(28):19670–6.

23. Marquardt U, Zettl F, Huber R, et al. The crystal structure of human alpha1-tryptase reveals a blocked substrate-binding region. J Mol Biol 2002;321(3): 491–502.

24. Selwood T, Wang ZM, McCaslin DR, et al. Diverse stability and catalytic properties of human tryptase alpha and beta isoforms are mediated by residue differences at the S1 pocket. Biochemistry 2002;41(10):3329–40.

25. Brown JK, Jones CA, Rooney LA, et al. Tryptase's potent mitogenic effects in human airway smooth muscle cells are via nonproteolytic actions. Am J Physiol Lung Cell Mol Physiol 2002;282(2):L197–206.

26. Chaisson MJ, Huddleston J, Dennis MY, et al. Resolving the complexity of the human genome using single-molecule sequencing. Nature 2015;517(7536):608–11.

27. Le QT, Lotfi-Emran S, Min HK, et al. A simple, sensitive and safe method to determine the human alpha/beta-tryptase genotype. PLoS One 2014;9(12):e114944.

28. Handsaker RE, Van Doren V, Berman JR, et al. Large multiallelic copy number variations in humans. Nat Genet 2015;47(3):296–303.

29. Doong JC, Chichester K, Oliver ET, et al. Chronic idiopathic urticaria: systemic complaints and their relationship with disease and immune measures. J Allergy Clin Immunol Pract 2017;5(5):1314–8.

30. Kucharewicz I, Bodzenta-Lukaszyk A, Szymanski W, et al. Basal serum tryptase level correlates with severity of hymenoptera sting and age. J Investig Allergol Clin Immunol 2007;17(2):65–9.

31. Sahiner UM, Yavuz ST, Buyuktiryaki B, et al. Serum basal tryptase may be a good marker for predicting the risk of anaphylaxis in children with food allergy. Allergy 2014;69(2):265–8.

32. Saito YA, Schoenfeld P, Locke GR 3rd. The epidemiology of irritable bowel syndrome in North America: a systematic review. Am J Gastroenterol 2002;97(8): 1910–5.

33. Sturm GJ, Kranzelbinder B, Schuster C, et al. Sensitization to Hymenoptera venoms is common, but systemic sting reactions are rare. J Allergy Clin Immunol 2014;133(6):1635–43.e1.

34. Bonadonna P, Zanotti R, Muller U. Mastocytosis and insect venom allergy. Curr Opin Allergy Clin Immunol 2010;10(4):347–53.

35. Haeberli G, Bronnimann M, Hunziker T, et al. Elevated basal serum tryptase and hymenoptera venom allergy: relation to severity of sting reactions and to safety and efficacy of venom immunotherapy. Clin Exp Allergy 2003;33(9):1216–20.
36. Rueff F, Przybilla B, Bilo MB, et al. Predictors of severe systemic anaphylactic reactions in patients with Hymenoptera venom allergy: importance of baseline serum tryptase-a study of the European Academy of Allergology and Clinical Immunology Interest Group on Insect Venom Hypersensitivity. J Allergy Clin Immunol 2009;124(5):1047–54.
37. Bernstein JA, Lang DM, Khan DA, et al. The diagnosis and management of acute and chronic urticaria: 2014 update. J Allergy Clin Immunol 2014;133(5):1270–7.
38. Frieri M, Alling DW, Metcalfe DD. Comparison of the therapeutic efficacy of cromolyn sodium with that of combined chlorpheniramine and cimetidine in systemic mastocytosis. Results of a double-blind clinical trial. Am J Med 1985;78(1):9–14.
39. Choi S, Na HS, Kim J, et al. Attenuated pain responses in mice lacking Ca(V)3.2 T-type channels. Genes Brain Behav 2007;6(5):425–31.
40. Marger F, Gelot A, Alloui A, et al. T-type calcium channels contribute to colonic hypersensitivity in a rat model of irritable bowel syndrome. Proc Natl Acad Sci U S A 2011;108(27):11268–73.

Association of Postural Tachycardia Syndrome and Ehlers-Danlos Syndrome with Mast Cell Activation Disorders

Rafael Bonamichi-Santos, MD[a],*, Kelly Yoshimi-Kanamori, MD[a], Pedro Giavina-Bianchi, MD, PhD[a], Marcelo Vivolo Aun, MD, PhD[a,b]

KEYWORDS

- Ehlers-Danlos syndrome • Postural tachycardia syndrome • Dysautonomia
- Mast cell activation disorders • Mastocytosis

KEY POINTS

- Mast cell activation disorders (MCADs) consist of episodic symptoms due to mast cell (MC) mediator release, even anaphylaxis, and diagnosis includes high levels of serum tryptase.
- Ehlers-Danlos syndrome (EDS) and postural tachycardia syndrome (POTS) frequently coexist in a single patient.
- Preliminary data suggest that patients with EDS and/or POTS can present symptoms compatible to MCADs, which could represent a specific phenotype.
- In terms of genetics, it seems there is a role for tryptase in the pathogenesis of MCADs, EDS, and POTS association.
- Studies with larger samples evaluating clinics, genetics, and histopathology are needed to determine if there really is a particular new disease cluster.

INTRODUCTION

Mast cells (MCs) are derived from myeloblasts, which are pluripotent hemopoietic progenitors in the bone marrow.[1] MC growth, differentiation, survival, migration, and functions are modulated by a transmembrane tyrosine kinase receptor (KIT) (also known as CD117) and its interaction with plasma stem cell factor.[1] Local tissue factors, such as interleukin (IL)-3, IL-4, IL-9, and IL-33, and transforming growth

Disclosure Statement: All authors having nothing to disclose in relation to this article.
[a] Clinical Immunology and Allergy Division, University of São Paulo, Av. Dr. Arnaldo, 455, Cerqueira César, São Paulo, São Paulo CEP 01246-903, Brazil; [b] Faculdade Israelita de Ciências da Saúde Albert Einstein, São Paulo, São Paulo, Brazil
* Corresponding author. Clinical Immunology and Allergy Division, University of São Paulo, Rua Florida 1901, 111BS, São Paulo, São Paulo 04565-001, Brazil.
E-mail address: rafaelbonamichi@hotmail.com

Immunol Allergy Clin N Am 38 (2018) 497–504
https://doi.org/10.1016/j.iac.2018.04.004
0889-8561/18/© 2018 Elsevier Inc. All rights reserved.
immunology.theclinics.com

factor $\beta1$, have been shown to influence the number and mediator content of MCs, leading to specific phenotypes.[2] MCs in the connective tissue, skin, and peritoneal cavity contain tryptase in their granules and express IL-5 and IL-6. MCs in the respiratory mucosa and gut contain tryptase and chymase and express IL-4.[3]

MC activation is triggered by the following: binding of KIT and stem cell factor; binding of bacterial peptidoglycan to complement receptors; corticotropin-releasing factor receptor 1 and corticotropin-releasing hormone; binding of Fc epsilon receptor I and specific antibodies, such as IgE, to antigens; binding of Fc gamma receptor I and specific antibodies, such as IgG, to worms; binding of Toll-like receptors to lipopolysaccharide and mold; binding of vasoactive intestinal peptide to vasoactive intestinal peptide receptor 1; binding of drugs to the MRGPRX2 receptor; nonsteroidal anti-inflammatory drugs; *Hymenoptera* venom; tumor necrosis factor α; and physical stimuli (pressure and temperature); among others.[4] Several mediators are released after MC activation, including histamine; proteoglycans (heparin); platelet-activating factor; prostaglandin (PG) D2; leukotrienes (LTs), such as LTC4, LTD4, and LTE4; cytokines, such as IL-1, IL-3, IL-8, IL-10, IL-13, IL-16, and tumor necrosis factor α; chemokines; and renin.[5]

MAST CELL ACTIVATION DISORDERS

In MC activation disorders (MCADs), MCs can be increased in number, activity, or both. They are classified as primary, secondary, or idiopathic (**Table 1**).[6] In MCADs, there are episodic symptoms consistent with MC mediator release and increased plasma levels of these mediators. These reactions can usually be successfully treated or prevented with antimediator therapy, such as H1 and H2 histamine receptor antagonists, LT antagonists, and MC stabilizers.[6]

The clinical presentation of MCADs is highly variable because multiple organs and systems, such as the skin (urticaria, angioedema, flushing, and pruritus), gastrointestinal tract (cramping, diarrhea, vomiting, reflux, and abdominal pain), neuromuscular tissues (osteopenia, bone fractures, headache, bone pain, and osteoporosis), airway (shortness of breath, wheezing, throat swelling, and nasal congestion), cardiovascular system (tachycardia, cardiovascular collapse, hypotension, and hypertension), and even the central nervous system (anxiety, shortened memory span, mixed organic brain syndrome, and depression),[5] can be compromised.

Table 1 Classification of diseases associated with mast cell activation	
Primary	Mastocytosis Monoclonal MCAS
Secondary	Allergic/atopic (IgE-mediated) disorders MC activation associated with chronic Inflammatory or neoplastic disorders Physical urticarias Chronic autoimmune urticaria
Idiopathic	Anaphylaxis Angioedema Urticaria MCAS

Adapted from Akin C, Valent P, Metcalfe DD. Mast cell activation syndrome: proposed diagnostic criteria. J Allergy Clin Immunol 2010;126(6):1101; with permission.

Unfortunately, only a few diagnostic tests are commercially available to clinicians. The measurement of serum tryptase is standardized and commercially available and is the most frequently used test for evaluating MC activity. The urinary (random and 24-h) histamine levels are measured at a few centers. Other tests are still under investigation, including measurements of PGs, such as PGD2 and 11β-PGF2α, LTE4, chromogranin A, plasma histamine, and N-methylhistamine.[5]

It is recommended that at least 2 elevated MC mediator levels be present for a diagnosis of a MCAD. In patients who have a clinical history that strongly suggests MCAD but who have normal levels of tryptase or urinary histamine, a clinician should repeat these tests when the patient is symptomatic.[4]

Several investigators have noted a possible association between MCAD, EDS, and/ or postural tachycardia syndrome (POTS).

EHLERS-DANLOS SYNDROME AND MAST CELL ACTIVATION DISORDERS

Ehlers-Danlos syndrome (EDS) is a heterogeneous group of heritable connective tissue disorders that are characterized by joint hypermobility, skin hyperextensibility, and tissue fragility.[7] The estimated frequency of EDS is 1 in 5000 individuals. Of the 13 subtypes, the hypermobility type of EDS (hEDS) is the most common.[7,8] The subtypes are distinct from each other, and the diagnosis is based on family history and clinical criteria, including the degree and nature of involvement of the skin, joints, skeleton, and vasculature.[8]

The genetic basis for the major types of EDS is known, except for the hEDS, which is still unknown (**Table 2**). Clinical classification prevails over genetic classification due to the low global availability of genetic screening.[7]

Some comorbidities have been frequently reported in EDS patients, such as asthma,[9] orthostatic intolerance,[10] eosinophilic gastrointestinal disorders,[11] osteoporosis,[12] and neuropsychiatric conditions.[13] In the past decade, several investigators have described a possible association between EDS and MCAD, particularly in patients with hEDS.[4] In 2011, Luzgina and colleagues[14] noted that patients who sought assistance in cosmetological clinics for connective tissue dysplasia syndrome had a higher density of chymase positive MCs in their undamaged skin. Two years later, Louisias and colleagues[15] noted that patients with joint hypermobility syndrome also had symptoms suggestive of MC degranulation, such as naso-ocular symptoms, asthma, and a history of anaphylaxis. Their study also showed that these patients had a positive response to classic MC/MC mediator antagonists, but the investigators did not observe high levels of tryptase or histamine. In the connective tissues, MCs are located close to peripheral nerves and blood vessels so they can modulate sympathetic activity, vascular tone, and angiogenesis.[16] EDS patients may suffer from peripheral neuropathy that consequently leads to autonomic dysfunction.[17,18]

In 2017, a review article regarding the association between MCAD and EDS was published.[4] The investigators postulated that migration and differentiation of MC progenitors, MC activation, and the pattern of mediators in the MC granules are affected by components of the extracellular matrix. Thus, they hypothesized that MC dysregulation might be associated with EDS.[4] Vengoechea[19] published a letter discussing that the scientific evidence supporting this association was too "weak" because it was a small case series, the study was not controlled, and the questionnaires used were not standardized.[19,20]

The management of EDS is highly variable, because it depends on different variants of the syndrome and a patient's clinical presentation and severity. The management of MCADs, however, is mainly based on the blockade of MC mediators. Chronic

Table 2
Clinical classification of the inheritance pattern and genetic basis of Ehlers-Danlos syndromes

Clinical Ehlers-Danlos Syndrome Subtype	Inheritance Pattern	Genetic Basis
Classical EDS	Autosomal dominant	Major: COL5A1, COL5A1 Rare: COL1A1 c.934C > T, p.(Arg312Cys)
Classic-like EDS	Autosomal recessive	TNXB
Cardiac-valvular	Autosomal recessive	COL1A2 (biallelic mutations that lead to COL1A2 nonsense-mediated mRNA decay and the absence of proa2[I] collagen chains)
Vascular EDS	Autosomal dominant	Major: COL3A1 Rare: COL1A1 c.934C > T, p.(Arg312Cys) c.1720C > T, p.(Arg574Cys) c.3227C > T, p.(Arg1093Cys)
hEDS	Autosomal dominant	Unknown
Arthrochalasia EDS	Autosomal dominant	COL1A1, COL1A2
Dermatosparaxis EDS	Autosomal recessive	ADAMTS2
Kyphoscoliotic EDS	Autosomal recessive	PLOD1 FKBP14
Brittle cornea syndrome	Autosomal recessive	ZNF469 PRDM5
Spondylodysplastic EDS	Autosomal recessive	B4GALT7 B3GALT6 SLC39A13
Musculocontractural EDS	Autosomal recessive	CHST14 DSE
Myopathic EDS	Autosomal dominant or Autosomal recessive	COL12A1
Periodontal EDS	Autosomal dominant	C1R C1S

Adapted from Malfait F, Francomano C, Byers P, et al. The 2017 international classification of the Ehlers-Danlos syndromes. Am J Med Genet C Semin Med Genet 2017;175(1):10; with permission.

glucocorticoid therapy is considered a poor choice for MCADs because of chronic toxicities, including the adverse effects of glucocorticoids on connective tissues. Thus, treatment with glucocorticoids may be an even worse treatment choice for MCAD patients who also have EDS.[4]

POSTURAL TACHYCARDIA SYNDROME AND MAST CELL ACTIVATION DISORDERS

POTS is defined as a chronic, multifactorial syndrome of orthostatic intolerance. Patients have recurrent increases in heart rate on standing without orthostatic hypotension and have other associated symptoms that also worsen on standing. For the diagnosis of POTS, clinicians should exclude other disorders, including prolonged bed rest, hyperthyroidism, medication use, and acute blood loss. The diagnostic criteria for POTS are described in **Box 1**.[21,22]

The evaluation of a patient suspected of having POTS should include a complete history and physical examination, orthostatic vital signs, and a 12-lead ECG.[21]

Box 1

Diagnostic criteria for postural tachycardia syndrome

- An increase in heart rate of ≥30 beats per minute on standing in adults (or ≥40 beats per minute in children) with no orthostatic hypotension (fall in systolic blood pressure of ≥20 mm Hg or diastolic blood pressure of ≥10 mm Hg)

- Associated symptoms that are worse with standing (light-headedness, fatigue, palpitations, and syncope) and better with recumbence

- Additional causes of tachycardia excluded, including prolonged bed rest, hyperthyroidism, medications, and acute blood loss

- Chronicity implying symptoms for longer than 6 months

Adapted from Freeman R, Wieling W, Axelrod FB, et al. Consensus statement on the definition of orthostatic hypotension, neurally mediated syncope and the postural tachycardia syndrome. Clin Auton Res 2011;21(2):69–72; with permission.

Selected patients might benefit from thyroid function testing and a hematocrit evaluation, 24-hour Holter electrocardiography, a transthoracic echocardiogram, and exercise stress testing. If a patient's orthostatic vital signs are normal and the clinical suspicion of POTS is high, a tilt-table test might be helpful because it can provide vital signs during longer periods than in a simple stand test.[21]

Some symptoms of autonomic dysregulation are common in both patients with POTS and those with EDS, such as lightheadedness, palpitations, presyncope, chest pain, and syncope.[23] Furthermore, autonomic testing in EDS patients shows sympathetic cardiovascular control similar to patients with POTS. With regard to patients with hEDS, studies of autonomic function confirmed a high prevalence of POTS-like orthostatic symptoms and orthostatic intolerance. These symptoms can be induced by exercise, meals, standing, or a hot environment.[17,18]

In a study of a POTS population, a prevalence of 18% was observed in patients who met the criteria for EDS, but its prevalence in the general population was approximately 0.02%.[24] It has been reported that hEDS is the most common disorder associated with POTS.[25] The exact relationship between POTS and hEDS is still unclear. Alterations in the connective tissue caused by EDS could lead to vascular laxity and predispose patients to orthostatic blood pooling in the lower extremities.[22,23] In conclusion, there is now more scientific evidence showing an association between EDS and dysautonomia/POTS.

In 2005, Shibao and colleagues[26] described a group of patients with POTS who were also suffering from episodes of flushing, shortness of breath, headache, lightheadedness, excessive diuresis, and gastrointestinal symptoms, such as diarrhea, nausea, and vomiting. They hypothesized that these individuals had abnormal MC activation beyond POTS and compared them with patients with isolated POTS and normal controls. The group of patients identified as "POTS plus MC activation" had higher levels of urine methylhistamine than did the other 2 groups, which suggested a probable role for MCs as the effector cell in this phenotype. They concluded that MC activation should be considered in patients with POTS presenting with flushing.[26] After this pivotal description, a few review articles[10,27] have replicated this information, citing the data first published by Shibao and colleagues.[26]

The management of POTS is complex. It is essentially based on nonpharmacologic approaches, such as a high amount of fluid intake and aerobic exercise. The US Food and Drug Administration has not approved any drug for treating POTS. Many medications have been used to improve the symptoms of POTS, mainly by decreasing the influence of sympathetic tone on the heart. One of these therapeutic agents is propranolol.[10] If a patient presents with POTS and features of MCAD, however, clinicians should avoid the use of β-blockers because they may increase the severity of bronchospasm or hypotension during an anaphylactic reaction and are associated with an increase in anaphylaxis fatalities.

EHLERS-DANLOS SYNDROME, POSTURAL TACHYCARDIA SYNDROME, AND MAST CELL ACTIVATION DISORDERS: A NEW DISEASE CLUSTER?

In 2015, Cheung and Vadas[28] presented a study during the annual meeting of the American Academy of Asthma, Allergy & Immunology. They used a screening questionnaire to look for symptoms compatible with MC activation syndrome (MCAS) and suggested a possible new disease cluster: MCAS, EDS, and POTS. Patients diagnosed as having POTS and EDS were asked to answer a questionnaire, and 66% of the respondents reported symptoms suggestive of MCAS, indicating an association among these 3 syndromes.[28] The investigators defined the study, however, as a pilot study because the sample size was small (15 individuals) and there was no control group.

With regard to the mechanisms involved in this new disease cluster, recent data involving familial cases with high levels of serum tryptase have become available. In 2014, it was demonstrated that familial hypertryptasemia could be associated with MCAS.[29] Moreover, another group described 9 families with an autosomal-dominant inheritance pattern of increased basal total serum tryptase levels and identified an association between MCAS symptoms and tryptase levels; however, none of the patients was diagnosed with monoclonal systemic mastocytosis.[30]

In 2016, the same group of researchers identified germline duplications and triplications in the *TPSAB1* gene, which encodes alpha-tryptase, that segregated with inherited increases in basal serum tryptase levels in 35 families presenting with associated multisystem complaints. Moreover, individuals harboring alleles encoding 3 copies of alpha-tryptase had higher basal serum levels of tryptase and were more symptomatic than were those with alleles encoding 2 copies, which suggested a gene-dose effect. They showed that of the 96 patients, 28% had EDS (2× higher than the general population incidence); 46% were orthostatic intolerant; 51% presented with urticaria, pruritus or flushing; and 16% had previously reacted to *Hymenoptera* venom (2×–3× higher than the general population incidence).[31]

SUMMARY

Preliminary data that were recently published suggest a possible association between MCAD, EDS, and POTS. Nonetheless, the studies had small samples and were based on epidemiologic associations without control groups. Moreover, it remains unclear how elevated basal serum tryptase levels could contribute to these multisystem disorders. The quality of life of patients who have these syndromes is usually low and might be decreased in patients who have several of these syndromes. A multidisciplinary approach, including the participation of allergists, dermatologists, neurologists, cardiologists, physical therapists, and nurses, is needed to better clarify the relationship among MCAD, EDS, and POTS and to find better management for these cases.

REFERENCES

1. Moon TC, St Laurent CD, Morris KE, et al. Advances in mast cell biology: new understanding of heterogeneity and function. Mucosal Immunol 2010;3(2):111–28.

2. Galli SJ, Borregaard N, Wynn TA. Phenotypic and functional plasticity of cells of innate immunity: macrophages, mast cells and neutrophils. Nat Immunol 2011; 12(11):1035–44.
3. Sigal LH. Basic science for the clinician 53: mast cells. J Clin Rheumatol 2011; 17(7):395–400.
4. Bonamichi-Santos R, Castells M. Mast cell activation syndromes. Curr Treat Options Allergy 2016;3(4):384–400.
5. Seneviratne SL, Maitland A, Afrin L. Mast cell disorders in Ehlers-Danlos syndrome. Am J Med Genet C Semin Med Genet 2017;175(1):226–36.
6. Akin C, Valent P, Metcalfe DD. Mast cell activation syndrome: proposed diagnostic criteria. J Allergy Clin Immunol 2010;126(6):1099–104.e4.
7. Malfait F, Francomano C, Byers P, et al. The 2017 international classification of the Ehlers–Danlos syndromes. Am J Med Genet C Semin Med Genet 2017;175(1): 8–26.
8. Beighton P, De Paepe A, Steinmann B, et al. Ehlers-Danlos syndromes: revised nosology, Villefranche, 1997. Ehlers-Danlos National Foundation (USA) and Ehlers-Danlos Support Group (UK). Am J Med Genet 1998;77(1):31–7.
9. Morgan AW, Pearson SB, Davies S, et al. Asthma and airways collapse in two heritable disorders of connective tissue. Ann Rheum Dis 2007;66(10):1369–73.
10. Garland EM, Celedonio JE, Raj SR. Postural tachycardia syndrome: beyond orthostatic intolerance. Curr Neurol Neurosci Rep 2015;15(9):60.
11. Abonia JP, Wen T, Stucke EM, et al. High prevalence of eosinophilic esophagitis in patients with inherited connective tissue disorders. J Allergy Clin Immunol 2013;132(2):378–86.
12. Deodhar AA, Woolf AD. Ehlers Danlos syndrome and osteoporosis. Ann Rheum Dis 1994;53(12):841–2.
13. Sinibaldi L, Ursini G, Castori M. Psychopathological manifestations of joint hypermobility and joint hypermobility syndrome/Ehlers-Danlos syndrome, hypermobility type: the link between connective tissue and psychological distress revised. Am J Med Genet C Semin Med Genet 2015;169C(1):97–106.
14. Luzgina NG, Potapova OV, Shkurupiy VA. Structural and functional peculiarities of mast cells in undifferentiated connective tissue dysplasia. Bull Exp Biol Med 2011;150(6):676–8.
15. Louisias M, Silverman S, Maitland A. Prevalence of allergic disorders and mast cell activation syndrome in patients with Ehlers Danlos syndrome. Ann Allergy Asthma Immunol 2013;111:A12–3.
16. Feoktistov I, Ryzhov S, Goldstein AE, et al. Mast cell-mediated stimulation of angiogenesis: cooperative interaction between A2B and A3 adenosine receptors. Circ Res 2003;92(5):485–92.
17. De Wandele I, Calders P, Peersman W, et al. Autonomic symptom burden in the hypermobility type of Ehlers-Danlos syndrome: a comparative study with two other EDS types, fibromyalgia, and healthy controls. Semin Arthritis Rheum 2014;44(3):353–61.
18. De Wandele I, Rombaut L, Leybaert L, et al. Dysautonomia and its underlying mechanisms in the hypermobility type of Ehlers-Danlos syndrome. Semin Arthritis Rheum 2014;44(1):93–100.
19. Vengoechea J. In reply to "mast cell disorders in Ehlers-Danlos syndrome". Am J Med Genet A 2017. https://doi.org/10.1002/ajmg.a.38518.
20. Seneviratne SL, Maitland A, Afrin LB. Response to: "in reply to: 'mast cell disorders in Ehlers-Danlos Syndrome' (Jaime Vengoechea, Department of Human Genetics, Emory University)". Am J Med Genet A 2018;176(1):251–2.

21. Freeman R, Wieling W, Axelrod FB, et al. Consensus statement on the definition of orthostatic hypotension, neurally mediated syncope and the postural tachycardia syndrome. Clin Auton Res 2011;21(2):69–72.

22. Sheldon RS, Grubb BP, Olshansky B, et al. 2015 heart rhythm society expert consensus statement on the diagnosis and treatment of postural tachycardia syndrome, inappropriate sinus tachycardia, and vasovagal syncope. Heart Rhythm 2015;12(6):e41–63.

23. Gazit Y, Nahir AM, Grahame R, et al. Dysautonomia in the joint hypermobility syndrome. Am J Med 2003;115(1):33–40.

24. Wallman D, Weinberg J, Hohler AD. Ehlers-Danlos syndrome and postural tachycardia syndrome: a relationship study. J Neurol Sci 2014;340(1–2):99–102.

25. Mathias CJ, Low DA, Iodice V, et al. Postural tachycardia syndrome–current experience and concepts. Nat Rev Neurol 2011;8(1):22–34.

26. Shibao C, Arzubiaga C, Roberts LJ, et al. Hyperadrenergic postural tachycardia syndrome in mast cell activation disorders. Hypertension 2005;45(3):385–90.

27. Raj SR. Postural tachycardia syndrome (POTS). Circulation 2013;127(23): 2336–42.

28. Cheung I, Vadas P. A new disease cluster: mast cell activation syndrome, postural orthostatic tachycardia syndrome, and Ehlers-Danlos syndrome. J Allergy Clin Immunol 2015;135(2):AB65.

29. Sabato V, Van De Vijver E, Hagendorens M, et al. Familial hypertryptasemia with associated mast cell activation syndrome. J Allergy Clin Immunol 2014;134(6): 1448–50.e3.

30. Lyons JJ, Sun G, Stone KD, et al. Mendelian inheritance of elevated serum tryptase associated with atopy and connective tissue abnormalities. J Allergy Clin Immunol 2014;133(5):1471–4.

31. Lyons JJ, Yu X, Hughes JD, et al. Elevated basal serum tryptase identifies a multisystem disorder associated with increased TPSAB1 copy number. Nat Genet 2016;48(12):1564–9.

Patient Perceptions in Mast Cell Disorders

Susan V. Jennings, PhD[a],*, Valerie M. Slee, RN, BSN[a], Rachel M. Zack, ScD, SM[a],
Srdan Verstovsek, MD, PhD[b], Tracy I. George, MD[c], Hongliang Shi, MS[d],
Philina Lee, PhD[d], Mariana C. Castells, MD, PhD[e]

KEYWORDS

- Mast cell disorder • Mast cell activation • Patient perceptions and experiences
- The Mastocytosis Society • Anaphylaxis • Quality of life • Support • Disability

KEY POINTS

- A wide range in frequency and intensity of mast cell activation symptoms exists among individual mast cell disorder patients and also collectively in this population.
- Mast cell disorder patients report both disruption and reduced quality of life, with possible financial repercussions, due to physical and/or neuropsychiatric symptoms, including anaphylaxis, and their unpredictable onset.
- Triggers of mast cell activation, some of which may be less recognized than others, vary widely and can include heat/cold, stress, fatigue, foods/beverages, alcohol, medications/contrast, venoms, odors, infections, and exercise.
- Patients report that treatment of mast cell disorders is primarily directed at symptom reduction rather than cure in all but the most advanced variants.

Disclosure Statements: The Mastocytosis Society, Research Committee Chair (S.V. Jennings). The Mastocytosis Society, Chair, Board of Directors (V.M. Slee). The Mastocytosis Society, Research Committee Member (R.M. Zack). Medical Advisory Board for The Mastocytosis Society (S. Verstovsek). Medical Advisory Board for The Mastocytosis Society; consulting fees, Blueprint Medicines (T.I. George). H. Shi and P. Lee are employees and stockholders at Blueprint Medicines. Medical Advisory Board for The Mastocytosis Society (M.C. Castells). Blueprint Medicines provides funds to help fund the Mast Cell Connect registry, and provides funds to The Mastocytosis Society, Inc.

[a] The Mastocytosis Society, Inc, PO Box 416, Sterling, MA 01564, USA; [b] Department of Leukemia, The University of Texas MD Anderson Cancer Center, 1515 Holcombe Boulevard, Houston, TX 77030, USA; [c] Department of Pathology, University of Utah, 15 N Medical Drive East, Suite 1100, Salt Lake City, Utah, 84112 USA; [d] Blueprint Medicines Corporation, 45 Sidney Street, Cambridge, MA 02139, USA; [e] Department of Medicine, Division of Rheumatology, Immunology, and Allergy, Mastocytosis Center, Brigham and Women's Hospital, Harvard Medical School, 60 Fenwood Road, Boston, MA 02115, USA
* Corresponding author.
E-mail address: susan.jennings@tmsforacure.org

Immunol Allergy Clin N Am 38 (2018) 505–525
https://doi.org/10.1016/j.iac.2018.04.006
0889-8561/18/© 2018 The Authors. Published by Elsevier Inc. This is an open access article under the CC BY-NC-ND license (http://creativecommons.org/licenses/by-nc-nd/4.0/).
immunology.theclinics.com

INTRODUCTION

The ability of health care professionals and industry representatives to understand the experiences, perceptions, and perspectives of patients plays a vital role in successful care, treatment, and informed development of novel therapies. Regulators increasingly recognize the patient's voice as critical to drug development, with the US Food and Drug Administration's 2009 Guidance on Patient-reported Outcomes, patient-focused drug development meetings, and the 21st Century Cures Act. Patients with a mast cell disorder (MCD), including mastocytosis, mast cell activation syndromes (MCAS), and hereditary α-tryptasemia, may experience daily physical, emotional, and social stressors, and awareness of these factors can help medical professionals provide more comprehensive care. Recognition that patient perceptions of their illness may differ from perceptions of treating physicians, especially related to quality of life, degree of disability, and chronicity of symptoms, is essential.

PATIENT POPULATION AND CHARACTERISTICS

MCDs, considered rare diseases, affect newborns to adults and are divided into clonal and nonclonal disorders. Clonal disorders include cutaneous mastocytosis (CM), systemic mastocytosis (SM), and monoclonal MCAS.[1–6] Nonclonal disorders include forms of MCAS that are secondary or idiopathic.[1,2,7] CM often presents in children less than 2 years old, and variants, most commonly maculopapular CM (urticaria pigmentosa), differ in size, shape, and pattern of skin rash, percentage of skin affected, and frequency of persistence into adulthood.[8] Cutaneous mastocytoma or mastocytomas, usually present at birth, may spontaneously regress during childhood.[3,5,8] SM, which may be associated with cutaneous lesions, is divided into indolent SM (ISM), smoldering SM (SSM), and the more advanced SM (AdvSM) categories: SM with associated hematologic neoplasm (SM-AHN), aggressive SM (ASM), and mast cell leukemia (MCL).[3–6] A separate category exists for mast cell (MC) sarcoma.[3,5] Progression from indolent to more aggressive disease is defined by strict diagnostic criteria.[3–6] A more recently described entity, hereditary α-tryptasemia, is associated with MC mediator release symptoms, dysautonomia, and connective tissue disorders, especially joint hypermobility.[9] Potential triggers of MC mediator release,[1,10,11] and resulting symptoms,[2,7,11,12] vary for each MCD patient (**Boxes 1** and **2**). Patients

---

Box 1
Common triggers for patients with a mast cell disorder

- Heat, cold, sudden temperature changes
- Emotional, physical, environmental stress
- Fatigue
- Exercise, friction, vibration, surgery
- Food, beverages, including alcohol
- Medications (opioids, NSAIDs, antibiotics, and anesthetics)/contrast dyes
- Hymenoptera venom
- Odors
- Infections

Data from Refs.[1,10,11]

Box 2
Common symptoms and signs for patients with a mast cell disorder

- Fatigue

- Flushing, itching, rashes

- Abdominal pain/bloating, reflux, diarrhea, nausea, vomiting

- Bone/musculoskeletal pain

- Osteopenia/osteoporosis

- Headache, brain fog/cognitive issues, anxiety/depression

- Chest pain, shortness of breath, lightheadedness/fainting, blood pressure changes

- Anaphylaxis

Data from Refs.[2,7,11,12]

---

with AdvSM can present with cytopenias and organ enlargement/dysfunction from MC infiltration.[3,4,6,13]

OVERVIEW OF STUDIES AND SURVEYS REVIEWED

Patients' perceptions, experiences, and perspectives have been reported using a variety of data-gathering mechanisms, including patient-related observations, quality-of-life measurements, and patient-reported studies. A limited number of articles related to or containing responses from MCD patients are currently available (**Table 1**).

Two studies that yielded critical insight resulted from questionnaire validation processes, both of which reported mean importance (MI) scores.[16,17] The Mastocytosis Quality-of-Life Questionnaire (MQLQ) and Mastocytosis Symptom Assessment Form (MSAF) validations noted the percent of patients reporting an item, along with an item's MI score,[16] noted herein as MQLQ-MI and MSAF-MI, respectively. The Mastocytosis Quality of Life Questionnaire (MC-QoL) validation of a different set of questions developed by a separate group, noted the frequency of patients reporting an item experienced over the previous 2 weeks, along with an item's MI score,[17] noted herein as MC-QoL-MI. An MI score denotes the average importance rating level chosen for a given item. Each questionnaire validation reported MI scores based on a different scale:

- MQLQ validation (importance range, 0–6) included an MQLQ-MI score that ranged from 1.5 to 3.4;
- MSAF validation (importance range, 0–10), included an MSAF-MI score that ranged from 3.25 to 5.42;
- MC-QoL validation (importance range, 1–5) included an MC-QoL-MI score that ranged from 2.20 to 3.51.[16,17]

Higher MI scores and items with higher frequency are generally noted in this article.

Online surveys, including patient-reported diagnoses, have facilitated wider-based data collection, albeit with the limitation that actual diagnoses may differ from those reported. Also, given general unfamiliarity with MCDs, in some cases physician diagnoses may not necessarily be accurate. Nevertheless, online surveys provide a collective voice and picture of patients seen by physicians for diagnosis or treatment. The Mastocytosis Society, Inc (TMS) Patient Survey (TMS Survey) (Russell N, Jennings S, Jennings B, et al. The mastocytosis society survey on mast cell disorders: part 2—clinical

Table 1
Studies and surveys reporting data on perceptions of patients with a mast cell disorder

Author, Year	Study Period	Country	N	Design	Data Collection Tool	Population/Disease Types
Heinze et al,[14] 2017	2002–2015	US	39	Cohort	CDLQI	Pediatric CM (aged ≥4 y)[a]
Gotlib et al,[15] 2016	2009–2013	Not reported	79	Open-label drug trial	MSAS	Adult ASM, SM-AHN, or MCL (AdvSM) (aged ≥18 y)[b]
van Anrooij et al,[16] 2016	Not reported	Netherlands	164	Cross-sectional	MQLQ[c] and MSAF[d] validation study	Adult ISM[e]
Siebenhaar et al,[17] 2016	Not reported	Germany	158	Cross-sectional	MC-QoL[f] validation study	Adult CM and ISM[g]
Lee et al,[18] 2016 and this article	2015–2016 and 2015–2017	Majority US; other countries	137 with SM[18] 228 with SM or CM (this article)	Cross-sectional	Patient-reported online registry	Adult and pediatric mastocytosis (any form)[h] (patient-reported)
Jennings et al,[19] 2014; Russell et al, submitted	2010	Majority US; other countries	420	Cross-sectional	Patient-reported survey (online or paper)	Adult and pediatric mastocytosis (any form) and MCAS (patient-reported)[i]

Valent et al,[2] 2012	2010	US and EU	Not reported	Cross-sectional	Patient-reported surveys	Mastocytosis and MCAS (patient-reported; further details not reported)
Nowak et al,[20] 2011	Patients hospitalized between 2005 and 2008	Germany	50	Cross-sectional	Mailed questionnaire following hospitalization for mastocytosis	Adult mastocytosis (CM and SM)[j]
Moura et al,[12] 2011	Patients tested between 2003 and 2007	France	288	Cross-sectional	Ham-D17	Adult mastocytosis (aged >18 y)[k]
Hermine et al,[21] 2008	1999–2004	France	363 cases, 90 controls	Case-control	Questionnaire on perceived disability	Adult mastocytosis (any form) (aged >18 y)[l]

Abbreviations: CDLQI, Children's Dermatology Life Quality Index; Ham-D17, Hamilton Depression Scale; MC-QoL, Mastocytosis Quality of Life; MSAS, memorial symptom assessment scale.

a Patients with 3 or more mastocytomas who visited Children's Hospital of Wisconsin Dermatology Clinic.
b Patients enrolled in a trial of midostaurin (baseline data).
c MQLQ data reported as percent experiencing item and MI (range, 0–6, representing responses of "none, or not applicable" [0] through "worst possible" [6]; MQLQ-MI).
d MSAF data reported as percent experiencing item and MI (range, 0–10, representing responses of "absent" [0] through "very severe" [10]; MSAF-MI).
e Patients with SM diagnosis according to World Health Organization criteria and at least 1 y of follow-up at the University Medical Center Groningen.
f MC-QoL Questionnaire data reported as frequency experiencing an item and MI (range, 1–5, representing responses of "never" [1] through "very often" [5]; MC-QoL-MI).
g Patients from 4 mastocytosis specialist centers in Germany.
h Participants in the Mast Cell Connect Mastocytosis Patient-Reported Registry.
i TMS members and others who were made aware of the survey through TMS publication, Web site, MCD blogs, and notices in specialty clinics.
j Patients hospitalized for mastocytosis at PsoriSol Clinic for Dermatology, Hersbruck/Nuremberg.
k Patients diagnosed according to WHO criteria, identified by the French mastocytosis organization AFIRMM.
l Patients identified by the French mastocytosis organization AFIRMM.

experiences and beyond, manuscript submitted.)[19] evolved from a pilot project, presented independently but in parallel to US and European Union (EU) MCD patients, that yielded a list of "Top 10 issues raised by patients in the US and EU."[2] In addition, some commentary herein derives from more than 20 years of TMS direct experience supporting patients affected by MCDs, their families, caregivers, and physicians.

Mast Cell Connect (MC Connect; NCT02620254, www.mastcellconnect.org),[18] a patient-reported registry, was developed to advance understanding of mastocytosis and its impact on patients, and to facilitate development of new therapies. Participants register on a secure online portal and complete a 25-item survey to provide demographic, disease, and treatment information. Enrollment began December 1, 2015 and has been enabled by TMS, expert physicians, and media coverage. The registry includes participants with SM or CM. Diagnoses are self-reported, and participants are asked to provide medical reports that can be used to confirm diagnoses in the future. The study is institutional review board–approved (Chesapeake), and informed consent is required. At time of data cutoff (July 31, 2017), 264 participants had consented to join MC Connect, of whom 251 participants had completed the survey (**Table 2**). Participant-reported disease subtypes are shown in **Fig. 1**. Subsequent analyses focus on participants who reported a diagnosis of SM or CM.

MEDICAL CARE EXPERIENCES AND PERCEPTIONS

Multiple challenges for diagnosis, care, and treatment of MCD patients exist. Heterogeneous presentation, unfamiliarity with MCDs, and evolution of newly recognized variants may prolong time from symptom onset to diagnosis. Considering reported average durations of 4 to 12 years (**Table 3**),[13,19,22] it is important to consider patient perceptions of the diagnostic process. Frustration with this process is a major topic during support group discussions.

Table 2
Mast cell connect registry: participant demographics

	All[a] (n = 251)	SM[b] (n = 163)	CM[c,d] (n = 65)
Age, median (range)	47 (1–79)	50 (3–79)	34 (1–69)
Gender, n (%)	n = 250	n = 162	n = 65
Male	67 (27)	34 (21)	30 (46)
Female	183 (73)	128 (79)	35 (54)
Race, n (%)	n = 247	n = 161	n = 63
White	231 (94)	155 (96)	55(87)
Country, n (%)	n = 251	n = 163	n = 65
US	224 (89)	146 (90)	56 (86)
Canada	11 (4)	6 (4)	4 (6)
Other[e]	16 (6)	11 (7)	5 (8)

[a] Fourteen participants reported diagnoses other than SM or CM; 9 participants did not report their diagnosis.
[b] Fifty percent (81 out of 163) of SM participants reported concomitant CM and were categorized as SM participants.
[c] All CM participants did not answer all demographic questions. Percentages were calculated based on the total number of respondents.
[d] Of those who reported CM only, 69% (45 out of 65) were greater than 18 y old, and some may have undiagnosed SM.
[e] Other countries include the United Kingdom (n = 3), Australia (n = 3), Brazil (n = 2); Belgium, Denmark, France, Italy, New Zealand, Switzerland, Taiwan, and Turkey (n = 1).

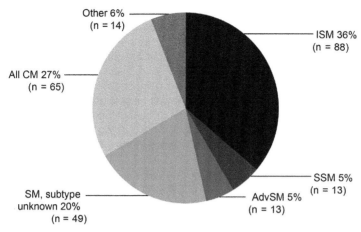

Fig. 1. Mast cell connect registry: participant-reported disease subtypes.

Mastocytosis patients visited a median of 3 specialists before a diagnosis was made,[18] and nearly half consulted 3 to 6 physicians while seeking a diagnosis.[20] Slightly more than one-third noted more than one specialist type, with dermatology, allergy/immunology, hematology/oncology, and general practice/internal medicine physicians most commonly involved in MCD diagnosis (Russell N, Jennings S, Jennings B, et al. The mastocytosis society survey on mast cell disorders: part 2—clinical experiences and beyond, manuscript submitted.)[18]

Challenges for patients seeking an evaluation for an MCD include the following:

- Obtaining a bone marrow biopsy, evaluated by pathologists familiar with mastocytosis
- Obtaining *KIT* mutation testing in bone marrow samples and/or peripheral blood, with appropriate test sensitivity
- Obtaining accurate mastocytosis disease subtyping
- Capturing an MC mediator rise (serum tryptase, for SM minor criterion, along with other urinary mediators for nonclonal MCDs)[2]
- Developing an ongoing plan to seek a cause for symptoms of MC activation, and to treat symptoms,[2,23] while ruling out other diagnoses, if mediator testing is negative

Patients in the US and EU endure difficulties identifying and accessing health care professionals knowledgeable about MCDs.[2] ISM patients (82%) were troubled by

Table 3
Mast cell connect registry: time from symptom onset to diagnosis

	SM (n = 149)[a]	ISM (n = 80)[a]	SSM[b] (n = 13)	AdvSM[b] (n = 13)	CM (n = 61)[a]
Median (y)[c]	7	9	9	3	1
Mean (SD)[c]	12 (13)	12 (12)	12 (11)	11 (14)	7 (14)

Abbreviation: SD, standard deviation.
  [a] Number of participants who responded to this question.
  [b] The numbers of participants who reported a diagnosis of AdvSM or SSM are small; hence, results should not be considered representative of patients with AdvSM or SSM in general.
  [c] Derived from the following questions: At what age did the participant first begin experiencing symptoms of mastocytosis? At what age was the diagnosis of mastocytosis made?

some physicians' lack of mastocytosis knowledge (MQLQ-MI, 2.9).[16] Nearly two-thirds of TMS Survey respondents receiving care in the US reported that it was not easy to access good care locally, and 37% had been denied care by a physician because of their MCD (Russell N, Jennings S, Jennings B, et al. The mastocytosis society survey on mast cell disorders: part 2—clinical experiences and beyond, manuscript submitted.) Although 39% were being treated by an MCD specialist, 80% noted the number of US MCD centers was insufficient; 83% reported comfort with the possibility of care managed locally, in conjunction with an MCD specialist (Russell N, Jennings S, Jennings B, et al. The mastocytosis society survey on mast cell disorders: part 2—clinical experiences and beyond, manuscript submitted.)

Although some patients are assertive in obtaining information and quality care, others are reluctant to "bother" their physicians. Sixty-six percent of US-treated TMS Survey respondents felt at least somewhat well informed by their physicians regarding diagnostic procedures, but fewer felt this way regarding follow-up investigations (58%), prognosis/future health (47%), and therapy options (53%) (Russell N, Jennings S, Jennings B, et al. The mastocytosis society survey on mast cell disorders: part 2—clinical experiences and beyond, manuscript submitted.)

Various terminologies have been used to describe forms of MCDs, including *mast cell disorders/diseases, clonal/monoclonal (primary), nonclonal (idiopathic or secondary),* with *MC activation disorders (MCAD)* and *MCAS* originally used interchangeably. Patients report confusion regarding these terms, compounded conceptually by occurrence of mastocytosis with or without MCAS.[2,24] Despite the availability of proposed diagnostic criteria developed by expert consensus,[2] confusion and disagreement regarding MCAS diagnosis exist among patients and physicians, with some physicians following alternate diagnostic criteria.[25] Patients often report to TMS resistance from physicians in accepting an MCAS diagnosis and that for any form of MCD, accurate diagnosis is essential for effective treatment. Studies suggest that most adults with mastocytosis skin lesions have SM, a diagnosis which requires a bone marrow biopsy.[4,26] However, only 40% of TMS Survey adults reporting a CM diagnosis recalled this assessment.[19]

ALLERGIES, SENSITIVITIES, AND TRIGGERS

More than half of patients in several studies reported foods and/or beverages as allergies, intolerances, or triggers, and the causative types varied considerably.[19–21] Alcohol, reported by 34% to 60%, posed a particular problem.[16,19,20] Obtaining adequate nutrition concerned approximately one-fifth of TMS Survey respondents (Russell N, Jennings S, Jennings B, et al. The mastocytosis society survey on mast cell disorders: part 2—clinical experiences and beyond, manuscript submitted.) Mastocytosis patients felt their nutrition was impacted (77%; MC-QoL-MI, 3.30) and 73% altered food/beverage choices (MC-QoL-MI, 3.14).[17] Allergies/intolerances to drugs were reported by roughly one-third to more than one-half of survey/study participants and to environmental substances and/or inhalants by more than half.[19–21] Nearly 38% of TMS Survey respondents noted insect venom ("stings") as an allergy, trigger, or problem,[19] reported for 18% of mastocytosis patients in another study.[20] Fear upon seeing a bee or wasp troubled 86% (MQLQ-MI, 3.4; highest MQLQ-MI in study).[16]

Heat (82%), stress (81%), and exercise (63%) were the most common triggers reported by TMS Survey respondents.[19] Temperature changes (76%; MQLQ-MI, 2.7) and cold (40%) were also problematic.[16,19] Stress is a potent trigger of MC activation[27] and a constant companion of living with an MCD. Managing physical symptoms of nausea, diarrhea, acute pain, bloating, or brain fog, while performing the most essential daily living activities, can be extremely stressful. Mental stress was a trigger for 71%.[16] Physical stresses (67%), such as friction, vibration, and environmental noise, while innocuous to others, can be significant threats.[16,19,28]

Patients struggle to identify triggers, especially those less commonly reported.[19] Others may be less willing to accept the concept of a physical, emotional, or temperature-related trigger, as opposed to more commonly known allergens. Patients and caregivers may feel the need to prove that the patient's reaction has a biological basis.

SYMPTOMS

A common denominator for many MCD patients is the unpredictable onset of symptoms arising from the cascade of MC mediator release, including life-threatening anaphylaxis. This concern was the greatest single cause of distress for one-quarter of TMS Survey respondents and affected more participants moderately/extremely (70.9%), or extremely (43.5%), than any other queried aspect of life related to having an MCD[19]; however, no other studies were found to address this issue in MCD patients.

There is a wide range in the frequency and intensity of any given symptom, individually and collectively[17,19]; some MCD patients are chronically disabled, whereas others may lead relatively normal lives.[19] Symptoms reported by registry participants are shown in **Table 4**, and by others, in **Table 5**. Patients commonly question whether a particular symptom is due to their MCD; this uncertainty troubled 89% of ISM patients (MQLQ-MI, 3).[16]

Fatigue and Sleep Difficulties

Mastocytosis patients commonly report fatigue, experienced by 48% to 84% (MC-QoL, 3.05; MQLQ-MI, 3.1; MSAF-MI, 5.42) (see **Table 5**),[16,17,19,20] and by a similar percentage of registry participants with SM (see **Table 4**). AdvSM patients reported lack of energy (86%) and feeling drowsy (72%).[15] Fatigue influenced general activities, mood/temper, and chores for 67% to 70% of ISM patients.[16] Some patients report to TMS that incorporating rest periods helps considerably. Approximately 70% of mastocytosis patients had difficulties with falling asleep and daytime fatigue due to poor sleep (MC-QoL-MI range, 3.01–3.12).[17] Difficulty sleeping was also reported by 60% of AdvSM patients.[15]

Skin

Itching was experienced by 60% to 83% of MCD patients, with higher MI scores (see **Table 5**).[14,16,17,19–21] However, registry percentages were generally lower (see **Table 4**). Mastocytosis patients were affected by skin redness/swelling (88%; MC-QoL-MI, 3.51; highest MC-QoL-MI in study)[17] and by erythematous crisis (81%).[21] Flushing was reported by 52% to 76% (see **Table 5**),[14,16,17,19,21] with slightly lower percentages for registry participants (see **Table 4**). Physically exhausting flushing attacks troubled 69% of ISM patients.[16] In addition to discomfort caused by the feeling of intense heat (75%; MQLQ-MI, 2.6),[16] patients report that heat and burning of flushing often indicate onset of a larger MC activation attack, such that flushing induces anxious feelings.

Gastrointestinal

TMS Survey respondents (66%) reported that gastrointestinal complaints moderately/extremely affected their lives.[19] Diarrhea, reported by 23% to 66%, when chronic and

Table 4
Mast cell connect registry: frequency (%) of participants experiencing moderately to severely bothersome symptoms within the past year

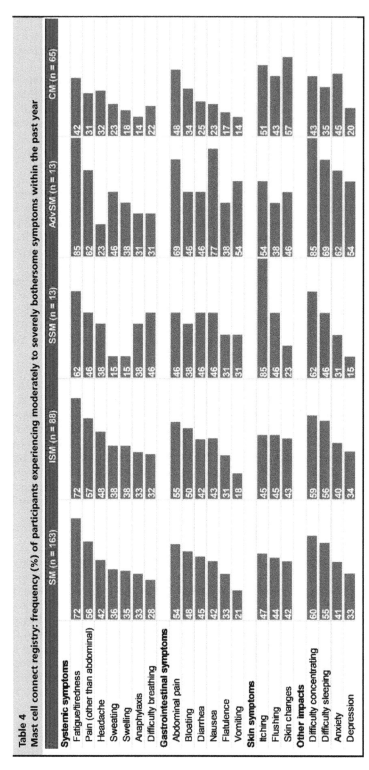

	SM (n = 163)	ISM (n = 88)	SSM (n = 13)	AdvSM (n = 13)	CM (n = 65)
Systemic symptoms					
Fatigue/tiredness	72	72	62	85	42
Pain (other than abdominal)	56	57	46	62	31
Headache	42	48	38	23	32
Sweating	36	38	15	46	23
Swelling	35	38	15	38	18
Anaphylaxis	33	33	38	31	14
Difficulty breathing	28	32	46	31	22
Gastrointestinal symptoms					
Abdominal pain	54	55	46	69	48
Bloating	48	50	38	46	34
Diarrhea	45	42	46	46	25
Nausea	42	43	46	77	23
Flatulence	33	31	31	38	17
Vomiting	21	18	31	54	14
Skin symptoms					
Itching	47	45	85	54	51
Flushing	44	45	46	38	43
Skin changes	42	43	23	46	57
Other impacts					
Difficulty concentrating	60	59	62	85	43
Difficulty sleeping	55	56	46	69	35
Anxiety	41	40	31	62	45
Depression	33	34	15	54	20

The number of participants who reported a diagnosis of AdvSM or SSM is small; hence, results should not be considered representative of patients with AdvSM or SSM in general.

Table 5
Percentage of patients with a mast cell disorder reporting specific symptoms

	Van Anrooij et al,[16] 2016	Siebenhaar et al,[17] 2016	Jennings et al,[19] 2014	Nowak et al,[20] 2011	Hermine et al,[21] 2008	Heinze et al,[14] 2017
Population and disease types	Adult ISM[a]	Adult CM and ISM[b]	Adult and pediatric mastocytosis (any form) and MCAS (patient-reported)[c]	Adult mastocytosis (CM and SM)[d]	Adult mastocytosis (any form) (aged >18 y)[e]	Pediatric CM (aged ≥4 y)[f]
Data presented	g,h	i	j	k	l	m
Symptom						
Fatigue	84% ("debilitating")[g] 81%[h] (during "last week")	77%	76%, 62%	48%	—	
Pruritis	81%[g] 83%[h]	78%	79%, 57%	66%	82%	60%
Flushing	75%[g] 59%[h] (per week)	56%	76%, 57%	40% ("hot flashes/flush") 32% (redness/face burning)	52%	63%
Diarrhea	64%[g]	58%	66%, 52%	42% ("frequent")	35%	23%
Nausea and/or vomiting	36%[h]	46%	54%, 37%	30% ("episodic")	49%	—
Abdominal pain/cramping	68%[g]	52%	56%, 46% ("lower") 46%, 36% ("upper") 73%, 60% (stomach)	22% ("frequent")	69% ("epigastric")	30%
Headache	72%[h]	60%	64%, 51%	46% ("frequent")	69%	42%
Brain fog/cognitive difficulties	70%–75%[g,h] 69%[h]	55%–59%[o]	67%, 46%	—	66% ("memory loss")	—
Depression	60%[h,p]	—	49%, 29%	—	57%	—
Anaphylaxis/anaphylactic shock	26% ("attacks", per month)	—	42%, 38%	36%	44%	—

(continued on next page)

Table 5
(continued)

	Van Anrooij et al,[16] 2016	Siebenhaar et al,[17] 2016	Jennings et al,[19] 2014	Nowak et al,[20] 2011	Hermine et al,[21] 2008	Heinze et al,[14] 2017
Bone pain	80%[h] (bone/muscle)	—	56%, 45%	22%	54%	44%
Muscle and joint pain/ cramps	—	71%	50%, 40% ("muscle, nerve, connective tissue") 61%, 46% (joint)	—	76%	—
Chest pain/palpitations	61%[h]	56%	37%, 23% (chest pain)	—	—	—
Dyspnea/ bronchoreactivity	58%[h]	48%	44%, 26% (wheezing, asthma)	—	43%	12% (asthma)
Dizziness	69%[h]	51%	61%, 44% ("lightheadedness/ syncope")	—	—	—

[a] Patients with SM diagnosis according to World Health Organization criteria and at least 1 y of follow-up at the University Medical Centre Groningen, Netherlands.
[b] Patients from 4 mastocytosis specialist centers in Germany.
[c] TMS members and others who were made aware of the survey through TMS publication, Web site, MCD blogs, and notices in specialty clinics.
[d] Patients hospitalized for mastocytosis at PsoriSol Clinic for Dermatology, Hersbruck/Nuremberg, Germany.
[f] Patients identified by the French mastocytosis organization AFIRMM.
[g] Patients with 3 or more mastocytomas who visited Children's Hospital of Wisconsin Dermatology Clinic.
[g] MQLQ[16]; symptom time period not noted.
[h] MSAF[16]; symptom time period not noted unless specified.
[i] Symptoms in the last 2 wk.
[j] Data reported for "any severity" and "moderate or extreme severity," both with any timing frequency, related to survey participants' MCD.
[k] Responses to query regarding symptoms patient or their physician first observed.
[l] Data reported for "any disability"; symptom time period not reported.
[m] Symptom time period not reported.
[n] "Clouding of consciousness," "reduced ability to concentrate," "inability to pay attention to conversations," "impaired short-term memory."
[o] "Forgetfulness," "difficulty in concentrating."
[p] "Depression, somberness."

associated with other gastrointestinal symptoms, especially nausea/vomiting (30%–54%), and abdominal/epigastric pain (22%–73%) (see **Tables 4** and **5**),[14,16,17,19–21] can be disabling and disrupting of daily lives. Diarrhea, nausea, and vomiting, with frequencies approximately 50%, 45% and 20%, respectively, were also reported for AdvSM patients.[15]

Pain

TMS Survey respondents (53%) were moderately/extremely affected by pain,[19] as were nearly 60% of AdvSM patients,[15] and 31% to 62% of registry participant groups (see **Table 4**). Muscle, joint, and bone pain were reported by many with an MCD (see **Table 5**), with high MI scores (muscle/joint pain, 71%, MC-QoL-MI, 2.97[17]; bone/muscle pain, 80%, MSAF-MI, 5.17).[16] Lower back pain was reported by 77% of ISM patients (MQLQ-MI, 2.4).[16] Headaches were recalled by 42% to 72% (see **Table 5**).[14,16,17,19–21] Some patients report to TMS that unrelieved pain triggers additional symptoms.

Anaphylaxis

Anaphylaxis affected 26% to 44% of those with MCD (see **Table 5**),[19–21] similar to registry participants with SM (see **Table 4**). Mastocytosis patients experienced fear of anaphylaxis (74%; MC-Qol-MI, 3.39),[17] worried about anaphylaxis treatment while traveling (81%; MQLQ-MI, 2.8), and were troubled by needing to rely on family during anaphylaxis (68%; MQLQ-MI, 2.4).[16] Seventy-seven percent of TMS Survey participants were prescribed self-injectable epinephrine, and 60% always carried the medication.[19]

Mental Health: Cognitive Issues, Depression, and Anxiety

Cognitive problems ("brain fog"), including memory impairment and difficulty focusing/processing, can hinder productivity at home, school, and work, and affect patients' ability to manage their disease. Such cognitive difficulties were reported by 43% to 85% (see **Tables 4** and **5**),[16,17,19,21] and concentration problems were specifically reported by mastocytosis patients with higher MI scores (59%; MC-QoL-MI, 2.88[17]; 69%; MSAF-MI, 4.37).[16] In support group meetings, MCD patients report to TMS that as a consequence of cognition problems, they fear others may see them as incompetent, resulting in significant loss of self-esteem and confidence, and in depression.

Depression and anxiety may be due to MC mediator release[11,12] and/or stressors related to living with a chronic illness. Depression/somberness was reported by 29% to 60% (see **Table 5**),[16,19,21] and by 64% in an additional study,[12] but by lower percentages in some registry participant groups (see **Table 4**). Moderate or greater somatic anxiety was experienced by roughly 55% with mild to moderate depression and 83% with major depression.[12] Psychic anxiety with a score of ≥2 on the Hamilton Depression Scale was reported by 44% with mild to moderate depression and approximately 20% with major depression.[12] More generally, 37% to 45% of TMS Survey and MC Connect Registry participants reported moderate or extreme/severe anxiety (see **Table 4**).[19] Patients report to TMS that depression and anxiety can influence their abilities to manage their disease.

FEAR AND UNCERTAINTY OF FUTURE HEALTH/DISEASE PROGRESSION

Consideration of prognostic indicators can help prepare families of pediatric patients for the possibility of disease persisting into adulthood.[8] No data were identified regarding patient and family perceptions related to future disease status in children with MCDs. In TMS support groups, parents whose children demonstrate extensive skin or systemic symptoms often report extreme fear of disease progression for their child. Adult mastocytosis patients report fear of "worsening disease" (84%; MC-QoL-MI, 3.37)[17] and fear of "disease progression" (91%; MQLQ-MI, 2.6).[16] No data were identified on this topic for patients with other MCD forms.

TREATMENT

US and EU patients highlighted a need to develop improved MCD therapies, including curative rather than symptom-targeted, and to increase focus on holistic care approaches[2]; these concerns persist. US patients also continue to report to TMS needing assistance, including financial, to obtain medications.[2] Mastocytosis patients were frustrated by the absence of curative therapy (83%; MQLQ-MI, 2.5), noted fear of anaphylaxis triggered by prescribed medication (75%),[16] and were afraid inappropriate treatment might be given if they were unresponsive (70%; MC-QoL-MI, 3.27).[17] Patients and caregivers report concern to TMS regarding drug interactions and identifying which medications are most efficacious while minimizing side effects. Some patients use compounding pharmacies to eliminate reactions to unnecessary fillers. MCD patients may be triggered by nonsteroidal anti-inflammatory drugs (NSAIDs) and opioid narcotics, making pain management challenging.

Despite articles outlining various MCD treatments supported by consensus,[2,7,11,29] some patients reported to TMS having a confirmed ISM diagnosis and being offered aggressive treatment not recommended for indolent disease. Although not widely discussed in literature, approximately 10 SSM patients stated to TMS that they had signs of improvement with chemotherapy to reduce MC burden and slow disease progression, resulting in decreased tryptase and symptoms. Patients may tend to receive improved diagnosis and treatment at MCD centers,[30] and some reported to TMS being offered stem cell transplants for nonadvanced variants at nonspecialized centers and this treatment as the *only* option for SSM, SM-AHN, and ASM, without attempting chemotherapy.

In contrast to current recommendations,[7] some MCD patients with nonclonal disease who have symptoms resistant to antimediator therapy have been offered tyrosine kinase inhibitors (TKIs), and have reported varying results. The authors are unaware of controlled studies involving large numbers of nonclonal MCD patients on TKIs. Another option reported by such patients seeking symptom relief is continuous diphenhydramine drip, with select patients self-reporting stabilization.[31] Significant concerns exist regarding long-term effects of antihistamine use on cognition; adding a continuous intravenous delivery route elevates concerns.[32] Both clonal and nonclonal MCD patients report to TMS success using omalizumab, an anti-immunoglobulin E monoclonal antibody, to control unprovoked anaphylaxis.[7]

IMPACTS ON DAILY LIFE AND QUALITY OF LIFE

Mastocytosis resulted in a moderate to extremely severe reduction in quality of life for 64% of patients[20] and impacted daily living for registry participants (**Fig. 2**). TMS Survey respondents (76%) reported moderate/extreme emotional impact on their life,[19] and 72% of mastocytosis patients reported psychological impact.[21] Disability experienced by mastocytosis patients due to symptoms occurred independent of diagnosis type, *KIT* mutation status, and elevated tryptase level.[21] Registry participants worried and felt irritable and depressed (see **Fig. 2**); more than 50% of AdvSM patients also reported worrying and feeling nervous.[15] Feelings of sadness, concern, lack of

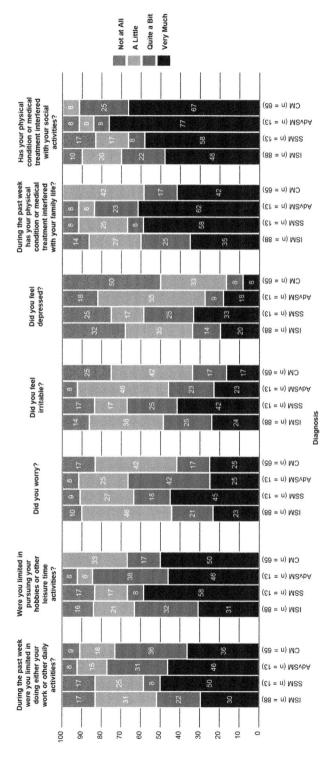

Fig. 2. Mast Cell Connect Registry: impacts on daily living. The number of participants who reported a diagnosis of AdvSM or SSM are small, hence results should not be considered representative of patients with AdvSM or SSM in general.

motivation, discouragement, frustration, or reduced capability were identified for approximately two-thirds of mastocytosis patients.[17] Fear of being a burden to others (62%) and fear of the future (78%; MC-QoL-MI, 3.07) were also concerns.[17] ISM patients reported being troubled by lack of cosmetic appeal, embarrassment, and increased visibility over time of their skin abnormalities (64%–71%).[16] In TMS's experience, there is great variability in how bothersome visibility of skin lesions is to patients; personality, age, and culture may be influencing factors.

Work, Daily Activity, and Leisure Time Aspects

More than half of MC Connect participants were at least "quite a bit" limited in performing daily work or other activities, or in pursuing hobbies/leisure activities (see **Fig. 2**). TMS Survey respondents (49%) were moderately/extremely affected by inability to work or participate in daily living activities,[19] and 52% of mastocytosis patients reported disability related to performance status.[21] Mastocytosis patients were limited in their school/university/work (62.1%), leisure time (68.4%), and sport/physical activities (80.0%) (MC-QoL-MI, 2.86–2.97).[17] Severity of depression may influence these aspects of life, because 97% of mastocytosis patients with major depression and 40% with mild to moderate depression had work and interests affected.[12] The sudden onset of gastrointestinal, cognitive, and anaphylactic symptoms, coupled with the need to inject epinephrine, makes it difficult or impossible for many patients to perform any job.

Financial Pressures/Disability

Patients report to TMS that loss of income from an inability to work affects their financial stability and their ability to manage their disease. Loss of health insurance impacts access to medications and health care. The unpredictable onset of acute symptoms is a primary reason MCD patients qualify for disability support in TMS's experience. In addition, patients report to TMS that accessing health care can become prohibitive when ancillary costs (travel, parking, and so forth) are considered.

Social Interactions

Mastocytosis patients commonly perceived negative effects on their family and social life (see **Fig. 2**). Fifty-five percent reported difficulty with social interactions.[21] Mastocytosis limited activities with other people (63%) and social relationships (72%).[17] Social life suffering from mastocytosis troubled 69%, and 68% reported being troubled by incomprehension of mastocytosis by family, friends, and colleagues.[16]

Patients reported a discomfort with being in public places because of their mastocytosis, with feelings of being watched in public (69%), being ashamed to visit public places (72%), and being uncomfortable in public (73%) (MC-QoL-MI, 2.85–2.96).[17] Reduced sexual relations (36%) and limited love life (56%) were also reported by mastocytosis patients.[17,21]

Children's Experiences and School-Related Aspects

Few data exist on quality of life in children with MCDs. One study of 39 pediatric patients with urticaria pigmentosa found that, although a majority reported their quality of life was mildly or not affected, and none were affected severely, 15 reported their quality of life was affected by "teasing, bullying, or asking questions."[14] Embarrassment, self-consciousness, and "being upset" were reported because of skin lesions by 12 patients.[14] Teens in TMS support group sessions discuss embarrassment about skin lesions, flushing, gastrointestinal symptoms, and dietary limitations when socializing; no formal studies were identified.

Parents report to TMS success with keeping children in school if a comprehensive plan is established to educate all adults with whom the child will interact, regarding triggers, presenting symptoms, and appropriate interventions. Parents also relay that children given a pivotal role in educating classmates/peers report feeling more confident and peer-supported. In support groups, parents report subtle triggers, like physical contact with other children, classroom temperature, and noise, result in fatigue, inattention, and flushing/itching. Because of stress from the school setting's social and emotional climate, some parents report their children were more stable during school vacations, leading some to opt for home schooling. Others report that with a medical/educational plan in place, children were able to thrive in a school setting.

OTHER CONSIDERATIONS
Importance and Identification of Support

Patients and their caregivers seek support to address challenges faced when confronting life with an MCD, including interactions with family and friends, attending support groups, and participating in online social media forums. Because mastocytosis patients felt isolated (76%; MC-QoL-MI, 3.06),[17] availability of easily accessed support, including social media, is vital. Physical and psychological effects of MCDs may lead patients to use a variety of coping mechanisms; seeking social support was a key coping strategy.[33] Patients often leave support meetings reporting to TMS that they no longer feel alone with their illness.

Concerns Regarding Possible Familial Disease

Patients desired further research into the existence of familial forms of MCDs.[2] TMS Survey respondents (23%) indicated *possible* MCDs in their family, with higher frequencies of respondents who reported an MCAS or idiopathic anaphylaxis diagnosis indicating possible family members with MCDs than those who reported a mastocytosis diagnosis (Russell N, Jennings S, Jennings B, et al. The mastocytosis society survey on mast cell disorders: part 2—clinical experiences and beyond, manuscript submitted.)

Obtaining Accurate Disease Information

Availability of reliable and accessible MCD information for patients and caregivers has been a concern.[2] Medical and patient organizations, for example, the European Competence Network on Mastocytosis (ECNM; www.ecnm.net), American Academy of Allergy, Asthma, and Immunology (AAAAI; www.aaaai.org), TMS (www.tmsforacure.org), and the National Organization for Rare Disorders (www.rarediseases.org), provide online MCD informational materials.

Collaboration

Collaborations between patients, health care professionals, government, and industry have been particularly effective for rare diseases.[34] TMS has worked closely with physicians, industry, and others to ensure patient perceptions and experiences are shared, and has been an active participant in advancement of MCD community initiatives (**Box 3**).

FUTURE CONSIDERATIONS/SUMMARY

Although progress has been made on some issues raised by patients,[2] such as publication of international working group–derived definitions and criteria for MCAS,[2] more specific disease classifications,[2,8,29,37] development of a proposed

---

Box 3
Examples of patient collaborations in advancement of mast cell disorder community initiatives

- Development of documentation in collaboration with the AAAAI, resulting in implementation of the first *ICD-10-CM* codes for MCAS (2016) and revised codes for mastocytosis (2017)

- Organization of meetings with physicians, industry and patient group representatives, resulting in support and collaboration for the establishment of an American MCD network (the American Initiative in Mast Cell Diseases; AIM), similar to the ECNM[35,36]

- Establishment of an online, easily-accessed physician database

- Development and dissemination of educational material for patients and health care professionals

- Distribution of research announcements and of funds for international research

- Collaboration on global patient-driven projects and support networks

---

mastocytosis diagnostic algorithm,[38] improved diagnostic methods,[39] and advances in treatment,[15,29] unmet needs exist (**Box 4**).

Because identifying and accessing knowledgeable physicians remains a primary challenge for the MCD community, TMS recently established an online physician self-enrolled database (www.tmsforacure.org). This system is being expanded to accept international entries, with translation services, to allow patients, physicians, and others easier identification of *physicians of all specialties* involved in MCD patient care. A goal of this database is to contribute to the foundation for an organized network for MCDs within the Americas (the American Initiative in Mast Cell Diseases, AIM), similar to the ECNM,[35,36] geared toward addressing MCD community needs, with hope for global collaboration.

Box 4
Patient perceptions of unmet needs of the mast cell disorder community

- Further advances in curative, in addition to symptomatic, treatments and therapies

- Increased number of knowledgeable physicians willing to diagnose and treat patients with all MCD

- Establishment of more specialty centers to provide coordinated, multidisciplinary care for patients with all MCD

- Establishment of practice parameters for all forms of MCD

- Clarification with regard to diagnosis of MCAS variants

- Recognition and familiarity with MCD within all medical specialties

- Increased availability of easily accessible diagnostic and prognostic tests

- Increased assistance in obtaining medications

- Official establishment of an American network for MCD (the American Initiative in Mast Cell diseases, AIM), similar to the ECNM[35,36]

- Further research into possible familial forms of MCD

- Studies focused on perceptions and experiences of specific groups of patients with MCD (eg, children and teens with mastocytosis, and MCAS patients of all ages)

ACKNOWLEDGMENTS

The authors thank Deyaa Adib for discussions and feedback, the patients/participants who took part in the discussed studies and surveys, and the many health care professionals, researchers and others who have worked to improve the lives of MCD patients.

REFERENCES

1. Akin C, Valent P, Metcalfe DD. Mast cell activation syndrome: proposed diagnostic criteria. J Allergy Clin Immunol 2010;126(6):1099–104.e4.
2. Valent P, Akin C, Arock M, et al. Definitions, criteria and global classification of mast cell disorders with special reference to mast cell activation syndromes: a consensus proposal. Int Arch Allergy Immunol 2012;157(3):215–25.
3. Valent P, Horny HP, Escribano L, et al. Diagnostic criteria and classification of mastocytosis: a consensus proposal. Leuk Res 2001;25(7):603–25.
4. Valent P, Akin C, Escribano L, et al. Standards and standardization in mastocytosis: consensus statements on diagnostics, treatment recommendations and response criteria. Eur J Clin Invest 2007;37(6):435–53.
5. Valent P, Horny H-P, Li CY, et al. Mastocytosis. In: Jaffe ES, Harris NL, Stein H, et al, editors. World Health Organization (WHO) classification of tumours. Pathology and genetics. Tumours of haematopoietic and lymphoid tissues. Lyon (France): IARC Press; 2001. p. 291–302.
6. Horny HP, Akin C, Metcalfe DD, et al. Mastocytosis (mast cell disease). In: Swerdlow SH, Campo E, Harris NL, et al, editors. World Health Organization (WHO) classification of tumours. Pathology and genetics. Tumours of haematopoietic and lymphoid tissues. Lyon (France): IARC Press; 2008. p. 54–63.
7. Akin C. Mast cell activation syndromes. J Allergy Clin Immunol 2017;140(2): 349–55.
8. Hartmann K, Escribano L, Grattan C, et al. Cutaneous manifestations in patients with mastocytosis: Consensus report of the European Competence Network on Mastocytosis; the American Academy of Allergy, Asthma & Immunology; and the European Academy of Allergology and Clinical Immunology. J Allergy Clin Immunol 2016;137(1):35–45.
9. Lyons JJ, Yu X, Hughes JD, et al. Elevated basal serum tryptase identifies a multisystem disorder associated with increased TPSAB1 copy number. Nat Genet 2016;48(12):1564–9.
10. Castells M, Metcalfe DD, Escribano L. Diagnosis and treatment of cutaneous mastocytosis in children: practical recommendations. Am J Clin Dermatol 2011; 12(4):259–70.
11. Theoharides TC, Valent P, Akin C. Mast cells, mastocytosis, and related disorders. N Engl J Med 2015;373(2):163–72.
12. Moura DS, Sultan S, Georgin-Lavialle S, et al. Depression in patients with mastocytosis: prevalence, features and effects of masitinib therapy. PLoS One 2011; 6(10):e26375.
13. Lim KH, Tefferi A, Lasho TL, et al. Systemic mastocytosis in 342 consecutive adults: survival studies and prognostic factors. Blood 2009;113(23):5727–36.
14. Heinze A, Kuemmet TJ, Chiu YE, et al. Longitudinal study of pediatric urticaria pigmentosa. Pediatr Dermatol 2017;34(2):144–9.
15. Gotlib J, Kluin-Nelemans HC, George TI, et al. Efficacy and safety of midostaurin in advanced systemic mastocytosis. N Engl J Med 2016;374(26):2530–41.

16. van Anrooij B, Kluin-Nelemans JC, Safy M, et al. Patient-reported disease-specific quality-of-life and symptom severity in systemic mastocytosis. Allergy 2016;71(11):1585–93.

17. Siebenhaar F, von Tschirnhaus E, Hartmann K, et al. Development and validation of the mastocytosis quality of life questionnaire: MC-QoL. Allergy 2016;71(6): 869–77.

18. Lee P, George TI, Shi H, et al. Systemic mastocytosis patient experience from mast cell connect, the first patient-reported registry for mastocytosis. Blood 2016;128:4783.

19. Jennings S, Russell N, Jennings B, et al. The Mastocytosis Society survey on mast cell disorders: patient experiences and perceptions. J Allergy Clin Immunol Pract 2014;2(1):70–6.

20. Nowak A, Gibbs BF, Amon U. Pre-inpatient evaluation on quality and impact of care in systemic mastocytosis and the influence of hospital stay periods from the perspective of patients: a pilot study. J Dtsch Dermatol Ges 2011;9(7): 525–32.

21. Hermine O, Lortholary O, Leventhal PS, et al. Case-control cohort study of patients' perceptions of disability in mastocytosis. PLoS One 2008;3(5):e2266.

22. Hamilton MJ, Hornick JL, Akin C, et al. Mast cell activation syndrome: a newly recognized disorder with systemic clinical manifestations. J Allergy Clin Immunol 2011;128(1):147–52.e2.

23. Cardet JC, Castells MC, Hamilton MJ. Immunology and clinical manifestations of non-clonal mast cell activation syndrome. Curr Allergy Asthma Rep 2013;13(1):10–8.

24. Horny HP, Sotlar K, Valent P. Evaluation of mast cell activation syndromes: impact of pathology and immunohistology. Int Arch Allergy Immunol 2012;159(1):1–5.

25. Molderings GJ, Brettner S, Homann J, et al. Mast cell activation disease: a concise practical guide for diagnostic workup and therapeutic options. J Hematol Oncol 2011;4:10.

26. Berezowska S, Flaig MJ, Rueff F, et al. Adult-onset mastocytosis in the skin is highly suggestive of systemic mastocytosis. Mod Pathol 2014;27(1):19–29.

27. Theoharides TC. Neuroendocrinology of mast cells: challenges and controversies. Exp Dermatol 2017;26(9):751–9.

28. Boyden SE, Desai A, Cruse G, et al. Vibratory urticaria associated with a missense variant in ADGRE2. N Engl J Med 2016;374(7):656–63.

29. Valent P, Akin C, Hartmann K, et al. Advances in the classification and treatment of mastocytosis: current status and outlook toward the future. Cancer Res 2017; 77(6):1261–70.

30. Sanchez-Munoz L, Morgado JM, Alvarez-Twose I, et al. Diagnosis and classification of mastocytosis in non-specialized versus reference centres: a Spanish Network on Mastocytosis (REMA) study on 122 patients. Br J Haematol 2016; 172(1):56–63.

31. Molderings GJ, Haenisch B, Brettner S, et al. Pharmacological treatment options for mast cell activation disease. Naunyn Schmiedebergs Arch Pharmacol 2016; 389(7):671–94.

32. Theoharides TC, Stewart JM. Antihistamines and mental status. J Clin Psychopharmacol 2016;36(3):195–7.

33. Nicoloro-SantaBarbara J, Lobel M, Wolfe D. Psychosocial impact of mast cell disorders: pilot investigation of a rare and understudied disease. J Health Psychol 2017;22(10):1277–88.

34. Forsythe LP, Szydlowski V, Murad MH, et al. A systematic review of approaches for engaging patients for research on rare diseases. J Gen Intern Med 2014; 29(Suppl 3):S788–800.
35. Valent P, Arock M, Bischoff SC, et al. The European Competence Network on Mastocytosis (ECNM). Wien Klin Wochenschr 2004;116(19–20):647–51.
36. Valent P, Arock M, Bonadonna P, et al. European Competence Network on Mastocytosis (ECNM): 10-year jubilee, update, and future perspectives. Wien Klin Wochenschr 2012;124(23–24):807–14.
37. Valent P, Sotlar K, Sperr WR, et al. Refined diagnostic criteria and classification of mast cell leukemia (MCL) and myelomastocytic leukemia (MML): a consensus proposal. Ann Oncol 2014;25(9):1691–700.
38. Valent P, Escribano L, Broesby-Olsen S, et al. Proposed diagnostic algorithm for patients with suspected mastocytosis: a proposal of the European competence network on mastocytosis. Allergy 2014;69(10):1267–74.
39. Arock M, Sotlar K, Akin C, et al. KIT mutation analysis in mast cell neoplasms: recommendations of the European Competence Network on mastocytosis. Leukemia 2015;29(6):1223–32.

Tyrosine Kinase Inhibition in Mastocytosis
KIT and Beyond KIT

Siham Bibi, PhD[a], Michel Arock, PharmD, PhD[a,b],*

KEYWORDS

- Mast cells • Mastocytosis • KIT mutations • Advanced disease
- Tyrosine kinase inhibitors • Targeted drugs • Drug development

KEY POINTS

- Mastocytosis is a group of orphan diseases characterized by abnormal accumulation/proliferation of mast cells in one or several organs.
- In adults, mastocytosis is mostly systemic and chronic, affecting the bone marrow and other internal organs, with or without skin involvement.
- Indolent systemic mastocytosis (SM) is usually well controlled by symptomatic therapy, whereas, in advanced SM, cytoreductive drugs are needed.
- In most patients with SM, a recurrent activating KIT mutation (D816V) is found in the neoplastic mast cells.
- In advanced SM, patients may benefit from treatment by KIT-targeting tyrosine kinase inhibitors; but new targeted drugs or drug combinations are still needed to improve patients' outcome.

INTRODUCTION

Mast cells (MCs) are hematopoietic stem cells–derived tissue resident granulated cells found close to blood vessels, nerves, and mucosal surfaces, such as respiratory and gastrointestinal (GI) tracts.[1] The major growth and differentiation factor for the MC lineage is stem cell factor (SCF), which binds KIT, a transmembrane receptor with intrinsic tyrosine kinase (TK) activity (**Fig. 1**).[2]

Disclosure: S. Bibi has received research grants from Blueprint Medicines and from Deciphera Pharmaceuticals. M. Arock receives honorarium from Deciphera Pharmaceuticals.
[a] Cellular and Molecular Oncology, LBPA CNRS UMR8113, Ecole Normale Supérieure de Paris Saclay, 61, Avenue du Président Wilson, Cachan Cedex 94235, France; [b] Laboratory of Hematology, Pitié-Salpêtrière Hospital, 83, Boulevard de l'Hôpital, Paris 75013, France
* Corresponding author. Cellular and Molecular Oncology, LBPA CNRS UMR8113, Ecole Normale Supérieure de Paris Saclay, 61, Avenue du Président Wilson, Cachan Cedex 94235, France.
E-mail address: arock@ens-cachan.fr

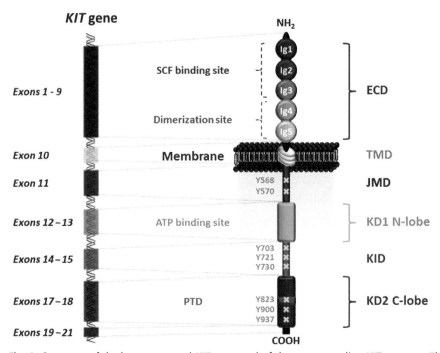

Fig. 1. Structure of the human normal *KIT* gene and of the corresponding KIT receptor. The *KIT* gene (*left*) contains 21 exons, encoding for a 145 kDa transmembrane protein, namely, the KIT receptor (*right*). KIT is represented in its monomeric form with its major structural and functional domains. The extracellular domain (ECD) is made by a longitudinal arrangement of 5 immunoglobulin-like (Ig-like) domains; the first 3 Ig-like domains of the ECD bind the SCF, whereas Ig-like domain 4 and 5 are involved in the dimerization process. The transmembrane domain (TMD) is composed of a hydrophobic α-helix allowing insertion of the receptor into the plasma membrane. The intracellular region contains the auto-inhibitory juxta-membrane domain (JMD) and a kinase domain (KD) divided by an insert region called kinase insert domain (KID) into a proximal N-lobe (KD1), which binds adenosine triphosphate (ATP) and a distal C-lobe, which contains the phosphotransferase domain (PTD). Yellow crosses indicate the position of the 8 tyrosine residues, which are phosphorylated upon activation of the receptor after ligation of SCF and dimerization.

Mastocytosis is a group of orphan diseases characterized by abnormal expansion of neoplastic MCs in at least one organ or tissue.[3] The most frequently affected organs/tissues are skin, bone marrow (BM), and GI tract.[3] Mastocytosis can affect both children and adults, with mostly pure cutaneous involvement in children, whereas systemic involvement is usually found in adults.[3] Most pediatric cases tend to resolve at adolescence, although some cases persist into adulthood.[3] By contrast, adult patients usually present with a chronic and indolent disease (indolent systemic mastocytosis [ISM]).[3] However, in some adult patients, more advanced subtypes of systemic mastocytosis (SM) may be diagnosed, for example, aggressive SM (ASM), SM with an associated hematologic neoplasm (SM-AHN), and MC leukemia (MCL).[3,4] Aggressive SM, SM-AHN, and MCL are collectively termed advanced SM (advSM). In ISM, clinical signs and symptoms are mostly related to increased mediator release by neoplastic MCs, whereas in advSM mediator–related symptoms are accompanied by organs damages following infiltration by neoplastic MCs.[3]

Most patients with mastocytosis (pediatric and adults) present *KIT* activating mutations in their neoplastic MCs.[5] Of note, a recurrent *KIT* mutation (D816V) located in the phosphotransferase domain (PTD) of the receptor is detectable in most patients with SM, including those with advSM.[5] Thus, it has been rapidly tempting to investigate the potential of KIT-targeted TK inhibitors (KIT-TKIs) for treatment. In this review, following a brief overview of the classification, physiopathology, and classic therapeutic options for SM, the authors focus on the present advances made to treat patients with advSM with KIT-TKIs. Because evidence suggest that such drugs might perhaps not be sufficient to cure patients with advSM, the authors finally discuss some future opportunities of alternative (combined) therapies.

CLASSIFICATION AND PHYSIOPATHOLOGY OF MASTOCYTOSIS

The World Health Organization (WHO) classifies mastocytosis into 3 broad categories: cutaneous mastocytosis (CM), SM, and MC sarcoma (MCS) (**Table 1**).[6]

Table 1
The 2016 updated World Health Organization's classification of mastocytosis, including criteria for diagnostic of systemic mastocytosis

Categories	Subtypes	Diagnostic Criteria	Prognosis
CM	• MPCM = UP[a] • DCM • Mastocytoma of skin	No systemic involvement (most patients are children)	+/− Good
SM[b]	ISM	• No B or C finding • Most patients are adults	Good
	SSM	• 2 or more B findings, no C findings	Good
	SM-AHN	• SM criteria and WHO diagnostic criteria for AHN are fulfilled • Frequently associated to myeloid AHNs (MPN, MDS, MPN/MDS), rarely to lymphoid AHNs	Depends on the type of SM and of the AHN
	ASM	• At least 1 C finding	Poor
	MCL	• BM smear >20% MCs • PB smear >10% MCs	Very poor
MCS		• Rare form of high-grade solid MC tumor • Very atypical MCs	Very poor

Abbreviations: DCM, diffuse CM; MDS, myelodysplastic syndrome; MPCM, maculopapular CM; MPN, myeloproliferative neoplasm; SSM, smoldering SM; UP, urticaria pigmentosa.

[a] A recently published consensus report of the European Competence Network on Mastocytosis, the American Academy of Allergy, Asthma & Immunology, and the European Academy of Allergology and Clinical Immunology recommends that the typical maculopapular cutaneous lesions (urticaria pigmentosa) should be subdivided into 2 variants, namely, a monomorphic variant with small maculopapular lesions, typically seen in adult patients, and a polymorphic variant with larger lesions of variable size and shape, typically seen in pediatric patients. Clinical observations suggest that the monomorphic variant, if it develops in children, often persists into adulthood, whereas the polymorphic variant may resolve around puberty.[79]

[b] According to the WHO, SM diagnosis requires the presence of both the major criterion and one minor criterion or at least 3 minor criteria. The major criterion consists of the presence of multifocal, dense infiltrates of aggregated MCs (>15 MCs) detected in BM and/or other extracutaneous organs. Minor criteria are the following: (1) atypical morphology in greater than 25% of MCs in infiltrates; (2) presence of an activating *KIT* point mutation at codon 816 of in BM, blood, or an extracutaneous organ; (3) aberrant expression of CD2 and/or CD25 by neoplastic MCs; and (4) elevated serum tryptase level (>20 ng/mL).

Data from Refs.[6–8]

Pure CM is the most common form of mastocytosis, generally affecting children. Several variants of CM are described (see **Table 1**).[7] Contrasting to CM, SM is detected mostly in adults. In SM, neoplastic MCs infiltrate internal organs, especially the BM, with or without skin involvement.[3] Diagnostic criteria for SM have been established by the WHO (see **Table 1**).[8]

Once the diagnosis of SM is established, the next step is to classify the disease into 5 subtypes (see **Table 1**). This classification is based on the presence or absence of B (borderline benign) findings and/or C (consider cytoreduction) findings, reflecting, respectively, a high MC burden and end-organ damages.[7] In the absence of B and C findings and of an AHN, patients are classified as having ISM. Such patients have a nearly normal life expectancy but may have MC mediator-related symptoms (pruritus, flush, gastrointestinal tract (GIT) symptoms, anaphylaxis, and so forth).[9] Besides, in patients with SM, the presence of 2 or more B findings but no C findings reflects a smoldering SM, a subtype of slowly progressive SM with high MC burden and intermediate prognosis.[10] By contrast, the presence of at least one C finding classifies the disease as ASM (MCs in BM smears <20% of nucleated cells) or MCL (MCs in BM smears >20% of nucleated cells), which share a poor prognosis.[11] Finally, SM-AHN is diagnosed when another hematological neoplasm is found associated with the different subtypes of SM.[12] In SM-AHN, the prognosis varies according to the aggressiveness of the SM component and to the one of the AHN.[11]

The pathophysiology of mastocytosis is governed by the presence of *KIT* activating mutations in neoplastic MCs.[13] Various *KIT* mutations have been described, firstly in patients with SM[14] and then in children with CM (**Table 2**).[15] In adults patients with SM, *KIT* mutations affect primarily exon 17 encoding for PTD, usually D816V (>80% of all patients) (see **Table 2**).[16] Other less frequent mutations affect exons 2, 8, and 9 encoding for the extracellular domain (ECD) or exons 13 and 14 encoding for Kinase Domain 1 (see **Fig. 1**, **Table 2**).[5] By contrast, in children, although a *KIT* mutation is found in 75% of skin biopsies, only 30% of the patients harbor the *KIT* D816V mutation.[15] The other mutations affect the ECD (codon 8 and 9) (see **Table 2**).[15] Finally, in the rare cases of familial mastocytosis, often represented by infant CM, most patients do not have *KIT* mutations or exhibit rare mutations, such as K509I, N835I, N835K, A533D, M835K, S841I, or K839E.[5]

The *KIT* D816V mutation induces KIT constitutive activation in the absence of the SCF (**Fig. 2**), the exact mechanism of which being not yet fully understood. The mutant receptor could either dimerize spontaneously with another mutant receptor or with a wild-type (WT) KIT receptor or could trigger a signaling cascade in its monomeric form.[17] Anyway, structural changes induced by the mutation affect normal KIT signaling and induce resistance to TKIs, such as imatinib.[18]

The development of neoplastic MCs is principally governed by the PI3K/AKT (phosphoinositide 3-kinase[PI3K]) and Janus kinase/Signal transducer and activator of transcription 5 (JAK/STAT5) signaling pathways activated downstream of the KIT mutant receptor (see **Fig. 2**).[19,20] AKT and STAT5 are constitutively activated in neoplastic MCs from patients with *KIT* D816V+ SM, and their specific inhibition induces growth arrest of such cells.[19,21] Besides, other intracellular pathways and molecules, such as the Feline sarcoma oncoprotein (FES),[22] or the mammalian target of rapamycin (mTOR) complex,[23] are also potential actors of oncogenesis linked to the KIT D816V mutant (see **Fig. 2**). In addition, the mutant can activate Extracellular signal-regulated kinase (ERK) independently of Sarcoma kinase (SRC), in contrast to KIT WT.[24] Finally, Lyn and Btk are found activated in neoplastic MCs, in a *KIT* D816V-independent manner.[25]

In ISM, the *KIT* D816V mutant seems to be the unique genetic abnormality found, which might explain the low incidence of progression.[26,27] By contrast, additional and recurrent somatic mutations of particular genes have been reported in advSM,

Table 2
Updated frequencies of the different *KIT* mutations found in mastocytosis

Mutation	KIT Domain	Frequency (Adults/Children) (%)
Y269C	ECD	<10
Del417–418–419insNA		<10
Del417–418–419insI		<10
Del417–418–419insY		<10
Del419		5–20 children
InsFF419		<10
C443Y		<10
S451C	TMD	<10
S476I		<10
ITD501–502		1–5 children
ITD502–503		1–5%children
Y503-504insAY		<10
ITD504		<10
ITD505–508		<10
K509I		5–20 children
F522C	JMD	<10
A533D		<10
K550N		<10
V559I		<10
V560G		<10
Del564–576		<10
D572A		<10
R633W	KD1	<10
K642E		<10
L799F	KD2	<10
InsVI815–816		<10
D816Y		Children < adults
D816F		<10
D816I		Children < adults
D816V		30 in children/90 in adults
D816H		<10
I817V		<10
V819Y		<10
D820G		<10
N822I/K		<10
E839K		<10
S840N		<10
S849I		<10

Abbreviations: Del, deletion; ECD, extracellular domain; ins, insertion; ITD, internal tandem duplication; JMD, juxta-membrane domain; KD, kinase domain; TMD, transmembrane domain.

Data from Arock M, Sotlar K, Akin C, et al. KIT mutation analysis in mast cell neoplasms: recommendations of the European Competence Network on Mastocytosis. Leukemia 2015;29(6):1223–32.

particularly in SM-AHN, the genes most frequently affected are *TET2*, *SRSF2*, *ASXL1*, *RUNX1*, *JAK2*, *N/KRAS*, and *CBL*.[26–30] By contrast, defects in *EZH2*, *IDH2*, *ETV6*, *U2AF*, or *SF3B1* are less frequent.[31] These defects usually contribute to aggressiveness of the disease, particularly in multi-mutated patients,[26,28–30] although a recent study led on 70 patients with *KIT* D816V[+] advSM has revealed that overall survival (OS) is influenced by *SRSF2*, *ASXL1*, and *RUNX1* (S/A/R) mutations but not by *TET2* or *JAK2* mutations.[27]

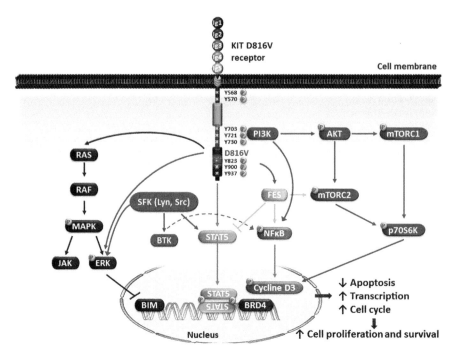

Fig. 2. Aberrant signaling pathways evoked by the KIT D816V mutant receptor. The D816V mutation activates constitutively the KIT receptor in the absence of SCF and alters the specificity of the protein, which shows substrate specificity that resembles that of SRC and ABL tyrosine kinases. The KIT mutant recruits downstream signaling pathways, though to be critical for the development of neoplastic MCs, such as PI3K/AKT and JAK/STAT5 signaling pathways. Indeed, AKT and STAT5 are constitutively activated in *KIT* D816V$^+$ neoplastic MCs, suggesting that these molecules play a crucial role in the pathogenesis of SM. Besides, some other intracellular TKs, such as the Feline sarcoma oncoprotein (FES), or the mammalian target of rapamycin (mTOR) complex, are also potential actors of oncogenesis linked to the KIT D816V mutant. In addition, the mutant can activate ERK independently of SRC. Of note, in advanced SM, Lyn and Btk are activated in neoplastic MCs in a KIT-independent manner. All these KIT-dependent and KIT-independent activated pathways and molecules combine to increase cell proliferation and decrease apoptosis of neoplastic MCs. BRD4, Bromodomain-containing protein 4; BTK, Bruton tyrosine kinase; ERK, Extracellular signal-regulated kinase; JAK, Janus kinase; MAPK, Mitogen Activated Protein Kinase; NFκB, nuclear factor-κ B; PI3K, phosphoinositide 3-kinase; SFK, Src family kinase; STAT5, Signal transducer and activator of transcription 5. (*Modified from* Bibi S, Langenfeld F, Jeanningros S, et al. Molecular defects in mastocytosis: KIT and beyond KIT. Immunol Allergy Clin North Am 2014;34(2):248; with permission).

NON-TARGETED TREATMENTS OF MASTOCYTOSIS

To date, there is no curative treatment of SM and caring is adapted depending on the case, the symptoms, and disease manifestations. Overall, SM treatments aim:

1. At counteracting mediator release symptoms (symptomatic treatments) and
2. In advSM, at reducing organ damage due to neoplastic MC infiltration (non-targeted cytoreductive drugs)

However, KIT-TKIs have recently emerged as promising agents to treat patients with advSM.

Symptomatic Treatments

Patients with ISM usually require only symptomatic treatments. The main objective is to reduce the symptoms of MC activation.[32] In case of pruritus or skin manifestations, antihistamines H1 (anti-H1) are used.[3,32] For GI tract manifestations, anti-H2 are effective alone or combined with anti-H1, disodium cromoglycate, or leukotriene inhibitors.[32] Besides, corticoids can suppress antihistamine recalcitrant symptoms.[9] Epinephrine is indicated for hypotension, which may be spontaneous or observed after an insect bite.[3] Indeed, some patients with SM may have a bee or wasp venom allergy.[33] In these patients, specific immunotherapy should be administered lifelong to ensure protection.[34] Finally, patients with SM with osteoporosis are treated with bisphosphonates together with supplementation of calcium and vitamin D.[35]

Non-targeted Chemotherapy and Allogeneic Stem Cell Transplantation

In advSM, symptomatic treatment is often associated with cytoreductive therapy. Interferon-α may be effective in a subset of patients, despite numerous side effects.[11] Cladribine provides high response rates together with long-lasting responses in some patients.[36,37] Besides, hydroxyurea (HU) is given in patients with SM-AHN, although HU is only active on the AHN component, but not on neoplastic MCs.[38] Of note, allogeneic stem cell transplantation (allo-SCT) is rarely used and reserved to fit patients with very aggressive, life-threatening advSM and a suitable donor.[39] Finally, allo-SCT provides more frequently good response rates and complete remissions in SM-AHN and ASM than in MCL.[40]

TYROSINE KINASE INHIBITORS FOR THE TREATMENT OF MASTOCYTOSIS

Recent approaches have concentrated on inhibitors targeting the KIT mutant receptor in patients with advSM. However, despite the fact that most patients with advSM harbor the imatinib-resistant *KIT* D816V mutant, it is of utmost importance to determine the *KIT* mutational status in each patient before applying KIT-TKIs, as some patients may present with *KIT* WT, or *KIT* mutant outside exon 17, potentially responsive to imatinib.

Major KIT-Targeted Tyrosine Kinase Inhibitors

Imatinib (STI571, Glivec) and masitinib (AB1010)

Imatinib and masitinib are structurally similar type I TKI (**Fig. 3**) active on some tyrosine kinases, including KIT WT and KIT mutants outside the exon 17 (**Table 3**).[41–43] In this respect, masitinib acts more potently than imatinib.[42] Although imatinib is devoid of effects on MC degranulation, masitinib inhibits this phenomenon, as a result of its activity on Lyn and Fyn.[42] Because imatinib has demonstrated clinical activity in single cases of patients with SM with *KIT* WT or *KIT* mutations outside exon 17 (reviewed in[44]), it has been approved by the Food and Drug Administration (FDA) in 2006 to treat *KIT* D816V-negative ASM or ASM with an unknown *KIT* mutational status.

By contrast, masitinib has been used in clinical trials in patients with SM, whatever their *KIT* mutational status, in the aim to decrease mediator-related symptoms. Indeed, in a phase III clinical trial published recently, 135 severely symptomatic patients with ISM not controlled by optimal antimediator therapies received either masitinib (6 mg/kg/d) or placebo.[45] After 24 weeks of treatment, masitinib induced a 75% improvement in at least one of the following symptoms: pruritus, flushes, depression, and severe fatigue (18.7% for the masitinib arm compared with 7.4% for the placebo arm), whatever the *KIT* mutational status. The most frequent adverse events were diarrhea (11%), rash (6%), and asthenia (6%).[45] Interestingly, the study also reported slightly decreased serum tryptase levels and improvement of skin lesions in the

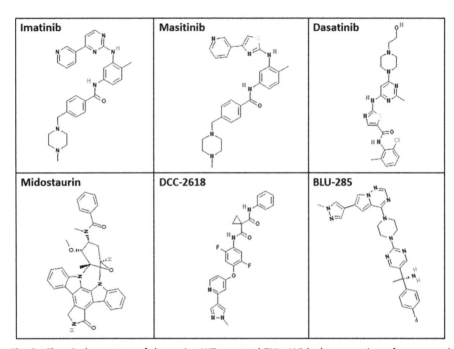

Fig. 3. Chemical structure of the major KIT-targeted TKIs. With the exception of compound DCC-2618, which targets the switch pocket of KIT, all the other KIT-targeted TKIs presented in this image are type I TKIs, which compete with adenosine triphosphate (ATP) for the ATP-binding site of the targeted kinase. Chemical formulas and molecular weights (MW) are as follows: imatinib: $C_{29}H_{31}N_7O$ (MW: 493.615); masitinib: $C_{28}H_{30}N_6OS$ (MW: 498.649); dasatinib: $C_{22}H_{26}ClN_7O_2S$ (MW: 488.007); midostaurin: $C_{35}H_{30}N_4O_4$ (MW: 570.649); DCC-2618: $C_{26}H_{21}F_2N_5O_3$ (MW: 489.483); BLU-285: $C_{26}H_{27}FN_{10}$ (MW: 498.57).

Table 3
Tyrosine kinase inhibitors of therapeutic interest in mastocytosis and their major molecular targets

TKIs	Major Molecular Targets
Imatinib	ARG, ABL, KIT WT, ECD and JMD KIT mutants, PDGFR
Masitinib	KIT WT, ECD and JMD KIT mutants, FMS, Lyn, Fyn
Dasatinib	ARG, ABL, KIT WT, KIT D816V, SRC, LCK, PDGFRβ
Midostaurin	PKC, KIT WT, KIT D816V, ECD and JMD KIT mutants, FLT3, PDGFR, FES, SYK, AURKA, AURKB, JAK2, JAK3, FGFR3, VEGFR2
DCC-2618	KIT WT, KIT D816V, ECD and JMD KIT mutants, PDGFR, KDR, FLT3, VEGFR2, TIE2, FMS
BLU-285	KIT WT, KIT D816V, KIT V560G, PDGFRα

Abbreviations: Abbreviations: AURK, aurora kinase; ECD; extracellular domain; FES, feline sarcoma; FGFR, fibroblast growth factor receptor; FLT3, Fms-like tyrosine kinase 3; FMS, M-CSF receptor; JAK, Janus kinase; JMD, juxta-membrane domain; KDR, Kinase insert domain receptor; LCK, lymphocyte-specific protein tyrosine kinase; PDGFR, platelet-derived growth factor receptor; SYK, Spleen tyrosine kinase; TIE2, tyrosine kinase with immunoglobulin and EGF homology domains; VEGFR, vascular endothelial growth factor receptor.

masitinib arm.[45] However, why masitinib is active only in a subset of patients independently of their *KIT* mutational status is still unclear and deserves further investigations.

Dasatinib (Sprycel)

Dasatinib (see **Fig. 3**) is a second-generation multi-kinase inhibitor acting on several targets (see **Table 3**).[46] It has in vitro efficacy against various KIT mutants, including KIT D816V.[47] By contrast, in a clinical study led with dasatinib given to 33 patients with SM,[48] an overall response rate (ORR) of 33% was achieved but short-lasting complete responses were only observed in 2 patients with *KIT* D816V-negative SM-AHN.[48] In addition, grade 3 toxicities were recorded in 58% of patients, with edema and pleural effusions.[48] In another trial, led on 4 patients with *KIT* D816V+, 2 patients had a major response with decreased BM MC burden but with severe cutaneous side effects.[49] Thus, because of numerous side effects and modest efficacy, dasatinib is not recommended in the treatment of patients with AdvSM.

Midostaurin (Rydapt)

Midostaurin (see **Fig. 3**), originally termed PKC412, is a potent TKI initially developed as a protein kinase C inhibitor.[50] In fact, midostaurin is a multi-kinase inhibitor (see **Table 3**). Unlike most TKIs, midostaurin inhibits not only the WT form of its targets but also their mutant forms. Particularly, midostaurin suppresses not only the kinase activity of WT KIT but also that of KIT mutants, including the D816V mutant.[47,51,52]

Indeed, midostaurin has in vitro growth-inhibitory activity on various cell lines expressing *KIT* WT, *KIT* V560G, or *KIT* D816V mutants, with half maximal inhibitory concentration (IC_{50}) ranging from 50 nM to 250 nM.[43,52] Of note, these growth-inhibitory effects are accompanied by inhibition of KIT phosphorylation and apoptosis.[43,52] Furthermore, midostaurin is also active on primary neoplastic MCs from patients with advSM.[52] Moreover, midostaurin produces synergistic growth-inhibitory effects when combined with dasatinib,[47] cladribine,[52] or JQ1 (a bromodomain 4 [BRD4] inhibitor).[53] Overall, these results have promptly encouraged the clinical use of midostaurin in patients with advSM.

Midostaurin was first used to treat a patient with *KIT* D816V+ MCL, resulting in a partial remission with a significant decrease in the percentage of circulating MCs, associated with decreased histamine level and *KIT* D816V mutation frequency in peripheral blood.[51] More recently, an international phase II clinical trial has been performed on 116 patients with advSM (all patients receiving 100 mg twice daily in 4-week continuous cycles).[54] Based on the presence of C findings, 89 patients (16 ASM, 57 SM-AHN, 16 MCL) were eligible for evaluation. Among them, 77 patients (87%) were positive for *KIT* D816V/Y/L mutation. The ORR for the whole cohort was 60% (53 of 89 patients), whereas the ORR for patients with MCL was 50% (8 of 16 patients).[54] The treatment significantly decreased the BM MC burden, serum tryptase levels, and spleen volume in most patients.[54] In addition, the median OS of responders was 44.4 months, whereas in MCL, OS was 9.4 months.[54] All grades' side effects mostly seen were anemia, neutropenia, thrombocytopenia, digestive toxicities, peripheral edema, fatigue, pyrexia, headache, back pain, and pruritus; but grade 3/4 toxicities were essentially hematologic.[54] The main conclusions of this study were that midostaurin induced frequently durable responses in patients with advSM, with an acceptable safety profile.[54] This favorable profile of activity was confirmed in another clinical study whereby 28 patients with advSM received midostaurin at a dosage of 100 mg twice daily.[55] Recently, the long-term potential therapeutic benefit of midostaurin given as a single agent to patients with advSM was confirmed by a 10-year median follow-up of a phase II trial conducted on 26 patients (3 ASM, 17 SM-AHN, and

6 MCL).[56] In this study, midostaurin produced a 50% or greater reduction in the BM MC burden and serum tryptase level in 68% and 46% of the patients, respectively. Of note, the median OS for the entire cohort was 40 months and 18.5 months for patients with MCL.[56] Based on these positive data, midostaurin has been approved in monotherapy to treat adult patients with advSM by the FDA (April 2017) and by the European Commission (September 2017) and is considered a major component of the first-line treatment in advSM.

DCC-2618 compound

Deciphera Compound-2618 (DCC-2618) (see **Fig. 3**) is a switch control type II inhibitor, which arrests KIT in an inactive state, regardless of the type of activating mutations, by targeting the switch pocket of the receptor that regulates its catalytic conformation.[57,58] Besides KIT, DCC-2618 recognizes several other oncogenic kinases (see **Table 3**).[58] DCC-2618 inhibits the proliferation and survival of human neoplastic MC lines expressing various *KIT* mutants, including *KIT* D816V, with IC_{50} less than 0.5 µM.[59] In addition, DCC-2618 suppressed endothelial cell proliferation, suggesting additional drug effects on disease-related angiogenesis.[59] Besides, DCC-2618 blocked immunoglobulin E–mediated histamine release by basophils and tryptase release by MCs.[59] Altogether, these data suggest that DCC-2618 might represent a promising drug to treat patients with advSM. Thus, a first clinical trial has been initiated with DCC-2618 in patients with advanced kinase-driven malignancies, including advSM (NCT02571036).

BLU-285 compound

Blueprint-285 compound (avapritinib) (see **Fig. 3**) is a novel TKI that potently inhibits selectively *KIT* exon 17 mutants, including KIT D816V (see **Table 3**).[60] BLU-285 also inhibits STAT3 and AKT phosphorylation in vitro in the Human MC line (HMC-1.2 cell line) and decreases tumor progression in vivo in mice grafted with murine mastocytoma cells P815.[60] Recently, a phase 1 clinical trial has been initiated to assess the safety, pharmacokinetics (PK), and preliminary clinical activity of avapritinib in patients with advSM (NCT02561988). Preliminary data analyzing the effects of BLU-285 on 30 patients (15 ASM; 9 SM-AHN; 3 MCL; 3 other D816V-mutant positive hematologic neoplasms) treated with BLU-285 in 7 cohorts at dosages of 30 to 400 mg daily have been recently reported.[61] Among these 30 patients, 24 had *KIT* D816V mutation, 2 had *KIT* D816Y mutation, 1 had *KIT* polymorphism M541L and 3 were *KIT* WT.[61] Twenty-four patients had 1 or more co-occurring mutations in BM, most frequently *TET2* (17), *DNMT3A* (9), *ASXL1* (7), *SRSF2* (6), and *GATA2* (6). Interestingly, in these patients, BLU-285 seemed well tolerated and demonstrated significant clinical (significant decrease in spleen volume) and biological (significant decrease in serum tryptase levels, BM MC and *KIT* D816V allele burden) activities in all AdvSM subtypes, including in those who have failed previous midostaurin treatment.[61] All in all, these are encouraging data that deserve long-term follow-up.

Other KIT-Targeted Tyrosine Kinase Inhibitors

Several TKIs have demonstrated in vitro efficacy on imatinib-resistant *KIT* mutants. Some of these drugs have been discontinued for safety issues, and others are already approved for the treatment of non–*KIT*-related malignancies, whereas the last drugs are still experimental. For instance, discontinued drugs comprise compound MLN518 (tandutinib),[62] purine inhibitors AP23464 and AP23848,[63] compound EXEL-0862,[64] and semaxanib (SU5416).[65] Besides, ponatinib (Iclusig) a TKI FDA approved to treat patients with imatinib-resistant CML, inhibited the kinase activity of various KIT mutant receptors, such as KIT Y823D,[66] KIT V560G, and KIT D816V.[67] In addition to its effects on the kinase activity of mutant KIT proteins, ponatinib inhibited in vitro the proliferation of *KIT* D816V$^+$-malignant MCs by inducing apoptosis and that, synergistically with midostaurin.[67] Nevertheless, ponatinib has still not been used clinically. More recently, nilotinib, a strong inhibitor of BCR-ABL1 approved as a first-line treatment in CML but that has some marginal activities in vitro on KIT mutants, has been administered to 61 patients with SM (including 37 with advSM) in a clinical trial, with low response rates not being in favor of its use in advSM.[68] Other compounds that are experimental are 2 thiazole amine derivatives: compound 126332, which inhibits the *KIT* D816V mutant in vitro in neoplastic MCs and in vivo in solid tumors generated by subcutaneous injection of cells of the KIT D816V+ human mast cell line (HMC-1.2),[69] and compound BPR1J373, which suppresses the KIT D816V phosphorylation.[70] Finally, about 40 new *KIT* D816V inhibitors have been developed by the Korea Advanced Institute of Science and Technology, 7 of which having significant in vitro activity on HMC-1.2 cells (IC$_{50}$ <1.0 μM).[71] However, to date, no clinical trials have been initiated with these experimental drugs.

Non–KIT-Targeted Kinase Inhibitors

As described earlier, the PI3K/AKT/mTOR and JAK/STAT pathways, and to a lesser extent the mitogen-activated protein kinase (MAPK) pathway, seem crucial for the proliferation of *KIT* D816V$^+$ malignant MCs.[20] These pathways might be alternative targets for specific inhibitors, used alone or in combination with KIT-TKIs. For instance, the pharmacologic inhibition of PI3K in vitro by NVP-BEZ235 induced a dose-dependent inhibition of HMC-1.2 cell proliferation, which was synergistically increased in combination with the MAPK inhibitor UO126.[72] In addition, treatment of *KIT* D816V$^+$ malignant MCs with AKT inhibitors reduced cell growth in vitro.[43] Besides, ruxolitinib, an inhibitor of JAK1 and JAK2, has been recently administered to 2 patients with SM, in 2 single case reports.[73,74] In both cases, ruxolitinib reduced symptoms and increased quality of life.[73,74] However, despite long-term treatment, no decrease in MC burden was recorded.[73,74] Of note, Lyn and Btk, are phosphorylated independently of KIT in neoplastic MCs in SM (**Fig. 4**).[47] Interestingly, bosutinib, an ABL-targeting TKI approved for the treatment of CML, inhibits also the phosphorylation of Lyn and Btk and exerts antiproliferative effects in vitro on *KIT* D816V$^+$ neoplastic MCs.[47] In addition, a combination with midostaurin provided synergistic antiproliferative and proapoptotic effects in vitro.[47] However, despite these promising data, bosutinib has been administered to one patient with advSM, without any clinical effects.[75]

SUMMARY AND FUTURE CONSIDERATIONS

Current therapeutic options for patients with SM are based on symptomatic treatment and, in advSM, on the use of cytoreductive agents and TKIs. However, in advSM, with the exception of allo-SCT applicable only to a minority of patients, none of these treatments, including midostaurin, has demonstrated true curative potential; the prognosis of these patients is still poor. Besides, knowledge on the pathophysiology of SM has increased dramatically these last years, highlighting the complexity of the processes leading to abnormal accumulation/proliferation of neoplastic MCs in SM, particularly in advSM. Indeed, in these patients, malignant MC proliferation is driven not only by *KIT* mutations but also by altered signaling pathways and additional genetic defects. Thus, new targets and alternative therapies are needed to achieve lifelong lasting remission. Alternative targets could be, for instance, aberrantly activated KIT-dependent and KIT-independent signal transduction pathways described earlier and members of the Bcl-2 family overexpressed in neoplastic MCs (see **Fig. 4**).[76] Besides,

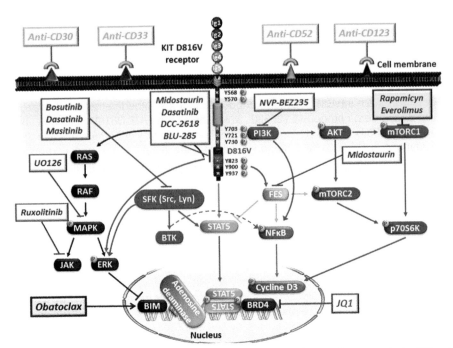

Fig. 4. Present and potential therapeutic targets in advanced systemic mastocytosis: *KIT* and beyond *KIT*. Several drugs can selectively inhibit the kinase activity of the KIT D816V mutant or some of the critical pathways aberrantly activated in a KIT-dependent or KIT-independent manner downstream of the mutant receptor, such as PI3-kinase/AKT/mTOR, MAPK, JAK/STAT and SFK pathways, the FES kinase, and the NFkB pathway. In addition, anti-apoptotic molecules, such as Mcl-1, Bcl-2, and Bcl-xL, may constitute potential targets since they are upregulated in *KIT* D816V+ neoplastic MCs[76] and because pan-Bcl-2 blockers can induce their apoptosis.[78] Besides, one promising class of targets within chromatin regulatory molecules are the BRD-containing proteins, such as BRD4, which is overexpressed in *KIT* D816V+ MCs in advanced SM and for which a specific inhibitor (JQ1) has proven efficacy on neoplastic MCs in vitro.[53] Finally, neoplastic MCs may express aberrantly some cell surface antigens, such as CD30, CD33, CD52, or CD123, which could be targeted by antibody-based toxin conjugates or other ligands. Kinase inhibitors are represented in blue, specific antibodies in green, Bcl-2 antagonist in black, inhibitor of BRD-containing proteins in brown, and mTOR inhibitors in purple. (*Modified from* Ustun C, Arock M, Kluin-Nelemans HC, et al. Advanced systemic mastocytosis: from molecular and genetic progress to clinical practice. Haematologica 2016;101(10):1137; with permission.)

other targets of potential interest should be cell surface antigens expressed by neoplastic MCs.[77] Some of these antigens are of particular interest (see **Fig. 4**), such as CD30, CD33, CD52, and CD123, for which targeted antibodies are already in clinical trials. All in all, these potential targets might serve as a basis for the development of new targeted therapies, which will be certainly used in combination with KIT-TKIs to improve the health outcome of patients with advSM.

REFERENCES

1. Krishnaswamy G, Ajitawi O, Chi DS. The human mast cell: an overview. Methods Mol Biol 2006;315:13–34.

2. Galli SJ, Tsai M, Wershil BK, et al. Regulation of mouse and human mast cell development, survival and function by stem cell factor, the ligand for the c-kit receptor. Int Arch Allergy Immunol 1995;107(1–3):51–3.
3. Carter MC, Metcalfe DD, Komarow HD. Mastocytosis. Immunol Allergy Clin North Am 2014;34(1):181–96.
4. Sperr WR, Horny HP, Valent P. Spectrum of associated clonal hematologic non-mast cell lineage disorders occurring in patients with systemic mastocytosis. Int Arch Allergy Immunol 2002;127(2):140–2.
5. Arock M, Sotlar K, Akin C, et al. KIT mutation analysis in mast cell neoplasms: recommendations of the European Competence Network on Mastocytosis. Leukemia 2015;29(6):1223–32.
6. Valent P, Akin C, Metcalfe DD. Mastocytosis: 2016 updated WHO classification and novel emerging treatment concepts. Blood 2017;129(11):1420–7.
7. Valent P, Akin C, Hartmann K, et al. Advances in the classification and treatment of mastocytosis: current status and outlook toward the future. Cancer Res 2017; 77(6):1261–70.
8. Valent P, Horny HP, Escribano L, et al. Diagnostic criteria and classification of mastocytosis: a consensus proposal. Leuk Res 2001;25(7):603–25.
9. Arock M, Akin C, Hermine O, et al. Current treatment options in patients with mastocytosis: status in 2015 and future perspectives. Eur J Haematol 2015;94(6):474–90.
10. Valent P, Akin C, Sperr WR, et al. Smouldering mastocytosis: a novel subtype of systemic mastocytosis with slow progression. Int Arch Allergy Immunol 2002; 127(2):137–9.
11. Pardanani A. Systemic mastocytosis in adults: 2017 update on diagnosis, risk stratification and management. Am J Hematol 2016;91(11):1146–59.
12. Valent P, Sotlar K, Blatt K, et al. Proposed diagnostic criteria and classification of basophilic leukemias and related disorders. Leukemia 2017;31(4):788–97.
13. Cruse G, Metcalfe DD, Olivera A. Functional deregulation of KIT: link to mast cell proliferative diseases and other neoplasms. Immunol Allergy Clin North Am 2014; 34(2):219–37.
14. Longley BJ, Tyrrell L, Lu SZ, et al. Somatic c-KIT activating mutation in urticaria pigmentosa and aggressive mastocytosis: establishment of clonality in a human mast cell neoplasm. Nat Genet 1996;12(3):312–4.
15. Bodemer C, Hermine O, Palmerini F, et al. Pediatric mastocytosis is a clonal disease associated with D816V and other activating c-KIT mutations. J Invest Dermatol 2010;130(3):804–15.
16. Orfao A, Garcia-Montero AC, Sanchez L, et al. Recent advances in the understanding of mastocytosis: the role of KIT mutations. Br J Haematol 2007;138(1):12–30.
17. Laine E, Chauvot de Beauchene I, Perahia D, et al. Mutation D816V alters the internal structure and dynamics of c-KIT receptor cytoplasmic region: implications for dimerization and activation mechanisms. PLoS Comput Biol 2011;7(6): e1002068.
18. Frost MJ, Ferrao PT, Hughes TP, et al. Juxtamembrane mutant V560GKit is more sensitive to Imatinib (STI571) compared with wild-type c-kit whereas the kinase domain mutant D816VKit is resistant. Mol Cancer Ther 2002;1(12):1115–24.
19. Harir N, Boudot C, Friedbichler K, et al. Oncogenic Kit controls neoplastic mast cell growth through a Stat5/PI3-kinase signaling cascade. Blood 2008;112(6): 2463–73.
20. Bibi S, Arslanhan MD, Langenfeld F, et al. Co-operating STAT5 and AKT signaling pathways in chronic myeloid leukemia and mastocytosis: possible new targets of therapy. Haematologica 2014;99(3):417–29.

21. Baumgartner C, Cerny-Reiterer S, Sonneck K, et al. Expression of activated STAT5 in neoplastic mast cells in systemic mastocytosis: subcellular distribution and role of the transforming oncoprotein KIT D816V. Am J Pathol 2009;175(6): 2416–29.

22. Voisset E, Lopez S, Dubreuil P, et al. The tyrosine kinase FES is an essential effector of KITD816V proliferation signal. Blood 2007;110(7):2593–9.

23. Smrz D, Kim MS, Zhang S, et al. mTORC1 and mTORC2 differentially regulate homeostasis of neoplastic and non-neoplastic human mast cells. Blood 2011; 118(26):6803–13.

24. Sun J, Pedersen M, Ronnstrand L. The D816V mutation of c-Kit circumvents a requirement for Src family kinases in c-Kit signal transduction. J Biol Chem 2009;284(17):11039–47.

25. Gleixner KV, Mayerhofer M, Cerny-Reiterer S, et al. KIT-D816V-independent oncogenic signaling in neoplastic cells in systemic mastocytosis: role of Lyn and Btk activation and disruption by dasatinib and bosutinib. Blood 2011; 118(7):1885–98.

26. Hanssens K, Brenet F, Agopian J, et al. SRSF2-p95 hotspot mutation is highly associated with advanced forms of mastocytosis and mutations in epigenetic regulator genes. Haematologica 2014;99(5):830–5.

27. Jawhar M, Schwaab J, Schnittger S, et al. Additional mutations in SRSF2, ASXL1 and/or RUNX1 identify a high-risk group of patients with KIT D816V(+) advanced systemic mastocytosis. Leukemia 2016;30(1):136–43.

28. Traina F, Visconte V, Jankowska AM, et al. Single nucleotide polymorphism array lesions, TET2, DNMT3A, ASXL1 and CBL mutations are present in systemic mastocytosis. PLoS One 2012;7(8):e43090.

29. Soucie E, Hanssens K, Mercher T, et al. In aggressive forms of mastocytosis, TET2 loss cooperates with c-KITD816V to transform mast cells. Blood 2012; 120(24):4846–9.

30. Damaj G, Joris M, Chandesris O, et al. ASXL1 but not TET2 mutations adversely impact overall survival of patients suffering systemic mastocytosis with associated clonal hematologic non-mast-cell diseases. PLoS One 2014;9(1):e85362.

31. Bibi S, Langenfeld F, Jeanningros S, et al. Molecular defects in mastocytosis: KIT and beyond KIT. Immunol Allergy Clin North Am 2014;34(2):239–62.

32. Worobec AS. Treatment of systemic mast cell disorders. Hematol Oncol Clin North Am 2000;14(3):659–87, vii.

33. Castells MC, Hornick JL, Akin C. Anaphylaxis after Hymenoptera sting: is it venom allergy, a clonal disorder, or both? J Allergy Clin Immunol Pract 2015; 3(3):350–5.

34. Niedoszytko M, Bonadonna P, Oude Elberink JN, et al. Epidemiology, diagnosis, and treatment of Hymenoptera venom allergy in mastocytosis patients. Immunol Allergy Clin North Am 2014;34(2):365–81.

35. Barete S, Assous N, de Gennes C, et al. Systemic mastocytosis and bone involvement in a cohort of 75 patients. Ann Rheum Dis 2010;69(10):1838–41.

36. Kluin-Nelemans HC, Oldhoff JM, Van Doormaal JJ, et al. Cladribine therapy for systemic mastocytosis. Blood 2003;102(13):4270–6.

37. Barete S, Lortholary O, Damaj G, et al. Long-term efficacy and safety of cladribine (2-CdA) in adult patients with mastocytosis. Blood 2015;126(8):1009–16 [quiz: 1050].

38. Lim KH, Pardanani A, Butterfield JH, et al. Cytoreductive therapy in 108 adults with systemic mastocytosis: outcome analysis and response prediction during treatment with interferon-alpha, hydroxyurea, imatinib mesylate or 2-chlorodeoxyadenosine. Am J Hematol 2009;84(12):790–4.

39. Ustun C, Gotlib J, Popat U, et al. Consensus opinion on allogeneic hematopoietic cell transplantation in advanced systemic mastocytosis. Biol Blood Marrow Transplant 2016;22(8):1348–56.

40. Ustun C, Reiter A, Scott BL, et al. Hematopoietic stem-cell transplantation for advanced systemic mastocytosis. J Clin Oncol 2014;32(29):3264–74.

41. Ma Y, Zeng S, Metcalfe DD, et al. The c-KIT mutation causing human mastocytosis is resistant to STI571 and other KIT kinase inhibitors; kinases with enzymatic site mutations show different inhibitor sensitivity profiles than wild-type kinases and those with regulatory-type mutations. Blood 2002;99(5):1741–4.

42. Dubreuil P, Letard S, Ciufolini M, et al. Masitinib (AB1010), a potent and selective tyrosine kinase inhibitor targeting KIT. PLoS One 2009;4(9):e7258.

43. Saleh R, Wedeh G, Herrmann H, et al. A new human mast cell line expressing a functional IgE receptor converts to tumorigenic growth by KIT D816V transfection. Blood 2014;124(1):111–20.

44. Alvarez-Twose I, Matito A, Morgado JM, et al. Imatinib in systemic mastocytosis: a phase IV clinical trial in patients lacking exon 17 KIT mutations and review of the literature. Oncotarget 2017;8(40):68950–63.

45. Lortholary O, Chandesris MO, Bulai Livideanu C, et al. Masitinib for treatment of severely symptomatic indolent systemic mastocytosis: a randomised, placebo-controlled, phase 3 study. Lancet 2017;389(10069):612–20.

46. Schittenhelm MM, Shiraga S, Schroeder A, et al. Dasatinib (BMS-354825), a dual SRC/ABL kinase inhibitor, inhibits the kinase activity of wild-type, juxtamembrane, and activation loop mutant KIT isoforms associated with human malignancies. Cancer Res 2006;66(1):473–81.

47. Gleixner KV, Mayerhofer M, Sonneck K, et al. Synergistic growth-inhibitory effects of two tyrosine kinase inhibitors, dasatinib and PKC412, on neoplastic mast cells expressing the D816V-mutated oncogenic variant of KIT. Haematologica 2007; 92(11):1451–9.

48. Verstovsek S, Tefferi A, Cortes J, et al. Phase II study of dasatinib in Philadelphia chromosome-negative acute and chronic myeloid diseases, including systemic mastocytosis. Clin Cancer Res 2008;14(12):3906–15.

49. Purtill D, Cooney J, Sinniah R, et al. Dasatinib therapy for systemic mastocytosis: four cases. Eur J Haematol 2008;80(5):456–8.

50. Tamaoki T, Nomoto H, Takahashi I, et al. Staurosporine, a potent inhibitor of phospholipid/Ca++dependent protein kinase. Biochem Biophys Res Commun 1986; 135(2):397–402.

51. Gotlib J, Berube C, Growney JD, et al. Activity of the tyrosine kinase inhibitor PKC412 in a patient with mast cell leukemia with the D816V KIT mutation. Blood 2005;106(8):2865–70.

52. Gleixner KV, Mayerhofer M, Aichberger KJ, et al. PKC412 inhibits in vitro growth of neoplastic human mast cells expressing the D816V-mutated variant of KIT: comparison with AMN107, imatinib, and cladribine (2CdA) and evaluation of cooperative drug effects. Blood 2006;107(2):752–9.

53. Wedeh G, Cerny-Reiterer S, Eisenwort G, et al. Identification of bromodomain-containing protein-4 as a novel marker and epigenetic target in mast cell leukemia. Leukemia 2015;29(11):2230–7.

54. Gotlib J, Kluin-Nelemans HC, George TI, et al. Efficacy and safety of midostaurin in advanced systemic mastocytosis. N Engl J Med 2016;374(26):2530–41.

55. Chandesris MO, Damaj G, Canioni D, et al. Midostaurin in advanced systemic mastocytosis. N Engl J Med 2016;374(26):2605–7.

56. DeAngelo DJ, George TI, Linder A, et al. Efficacy and safety of midostaurin in patients with advanced systemic mastocytosis: 10-year median follow-up of a phase II trial. Leukemia 2018;32(2):470–8.

57. Mol CD, Dougan DR, Schneider TR, et al. Structural basis for the autoinhibition and STI-571 inhibition of c-Kit tyrosine kinase. J Biol Chem 2004;279(30): 31655–63.

58. Smith BD, Molly MH, Wise SC, et al. DCC-2618 is a potent inhibitor of wild-type and mutant KIT, including refractory exon 17 D816 KIT mutations, and exhibits efficacy in refractory GIST and AML xenograft models. Cancer Res 2015;75(15 Supplement):2690.

59. Schneeweiss MA, Peter B, Blatt K, et al. The multi-kinase inhibitor DCC-2618 Inhibits proliferation and survival of neoplastic mast cells and other cell types involved in systemic mastocytosis. Blood 2016;128(22):1965.

60. Evans E, Gardino A, Hodous B, et al. Blu-285, a potent and selective inhibitor for hematologic malignancies with KIT exon 17 mutations. Blood 2015;126(23):568.

61. DeAngelo DJ, Quiery AT, Radia D, et al. Clinical activity in a phase 1 study of Blu-285, a potent, highly-selective inhibitor of KIT D816V in advanced systemic mastocytosis (AdvSM). Blood 2017;130(Suppl 1):2.

62. Corbin AS, Griswold IJ, La Rosee P, et al. Sensitivity of oncogenic KIT mutants to the kinase inhibitors MLN518 and PD180970. Blood 2004;104(12):3754–7.

63. Corbin AS, Demehri S, Griswold IJ, et al. In vitro and in vivo activity of ATP-based kinase inhibitors AP23464 and AP23848 against activation-loop mutants of Kit. Blood 2005;106(1):227–34.

64. Pan J, Quintas-Cardama A, Kantarjian HM, et al. EXEL-0862, a novel tyrosine kinase inhibitor, induces apoptosis in vitro and ex vivo in human mast cells expressing the KIT D816V mutation. Blood 2007;109(1):315–22.

65. Kosmider O, Denis N, Dubreuil P, et al. Semaxinib (SU5416) as a therapeutic agent targeting oncogenic Kit mutants resistant to imatinib mesylate. Oncogene 2007;26(26):3904–8.

66. Lierman E, Smits S, Cools J, et al. Ponatinib is active against imatinib-resistant mutants of FIP1L1-PDGFRA and KIT, and against FGFR1-derived fusion kinases. Leukemia 2012;26(7):1693–5.

67. Gleixner KV, Peter B, Blatt K, et al. Synergistic growth-inhibitory effects of ponatinib and midostaurin (PKC412) on neoplastic mast cells carrying KIT D816V. Haematologica 2013;98(9):1450–7.

68. Hochhaus A, Baccarani M, Giles FJ, et al. Nilotinib in patients with systemic mastocytosis: analysis of the phase 2, open-label, single-arm nilotinib registration study. J Cancer Res Clin Oncol 2015;141(11):2047–60.

69. Jin Y, Ding K, Wang D, et al. Novel thiazole amine class tyrosine kinase inhibitors induce apoptosis in human mast cells expressing D816V KIT mutation. Cancer Lett 2014;353(1):115–23.

70. Chen LT, Chen CT, Jiaang WT, et al. BPR1J373, an oral multiple tyrosine kinase inhibitor, targets c-KIT for the treatment of c-KIT-driven myeloid leukemia. Mol Cancer Ther 2016;15(10):2323–33.

71. Lee S, Lee H, Kim J, et al. Development and biological evaluation of potent and selective c-KIT(D816V) inhibitors. J Med Chem 2014;57(15):6428–43.

72. Buet D, Gallais I, Lauret E, et al. Cotargeting signaling pathways driving survival and cell cycle circumvents resistance to Kit inhibitors in leukemia. Blood 2012; 119(18):4228–41.

73. Yacoub A, Prochaska L. Ruxolitinib improves symptoms and quality of life in a patient with systemic mastocytosis. Biomark Res 2016;4:2.

74. Dowse R, Ibrahim M, McLornan DP, et al. Beneficial effects of JAK inhibitor therapy in systemic mastocytosis. Br J Haematol 2017;176(2):324–7.
75. Randall N, Courville EL, Baughn L, et al. Bosutinib, a Lyn/Btk inhibiting tyrosine kinase inhibitor, is ineffective in advanced systemic mastocytosis. Am J Hematol 2015;90(4):E74.
76. Aichberger KJ, Gleixner KV, Mirkina I, et al. Identification of proapoptotic Bim as a tumor suppressor in neoplastic mast cells: role of KIT D816V and effects of various targeted drugs. Blood 2009;114(26):5342–51.
77. Valent P, Cerny-Reiterer S, Herrmann H, et al. Phenotypic heterogeneity, novel diagnostic markers, and target expression profiles in normal and neoplastic human mast cells. Best Pract Res Clin Haematol 2010;23(3):369–78.
78. Peter B, Cerny-Reiterer S, Hadzijusufovic E, et al. The pan-Bcl-2 blocker obatoclax promotes the expression of Puma, Noxa, and Bim mRNA and induces apoptosis in neoplastic mast cells. J Leukoc Biol 2014;95(1):95–104.
79. Hartmann K, Escribano L, Grattan C, et al. Cutaneous manifestations in patients with mastocytosis: consensus report of the European Competence Network on Mastocytosis; the American Academy of Allergy, Asthma & Immunology; and the European Academy of Allergology and Clinical Immunology. J Allergy Clin Immunol 2016;137(1):35–45.

Moving?

Make sure your subscription moves with you!

To notify us of your new address, find your **Clinics Account Number** (located on your mailing label above your name), and contact customer service at:

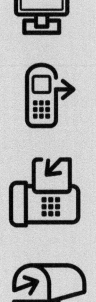

Email: journalscustomerservice-usa@elsevier.com

800-654-2452 (subscribers in the U.S. & Canada)
314-447-8871 (subscribers outside of the U.S. & Canada)

Fax number: 314-447-8029

Elsevier Health Sciences Division
Subscription Customer Service
3251 Riverport Lane
Maryland Heights, MO 63043

*To ensure uninterrupted delivery of your subscription, please notify us at least 4 weeks in advance of move.

Printed and bound by CPI Group (UK) Ltd, Croydon, CR0 4YY

07/10/2024

01040502-0004